Reducing Gun Violence in America

Reducing Gun Violence in America

Informing Policy with Evidence and Analysis

EDITED BY

Daniel W. Webster, ScD, MPH,
and Jon S. Vernick, JD, MPH

Center for Gun Policy and Research
Johns Hopkins Bloomberg School of Public Health

The Johns Hopkins University Press
Baltimore

© 2013 The Johns Hopkins University Press
All rights reserved. Published 2013
Printed in the United States of America on acid-free paper
9 8 7 6 5 4 3 2 1

The Johns Hopkins University Press
2715 North Charles Street
Baltimore, Maryland 21218-4363
www.press.jhu.edu

Library of Congress Control Number: 2013930408
A catalog record for this book is available from the British Library.

ISBN 13: 978-1-4214-1110-1 (pbk. : alk. paper)
ISBN 10: 1-4214-1110-5 (pbk. : alk. paper)
ISBN 13: 978-1-4214-1111-8 (electronic)
ISBN 10: 1-4214-1111-3 (electronic)

Special discounts are available for bulk purchases of this book.
For more information, please contact Special Sales at 410-516-6936 or
specialsales@press.jhu.edu.

The Johns Hopkins University Press uses environmentally friendly book
materials, including recycled text paper that is composed of at least 30
percent post-consumer waste, whenever possible.

ACC LIBRARY SERVICES AUSTIN, TX

*To victims of gun violence and
to those who work daily
to reduce it*

Contents

Foreword xi
Michael R. Bloomberg

Preface xix
Ronald J. Daniels and Michael J. Klag

Acknowledgments xxi

Introduction xxv
Daniel W. Webster and Jon S. Vernick

PART I: GUN POLICY LESSONS FROM
THE UNITED STATES: KEEPING GUNS
FROM HIGH-RISK INDIVIDUALS

1 Firearms and Violent Death in the United States 3
Matthew Miller, Deborah Azrael, and David Hemenway

2 The Limited Impact of the Brady Act: Evaluation
and Implications 21
Philip J. Cook and Jens Ludwig

3 Preventing Gun Violence Involving People with Serious
Mental Illness 33
*Jeffrey W. Swanson, Allison Gilbert Robertson, Linda K. Frisman,
Michael A. Norko, Hsiu-Ju Lin, Marvin S. Swartz, and Philip J. Cook*

4 Evidence for Optimism: Policies to Limit Batterers' Access
to Guns 53
April M. Zeoli and Shannon Frattaroli

5   Reconsidering the Adequacy of Current Conditions on
    Legal Firearm Ownership   65
    Katherine A. Vittes, Daniel W. Webster, and Jon S. Vernick

6   Broadening Denial Criteria for the Purchase and Possession
    of Firearms: Need, Feasibility, and Effectiveness   77
    Garen J. Wintemute

7   Comprehensive Background Checks for Firearm Sales:
    Evidence from Gun Shows   95
    Garen J. Wintemute

8   Preventing the Diversion of Guns to Criminals through
    Effective Firearm Sales Laws   109
    Daniel W. Webster, Jon S. Vernick, Emma E. McGinty, and Ted Alcorn

9   Spurring Responsible Firearms Sales Practices through Litigation:
    The Impact of New York City's Lawsuits against Gun Dealers
    on Interstate Gun Trafficking   123
    Daniel W. Webster and Jon S. Vernick

10 Curtailing Dangerous Sales Practices by Licensed Firearm
    Dealers: Legal Opportunities and Obstacles   133
    Jon S. Vernick and Daniel W. Webster

    PART II. MAKING GUN LAWS ENFORCEABLE

11 Enforcing Federal Laws against Firearms Traffickers: Raising
    Operational Effectiveness by Lowering Enforcement Obstacles   143
    Anthony A. Braga and Peter L. Gagliardi

    PART III. GUN POLICY LESSONS FROM
    THE UNITED STATES: HIGH-RISK GUNS

12 America's Experience with the Federal Assault Weapons Ban,
    1994–2004: Key Findings and Implications   157
    Christopher S. Koper

13 Personalized Guns: Using Technology to Save Lives   173
    Stephen P. Teret and Adam D. Mernit

PART IV. INTERNATIONAL CASE STUDIES
OF RESPONSES TO GUN VIOLENCE

14   Gun Control in Great Britain after the Dunblane Shootings   185
     Michael J. North

15   Rational Firearm Regulation: Evidence-based Gun Laws
     in Australia   195
     Rebecca Peters

16   The Big Melt: How One Democracy Changed after Scrapping
     a Third of Its Firearms   205
     Philip Alpers

17   Brazil: Gun Control and Homicide Reduction   213
     Antonio Rangel Bandeira

PART V. SECOND AMENDMENT

18   The Scope of Regulatory Authority under the
     Second Amendment   225
     Lawrence E. Rosenthal and Adam Winkler

PART VI. PUBLIC OPINION ON GUN POLICY

19   Public Opinion on Proposals to Strengthen U.S. Gun Laws:
     Findings from a 2013 Survey   239
     *Emma E. McGinty, Daniel W. Webster, Jon S. Vernick,
     and Colleen L. Barry*

     Consensus Recommendations for Reforms to Federal
     Gun Policies   259

     Biographies of Contributors   263
     Index   275

Foreword

On December 14, 2012, a deranged young man pulled into the parking lot of the Sandy Hook Elementary School in Newtown, Connecticut, and then shot his way into the building with a high-capacity semi-automatic rifle. The slaughter of 6 adults and 20 children really broke the country's heart, and for many Americans this is the straw that has broken the camel's back.

Since the Sandy Hook massacre, more than 100 mayors from across the country have joined the bipartisan coalition Mayors Against Illegal Guns. The total number of mayors involved is now more than 800. As of January 14, 2013, roughly one million Americans have signed on to the coalition's "I Demand a Plan" campaign against gun violence. Vice President Joe Biden will announce his recommendations for action to President Barack Obama this week. The vice president knows that as horrific as Sandy Hook has been, as have all the other seemingly endless episodes of mass violence, we experience that level of carnage, or worse, every single day across our country, *because every day of the year, an average of 33 Americans are murdered with guns.*

Here's another way to think about what that means. On January 21, 2013, President Obama took the oath of office for his second term. Unless we take action, during those four years some 48,000 Americans will be killed with guns—nearly twice as many people as were killed in combat during the entire Vietnam War. I have made it clear to the vice president that our bipartisan coalition of mayors is supporting seven measures—three that need legislation and four that require only executive action. We're hopeful that the vice president and president will support all seven.

First and most urgently, we need the president and Congress together to require background checks for all gun sales, including private sales at gun shows and online. These private sales now account for more than 40 percent of all gun sales nationally, which means that in 2012 alone, there were more than six million gun sales that happened with no background checks. Many of those guns are handguns, which are used in about 90 percent of all firearms murders. Across the United States, more than 80 percent of gun owners, and more than 90 percent of Americans, support requiring background checks for all gun sales. There's really no debate here. It's common sense. We have laws on the books that require a background check when dealers sell guns. It's time for the president and Congress to make that the law of the land for all sales. The forty percent to which the law does not apply means the law is basically a sham.

Second, Congress should make gun trafficking a federal crime. In New York City, 85 percent of the weapons that we recover from crime scenes come from out-of-state sources, but federal laws designed to curb illegal sales across borders are incredibly weak. Criminals who traffic in guns get a slap on the wrist. We've made New York the safest big city in the nation, in part by adopting tough gun laws and proactively enforcing them. Every state in the Union has citizens killed by guns coming from other another state, and every state is powerless to stop the mayhem. Until Congress gets tough on trafficking, guns will continue flowing to our streets from states with much looser gun laws.

The third legislative measure that the White House should support is limiting the availability of military-style weapons and of high-capacity magazines with more than 10 rounds. These guns and equipment are not designed for sport or home defense. They are designed to kill large numbers of people quickly. That's the only purpose they have. They belong on the battlefield, in the hands of our brave professionally trained soldiers, not on the streets of our cities, suburbs, or rural areas, as retired military leaders like Colin Powell and Stanley McChrystal have said.

Many of the weapons in this category were previously banned under the federal assault weapons law that expired in 2004. That law was, incidentally, first initiated and passed by Vice President Biden. He is the right person to have been appointed by the president to come up with what we should do next. Regulating assault weapons certainly falls within the bounds of the Second Amendment. So does everything else we're urging.

This is not a constitutional question; it's a question of political courage. The U.S. Supreme Court, the entity that defines what the Constitution means, has ruled that reasonable regulations are consistent with the Second Amendment. When the gun lobby raises concerns over protection of the Second Amendment, it is nothing but a red herring. And it's time for Second Amendment defenders in Congress to call them on it.

The three measures that I've discussed—requiring background checks for all gun sales, making gun trafficking a federal crime, and limiting military-style assault weapons and high-capacity magazines—will require leadership from both the president and members of Congress. But there are other steps President Obama can take without congressional approval—any time he chooses, with the stroke of a pen. Vice President Biden understands this, and we hope his recommendations will include at least these next four steps that we've urged him to take.

In the first of these four steps, the president can order all federal agencies to submit their relevant data to the national gun background check database. Every missing record is a potential murder in the making. If the data aren't in the database, those people that use the database don't get what they need, allowing gun sales to go ahead in cases where we all agree—and federal law says—they shouldn't.

Second, the president can direct the Justice Department to make a priority of prosecuting convicted criminals who provide false personal information during gun purchase background checks. Yes, even criminals buy from dealers, knowing there's going to be a background check, except that they lie when they do so. As a matter of fact, during 2010 there were more than 76,000 cases referred by the FBI to the Justice Department. Do you know how many were prosecuted out of 76,000 in 2010, the last year for which we have data? Forty-four. Not 44,000, but 44 out of 76,000. This is a joke. It's a sad joke, and it's a lethal joke.

These are felony cases involving criminals trying to buy guns, and yet our federal government is prosecuting less than one-tenth of one percent of them. It is shameful, and it has to end, and the president can do that by just picking up the phone and saying to the Justice Department: This is your job, go do it or I'll get somebody that will.

As a third step, the president can make a recess appointment to get someone to head the Federal Bureau of Alcohol, Tobacco, Firearms and Explosives. The ATF, as it's called, hasn't had a director for six years. Can you imagine how much outrage there'd be if we'd been without a Homeland Security Secretary for six years? You can't have an agency without somebody running it that's going to allow it to do the job for which it was, and that job is to protect everyone in this city, state, and country—including those we love the most, our children, and those we have the greatest responsibility to, the police officers who run into danger when the rest of us are running the other way.

The president, and this is our fourth recommendation, can stop supporting what's called the Tiahrt order. Todd Tiahrt is a congressman from Wichita who got the Congress to pass a law that keeps the public in the dark about who gun traffickers are and how they operate. There can be no excuse for shielding criminals from public view.

At the bidding of the gun lobby, Congress has tied the hands of the Bureau of Alcohol, Tobacco, Firearms and Explosive and has prevented it from releasing critical data to law enforcement authorities and to the public. Unfortunately, the ATF is not alone is being gagged by Congress when it comes to the issue of guns.

The bipartisan coalition of Mayors Against Illegal Guns released a report, "Access Denied" detailing how Congress, bowing to the gun lobby, has systematically denied the American people access to information about guns and gun violence. Most egregiously and outrageously, Congress has severely restricted the scientists at the Centers for Disease Control and Prevention from studying the epidemic of gun violence, and they've put similar restrictions on the scientists at the National Institutes of Health. Congress has no business dictating what public health issues scientists can and should study.

At Johns Hopkins the motto is, The truth shall make you free. When elected officials try to muzzle scientific research and bury the truth, they make our free society less free and less safe. Today, because of congressional restrictions, CDC funding for firearms injury research totals $100,000, out of an annual budget of nearly $6 billion. The National Institutes of Health is estimated to spend less than $1 million on firearms injury research, out of an annual budget of $31 billion. To put that in perspective, the NIH spends $21 million annually researching headaches. But it spends less than $1 million on all the gun deaths that happen every year. If that doesn't give you a headache, it should.

There are 31,000 gun deaths every year in America, including about 19,000 suicides, many of which are children—every parent's nightmare. In New York City, our suicide rate is less than half the national average, and one of the differences is that New York has tough gun laws. Nationally, 51 percent of suicides are by gun. In New York City, it is only 16 percent of suicides. The gun lobby callously says that someone who wants to kill him or herself will find a way to do it. In many cases, they are tragically wrong. We can prevent thousands of these senseless deaths with smart gun regulations, and we're proving it in New York City.

Unfortunately, American scientists are not the only people Congress has attempted to silence. In 2010, again at the gun lobby's bidding, Congress included language in a funding a bill that prevented military officers and doctors, as well as mental health counselors, from even discussing firearms ownership with severely depressed service members. There is a suicide crisis going on right now in our military. It's tough seeing and doing what we ask our soldiers to do. We have an all-volunteer army, but they come back and many of them really do have a problem. Congress, instead of trying to help, is just doing everything it can to make it worse. Our men and women in uniform deserve better. Thankfully, after mayors and retired military leaders urged Congress to rescind this prohibition, they did—but not until December of 2012, and only after too many men and women in uniform had taken their own lives with guns.

Enough is enough. It's time for Congress and the White House to put public health above special interest politics. And it's time for Congress to stop gagging our scientists, military leaders, and law enforcement officers—and stop trying to hide the truth from the American people. That's why this summit was so important. It is especially fitting that it was hosted at the Johns Hopkins Bloomberg School of Public Health, where so much outstanding and important work is being done, in areas ranging from malaria research and environmental health to tobacco control and road safety. It's all designed around the school's motto, Protecting Health, Saving Lives—Millions at a Time. Reducing gun violence will have that kind of an impact, too.

A few years ago, Daniel Webster, director of the School's Center for Gun Policy and Research, conducted a study of an initiative in New York City that aimed to identify the most problematic out-of-state gun dealers, based on crime data, conducting undercover investigations of their sales practices and suing those who sold guns to our straw purchasers. Straw purchasers are those who lie about who is the actual purchaser of the gun, standing in for somebody who could not pass a background check. Twenty-four of the most problematic dealers settled or were put under a court monitor. Dr. Webster found that in New York City the likelihood of recovering a gun at a crime scene from one of these dealers dropped almost overnight by 84 percent.

Ninety-nine percent of the gun dealers in our country do obey the law; one percent do not, and those are the ones that we have to go after. And the results are dramatic and almost instantaneous. Our investigation never would have happened without the data that allowed us to identify the problematic dealers. And yet, if it were up to the NRA, we would never have had access to it. More guns would have flowed onto our streets and, in all likelihood, more people would have been murdered.

The undercover investigations we've conducted are just one example of how we've worked to crack down on gun violence. At our urging, the New York state legislature enacted the toughest penalties in the nation for illegal possession of a handgun: a 3½-year mandatory minimum prison sentence. We have also worked with our city council to adopt a law enabling the NYPD to keep tabs on gun offenders in our city, in the same way that they track sex offenders. We enforce those laws and other laws rigorously, which is an important reason New York is the safest big city in the country. In 2012, New York City had the fewest murders in nearly half a century (comparable records started to be kept back in 1963). We've never had a year remotely as safe as this past one.

As hard as we've worked, however, and as much as we've achieved, the reality remains that, in New York during 2012, there were still 418 murders in the City, and a lot of the people that were killed were kids. While shooting incidents are down in New York City, as well as murders, I recently visited three NYPD officers who'd been shot by criminals in two separate incidents on the same night. Thankfully, the officers are all expected to fully recover. But I think the events of that night really do demonstrate a flaw in an argument we've heard lately. That argument is that the solution to "bad guys with guns is good guys with guns." The problem is that sometimes the good guys get shot. Sometimes, in fact, they get killed. And I think the hardest part of my job, the part that I dread the most as mayor, is talking to the family of a police officer at a hospital to tell them that their husband, wife, mother, father, son or daughter won't ever be coming home again.

The tragic fact is that all across America today, fathers and mothers, wives and husbands, friends and neighbors will experience that kind of pain and loss in their lives because of gun violence. The rate of firearms homicides in America is 20 times higher than it is in other economically advanced nations. We have got to change that—and it has to start now, with real leadership from the White House.

If you haven't done so, go to DemandAPlan.org and join the campaign for gun safety reform, or call your senators or your congressmen and say, "We're not going to take this. Even if *you* vote the right way, your associates in Congress aren't voting the right way. And since I don't get a chance to influence them, but you want my vote, you do something about it. It is your responsibility to do it as much as it is the responsibility of the other senators and the other congressmen." Let us hope that Washington gives the issue the attention that it deserves. This is going to make a real difference between what our lives are like today and a safe future for our kids.

Michael R. Bloomberg, Mayor of New York City
Excerpted from opening remarks given at the Summit on
Reducing Gun Violence in America at the Johns Hopkins
Bloomberg School of Public Health, January 14, 2013

Preface

One month—to the hour—after the harrowing and unfathomable massacre of 20 children and 6 adults in a Newtown, Connecticut, elementary school, Johns Hopkins University convened a summit that brought together preeminent researchers on gun violence from across the country and around the world. This was a moment when advocates, lobbyists, and politicians on both sides of the gun-control debate were beginning to mobilize and spar. In this unruly mix, Johns Hopkins seized the opportunity to discharge a critical role of research universities and provided principled scaffolding for the debate. We wanted to use the opportunity to cut through the din of the shrill and the incendiary, the rancorous and the baseless, and provide rigorous, research-based considerations of the most effective gun regulations and the appropriate balance between individual rights and civic obligation.

At Johns Hopkins, our scholars and researchers have been investigating the public health effects of gun violence for well over two decades. For the past seventeen years, the Center for Gun Policy and Research has provided a home for that study, producing nationally recognized research and recommendations aimed at understanding and curtailing the impact of gun violence.

Given the national historical backdrop of a bleak record of stunted policy reform in this area, some may have considered this summit to be another exercise in futility. The skeptic's fear is that good ideas for gun-policy reform are no match for the formidable interests that oppose gun control legislation—even after an event as cataclysmic as Newtown.

But our decidedly more optimistic view is predicated on the belief that this country is not slavishly tethered to the current matrix of inadequate national gun laws. Rather, despite a long history of failed legislative and policy reform and of opportunities inexplicably squandered, progress is possible. This view is illustrated both by the experiences of other countries and those of the United States.

At the summit, speakers from Australia, Scotland, and Brazil discussed the adoption of significant new policies in the wake of horrific moments of gun violence. These nations have never had constitutional guarantees protecting individuals' rights to bear arms, their political institutions vary greatly from those in the United States, and "gun culture" is an alien concept. But there are telling lessons to be gleaned from the approaches these countries took to address the wanton loss of life from gun violence.

In the United States, there is no denying the sea change in public sentiment that has buttressed public health reforms in areas as diverse as seat belt usage, drunk driving, and lead exposure. From the passage of civil rights legislation to the regulation of tobacco products, we have observed enough nontrivial policy change in recent decades to recognize that the apparent iron grip of status quo forces can be shattered and our policy can progress.

We owe great appreciation to Daniel Webster and Jon Vernick, of the Johns Hopkins Center for Gun Policy and Research, who framed the questions at the heart of this issue, organized the summit, and edited this book, all with extraordinary sophistication and speed. They were supported by a team of committed Johns Hopkins staff who set aside daily obligations to support this urgent cause. To each of them, and to the Johns Hopkins University Press, which published this book in unprecedented time, we are grateful.

Ronald J. Daniels, President, Johns Hopkins University

Michael J. Klag, Dean, Johns Hopkins Bloomberg
School of Public Health

Acknowledgments

This book—published in only ten days—would be nothing more than an ambitious wish without the extraordinary efforts of many people.

We owe an immense debt of gratitude to Johns Hopkins University President Ron Daniels, who, in the wake of the Newtown tragedy, urged us to seize the moment and bring the depth and rigor of empirical research to one of the most complex and fractious issues our country has ever faced. His leadership and vision epitomize the spirit of Johns Hopkins and our obligation to spread knowledge beyond the realm of academe and into the streets, where everyday citizens live the public health challenges we study.

We are grateful also to Dean Michael Klag of the Bloomberg School of Public Health, who has been an unflagging supporter of the Center for Gun Policy and Research for many years, even and especially when public attention for our research was in short supply. His enthusiastic support for the Summit and the book proved essential to making both a reality.

A few days before the December holidays, we contacted more than twenty of the world's top experts on gun policy, some scattered around the globe, and asked them to present their research and experience at a January summit that would inform important policy decisions and to write chapters for a companion volume that would be published the same month. These colleagues and friends—many of whom have devoted their careers to the study of violence and gun policy—answered the call without hesitation, interrupting family time during the holidays to join us in this important work.

We appreciate the valuable guidance provided by Stephen Teret, the founding director of the Johns Hopkins Center for Gun Policy and Research, in addition to his important chapter in the book. Thank you to Alicia Samuels, our Center's communications director, for ensuring the outcomes of this Summit reached key audiences. We are also grateful to the work of the many Center faculty who contributed valuable chapters to the book. And we are in awe of Colleen Barry's and Emma McGinty's exceptional effort to design and carry out a survey of public opinion on gun policy of such exceptional depth and quality during the first two weeks of January 2013.

Our sincere thanks to New York City Mayor Michael R. Bloomberg, whose powerful opening remarks at the Johns Hopkins Summit on Reducing Gun Violence in America inspired courage and conviction. We are likewise grateful to Maryland Governor Martin O'Malley, who cleared his calendar to speak at the Summit in the opening days of the legislative session.

Our colleagues at the Bloomberg School rose to the considerable challenge of organizing a high-profile event with short notice. We express our deepest gratitude to Josh Else, Jim Yager, Jane Schlegel, Felicity Turner, Susan Sperry, and Susan Murrow, who set aside the considerable demands of their daily work to make the Summit happen, along with their colleagues David Croft, Brian Simpson, Lauren Haney, Chip Hickey, Rachel Howard, Scott Klein, Ross McKenzie, Robert Ollinger, Tim Parsons, Maryalice Yakutchik, Mike Smith, Jackie Powder Frank, John Replogle, Yolanda Tillett, Alyssa Vetro, and Natalie Wood-Wright. And thank you to the countless other faculty, staff, and students for their support and interest in our work.

We received incredible support from our colleagues on the Homewood Campus, especially Lois Chiang, Glenn Bieler, Tom Lewis, Eileen Fader, Dennis O'Shea, and Jill Williams. They, along with their colleagues Beth Felder, Melisa Lindamood, Dave Alexander, Doug Behr, Lauren Custer, Lisa DeNike, Amy Lunday, Erin Oglesby, Tracey Reeves, Greg Rienzi, Hilary Roxe, Tricia Schellenbach, Gus Sentementes, Glenn Simmons, Phil Sneiderman, and others, demonstrated the spirit of "One Hopkins" by traveling between various campuses and offices to get the job done.

The Johns Hopkins University Press director Kathleen Keane and editorial director Greg Britton welcomed this project from the moment it was proposed, and we extend special thanks to our editor Kelley Squazzo, who embraced the challenges of working with multiple contributors over thousands of miles to produce a book in record time. We thank the peer reviewers for their very helpful feedback on the chapters in this book. Editorial, design, and production colleagues Julie McCarthy, Martha Sewall, John Cronin, Sara Cleary, Michele Callaghan, Mary Lou Kenney, and Carol Eckhart tended this project with extraordinary care under immense time constraints. Marketing staff Becky Brasington Clark, Tom Lovett, Karen Willmes, Kathy Alexander, Claire McCabe Tamberino, Brendan Coyne, Robin Rennison, Robin Noonan, Jack Holmes, Susan Ventura, Alexis de la Rosa, Cathy Bergeron, and Vanessa Kotz did an extraordinary job with promotion.

Our deepest thanks go to our families, who sustain us and support this important work.

Daniel W. Webster, ScD, MPH

Jon S. Vernick, JD, MPH

Introduction

The role of guns in violence, and what should be done, are subjects of intense debate in the United States and elsewhere. But certain facts are not debatable. More than 31,000 people died from gunshot wounds in the United States in 2010.[1] Because the victims are disproportionately young, gun violence is one of the leading causes of premature mortality in the United States. In addition to these deaths, in 2010, there were an estimated 337,960 nonfatal violent crimes committed with guns,[2] and 73,505 persons were treated in hospital emergency departments for nonfatal gunshot wounds.[3,4] The social and economic costs of gun violence in America are also enormous.

Despite the huge daily impact of gun violence, most public discourse on gun policy is centered on mass shootings in public places. Such incidents are typically portrayed as random acts by severely mentally ill individuals which are impossible to predict or prevent. Those who viewed, heard, or read news stories on gun policy might conclude the following: (1) mass shootings, the mentally ill, and assault weapons are the primary concerns; (2) gun control laws disarm law-abiding citizens without affecting criminals' access to guns;

(3) there is no evidence that gun control laws work; and (4) the public has no appetite for strengthening current gun laws. Yet all of the evidence in this book counters each of these misperceptions with facts to the contrary.

As Miller et al. point out in their essay, gun availability greatly increases the risk of violent death in America because many acts of gun violence involve spontaneous altercations that result in death or serious injury when a gun is readily available. Vittes et al. explain in their call for expanding disqualifying conditions for having handguns that this is especially true when these conflicts involve individuals with criminal histories, perpetrators of domestic violence, substance abusers, and youth.

Cook and Ludwig's essay reveals disappointing but not surprising findings of their evaluation of the Brady Law given that it leaves a substantial gap in federal gun control laws by omitting private transactions from background check and record keeping requirements. Papers by Webster et al. and Wintemute provide evidence that state laws that fill this gap by requiring universal background checks reduce diversions of guns to criminals.

Addressing gaps in the background check system are important because prohibiting firearm purchase and possession by high-risk groups appears to decrease violence. Swanson et al. document beneficial effects from prohibiting firearms for individuals with certain mental illnesses as long as appropriate records are shared with law enforcement agencies that screen gun buyers. Zeoli and Frattaroli share evidence that some firearm prohibitions for domestic violence offenders are saving lives, and Wintemute provides evidence that preventing violent misdemeanants from purchasing handguns reduces violence.

Some elected officials claim that they are looking out for gun owners when they pass measures deceptively named "Firearm Owners' Protection Act" or "Protection of Lawful Commerce in Arms Act." But essays by Vernick and Webster and by Braga and Gagliardi demonstrate that these laws and others like them are designed solely to protect gun sellers against measures that would otherwise hold them accountable for practices that divert guns to criminals. Current federal laws make it very difficult to prosecute, sue, revoke the licenses of rogue gun dealers, or even share data about which gun manufacturers and retailers are connected to unusually large numbers of guns used by criminals. Studies have shown that when gun dealers experience greater regulation and oversight by law enforcement and are vulnerable to lawsuits for illegal sales practices, far fewer of the guns they sell end up in the hands of criminals.

Koper reviews his evaluation of the 1994 federal ban on assault weapons and high-capacity ammunition magazines. That ban was designed to remove military-style weapons and make it harder for multiple rounds to be fired without reloading. Unfortunately, the assault weapon ban was easy to evade and millions of existing high-capacity ammunition magazines were grandfathered. The law was allowed to expire in 2004, but Koper's findings can teach us how to improve such laws in the future.

Firearms themselves can also be made safer. Teret and Mernit describe the benefits of safe gun designs, particularly personalized guns designed to be operable only by an authorized user. They discuss the history of these technologies, their present-day feasibility, and ways to promote their adoption.

The United States is not the only nation to have suffered from mass shootings or to address an endemic gun violence problem. Mass shootings in Dunblane, Scotland, and Port Arthur, Tasmania, led to major changes in the gun laws of the United Kingdom and Australia. Essays by North, Peters, and Alpers describe these new laws. Brazil had some of the highest rates of gun violence in the world. Yet here, too, comprehensive changes to gun laws were associated with reductions in rates of violence. Bandeira discusses this success story Although bans on certain handguns (as in the UK) or bans and mass buybacks of specific long guns (in Australia) are unlikely to occur in the United States, the authors discuss the lessons U.S. advocates and policymakers can learn from these successes in other nations.

For many years, some groups have claimed that the Second Amendment to the U.S. Constitution stands as an obstacle to most gun laws. Rosenthal and Winkler debunk this myth with careful legal analysis of recent U.S. Supreme Court and lower court opinions. The recommendations provided in this book should withstand constitutional scrutiny.

Public opinion is also an important determinant of whether any particular evidence-based policy becomes law. McGinty et al. report on a newly conducted national public opinion poll of 33 different policies. Most were supported by strong majorities of the public, including a majority of gun owners.

The book concludes with consensus recommendations from the book's contributors. These recommendations address the full range of topics covered in this book. If implemented, these recommendations have the potential to dramatically reduce the number of gun deaths in the United States, enhancing the quality of life for all Americans.

Daniel W. Webster, ScD, MPH

Jon S. Vernick, JD, MPH

NOTES

1. Centers for Disease Control and Prevention. Web-based Injury Statistics Query and Reporting System (WISQARS) [Online]. National Center for Injury Control and Prevention, Centers for Disease Control and Prevention (producer). Available from: URL: http://www.cdc.gov/injury/wisqars/index.html. [2012, Mar. 15].

2. Truman JL. Criminal Victimization, 2010. National Crime Victimization Survey. NCJ 235508, Washington, DC: United States Department of Justice, Bureau of Justice Statistics, Sept. 2010.

3. Centers for Disease Control and Prevention. Web-based Injury Statistics Query and Reporting System (WISQARS) [Online]. National Center for Injury Control and Prevention, Centers for Disease Control and Prevention (producer). Available from: URL: http://www.cdc.gov/injury/wisqars/index.html. [2012, Mar. 15].

4. Vyrostek SB, Annest JL, Ryan GW. Surveillance for Fatal and Non-Fatal Injuries—United States, 2001. *MMWR.* 2004; 53(SS07):1–57.

Part I / Gun Policy Lessons from the United States

Keeping Guns from High-Risk Individuals

Firearms and Violent Death in the United States

Matthew Miller, Deborah Azrael, and David Hemenway

Firearm-Related Deaths in the United States

In 2010, there were more than 31,000 firearm deaths in the United States: 62% were suicides, 36% were homicides, and 2% were unintentional (2%) (CDC 2012a). Almost as many Americans die from gunfire as die from motor vehicle crashes (almost 34,000 in 2010). Americans under age 40 are more likely to die from gunfire than from any specific disease (CDC 2012a).

Homicide

The United States is not a more violent country than other high-income nations. Our rates of car theft, burglary, robbery, sexual assault, and aggravated assault are similar to those of other high-income countries (van Kesteren, Mayhew, and Nieuwbeerta 2001); our adolescent fighting rates are also similar (Pickett

Matthew Miller, MD, ScD, MPH, is deputy director of the Harvard Injury Control Research Center and associate professor of Injury Prevention and Health Policy at the Harvard School of Public Health. Deborah Azrael, PhD, has been a member of the firearms research group at the Harvard School of Public Health for more than 20 years. David Hemenway, PhD, is an economist and professor at the Harvard School of Public Health and director of the Harvard Injury Control Research Center.

Table 1.1 Homicide, suicide, and unintentional gun
deaths among 5–14 year olds: The United States versus
25 other high-income populous countries (early 2003)

	Mortality rate ratio
Homicides	
Gun homicides	13.2
Non-gun homicides	1.7
Total	3.4
Suicides	
Gun suicides	7.8
Non-gun suicides	1.3
Total	1.7
Unintentional firearm deaths	10.3

Source: Richardson and Hemenway 2011

et al. 2013). However, when Americans are violent, the injuries that result are more likely to prove fatal. For example, the U.S. rate of firearm homicide for children 5 to 14 years of age is thirteen times higher than the firearms homicide rate of other developed nations, and the rate of homicide overall is more than three times higher (Table 1.1).

U.S. homicide rates vary cyclically over time. Current rates are at a 30-year low, but as recently as 1991 rates were nearly twice as high (CDC 2012a). Changes in homicide rates over the past several decades are largely attributable to changes in firearm homicide rates, mostly driven by changes in firearm homicide rates among adolescent and young men in large cities (Hepburn and Hemenway 2004, Blumstein and Wallman 2000, Cork 1999, Cook and John 2002).[1]

The U.S. homicide rate is much higher in urban than in rural areas, as are rates of all violent crime. Nine out of ten homicide offenders are male, and 75% of victims are male. African Americans are disproportionately represented among both perpetrators and victims.[2]

Suicide

Compared with other high-income countries, the U.S. adult suicide rate falls roughly in the middle. Among younger persons, however, our suicide mortality is relatively high: for children under 15 years of age, the overall suicide rate in the United States is 1.6 times that of the average of other high-income countries, largely accounted for by a firearm suicide rate eight times that of the average of these countries (Richardson and Hemenway 2011).

Over the past several decades, suicide rates have been more stable than have rates of homicide (Miller, Azrael, and Barber 2012). Nevertheless, after declining from a peak of 12.9/100,000 in 1986 to 10.4 in 2000, driven largely by a decline in the rate of firearm suicide, the suicide rate has increased over the past decade to 12.4/100,000 in 2010, mostly due to an increase in suicide by hanging (Miller, Azrael, and Barber 2012, CDC 2012a).

Age, sex, race, and other demographic characteristics—including marital status, income, educational attainment, and employment status—all influence suicide mortality (Nock et al. 2008). Suicide rates are higher, for example, for white and Native Americans than for black, Hispanic, and Asian Americans (CDC 2007). A consistent finding across numerous studies is that the strongest individual-level risk factor for a fatal suicidal act is having previously attempted suicide; other strong risk factors include psychiatric and substance abuse disorders (Shaffer et al. 1996).

In contrast to homicide rates, suicide rates are higher in rural than in urban areas almost entirely due to higher rates of firearm suicide in rural areas.

Unintentional Firearm Deaths

Approximately 675 Americans per year were killed unintentionally with firearms between 2001 and 2010 (CDC 2007). Data from the National Violent Death Reporting System show that two-thirds of the accidental shooting deaths occurred in someone's home, about half of the victims were younger than 25 years, and half of all deaths were other-inflicted. In other-inflicted shootings, the victim was typically shot accidentally by a friend or family member—often an older brother (Hemenway, Barber, and Miller 2010).

Firearm Ownership in the United States

The United States has more private guns per capita (particularly more handguns) and higher levels of household gun ownership than other developed countries (Killias 1993, SAS 2007).

Most of what we know about gun ownership levels in the United States over the past several decades comes from the General Social Survey (GSS 2010), a relatively small biannual survey of U.S. adults. Data from the GSS show that the percentage of households with firearms has fallen from approximately 50% in the late 1970s to 33% today. Changing household demographics are believed to explain the decline in the household ownership of guns chiefly due to a fall in the number of households with an adult male (Smith 2000). Notably, however, the percentage of individuals owning firearms has remained relatively constant over the past several decades (GSS 2010).

The GSS does not speak to the number of guns in civilian hands or the distribution of guns within households. For this information, researchers have turned to data from two medium-sized national surveys conducted a decade apart. These surveys suggest that the number of guns in civilian hands grew from approximately 200 million in 1994 to 300 million in 2004—and that the average gun owner now owns more guns than previously (Hepburn et al. 2007, Cook and Ludwig 1997).

Compared with other Americans, gun owners are disproportionately male, married, older than 40, and more likely to live in nonurban areas. Their long guns (rifles, shotguns) are owned mainly for sport (hunting and target shooting). People who own only handguns typically own the guns for protection against crime (Hepburn et al. 2007, Cook 1979).

In 2001, 2002, and 2004, but not before or since, information on household gun ownership from the General Social Survey was supplemented by information from the National Behavioral Risk Factor Surveillance System (CDC 1997). The BRFSS is of sufficient size (more than 200,000 respondents annually) that household gun ownership could, for the first time, be determined at the state level for all 50 states and for some Metropolitan Statistical Areas.

Prior to these three iterations of the BRFSS, researchers generally used proxies to measure firearm ownership rates at the state and sub-state level. A validation study by Azrael, Philip, and Miller (2004) found that from among all proxies, the fraction of suicides that are committed with firearms (FS/S) correlates most strongly and consistently with cross-sectional survey-based measures of household firearm ownership at the county, state, and regional levels.

Household firearm ownership is probably a good measure of the accessibility of guns used in suicides, since most suicides involving firearms occur in the home (Kellermann et al. 1992, CDC 2012b) and involve a firearm owned by a member of the household (Kellermann et al. 1992). Household gun ownership levels seem also to be the key exposure variable for firearm homicides that take place in the home, where women, children and older adults are particularly likely to be killed. The most common perpetrator in such instances is a family member (CDC 2012b). By contrast, older adolescent and young adult males are more often killed outside the home by guns owned by a non-family member.[3]

In this essay, we focus on studies that assess the relationship between gun prevalence and violent death. As such, the essay does not examine studies of gun carrying nor any literature on illegal gun markets. It also does not address research that investigates the relationship between firearm regulations and violent death. Note, however, that firearm prevalence and firearm regulation are highly collinear. Strong regulations may limit firearm ownership, and low levels of firearm ownership make it easier to pass stronger regulations.

This essay is also not an exhaustive review of the literature examining the association of firearm availability and violent death. (For more comprehensive reviews, see Hepburn and Hemenway 2004, Miller and Hemenway 1999, and Brent 2001.) Rather, it briefly summarizes (a) international ecologic studies comparing the United States to other countries, (b) ecologic studies of U.S. regions, states, and metropolitan areas, and (c) individual case-control and cohort studies.

Studies included in this brief review met a minimal threshold of attempting to control for important confounders: studies had to compare likes to likes. For case-control studies of homicide, that means—at a minimum—controlling for age, gender, and neighborhood; in suicide studies, for age, sex, and psychiatric risk factors for suicidal behavior. For international studies of homicide, it means comparing high-income countries to high-income countries. International comparisons of adult suicide rates are confounded by large differences in religion, culture and recording practices (i.e., the social meaning and cultural acceptance of adult suicide), as evidenced by tenfold differences in suicide rates across high-income nations. Thus, the only international studies of suicide included focus on the suicides of children—which all countries hold to be tragedies. For ecologic studies in the United States, making "like to like" comparisons means comparing states to states with similar levels of urbanization (or, for homicide, similar crime rates), cities to cities, and rural areas to rural areas.[4]

Firearms and Homicide
Ecologic Studies

Killias (1993) evaluated rates of violence in 14 developed countries: 11 in Europe, along with the United States, Canada, and Australia. He used data from the 1989 International Crime Survey, a telephone survey of 14 countries and 28,000 respondents, to measure firearm prevalence. Respondents were asked whether there were any firearms in their household and, if so, whether any were a handgun or a long gun. Military firearms were excluded. In this study, which did not include control variables, rates of firearm ownership and homicide were positively correlated, while rates of firearm ownership and non-firearm homicide were not.

A study by Hemenway and Miller (2000) included 26 high-income nations with populations greater than one million. To measure gun availability, the authors used two proxies, including FS/S. No control variables were included in the analysis. Firearm availability was strongly and significantly associated with homicide across the 26 countries.

A follow-up study (Hemenway, Shinoda-Tagawa, and Miller 2002) examined homicide rates among women across high-income countries. The validated proxy (FS/S, or the percentage of suicides committed with a firearm) was used to estimate firearm ownership in each country. Urbanization and income inequality were included as control variables. The United States accounted for 70% of all female homicide victims in the study and had the highest firearm ownership rates. The U.S. homicide rate for women was five times higher than that of all of the other countries combined; its female firearm homicide rate was eleven times higher.

U.S. Studies

Cook (1979) conducted a cross-sectional analysis of 50 large cities in the United States to explore the relationship between gun availability and robbery, including robbery-murder. Using data on the number of robberies in 1975, Cook examined how firearm availability (as proxied by Cook's index) was related to robbery and robbery-murder rates, controlling for measures of the effectiveness of the criminal justice system, population density, and other regional and state differences. Increased gun availability was not associated with overall robbery rates, but it was positively associated with the proportion of robberies that involved a gun—and with the per capita robbery-murder rate, through an increased rate of gun robbery.

Miller et al. (2002) evaluated the relationship between levels of firearm ownership at the state and regional level and the incidence of homicide from 1988 to 1997 for 50 states and 9 regions. At the state level, they used the percentage of suicides with a firearm as a proxy for ownership and they measured gun availability at the regional level with data from the GSS. Five potential confounders were included: poverty, urbanization, unemployment, alcohol consumption, and (non-homicide) violent crime rates. In the multivariate analyses, a positive and significant association between gun ownership and homicide rates was found for the entire population and for every age group (except ages 0–4), primarily due to higher firearm homicide rates.

A similar study (Miller et al. 2007) used survey estimates of household gun ownership for each state from the Behavioral Risk Factor Surveillance System. It examined data from 2001 to 2003 and controlled for state-level rates of aggravated assault, robbery, unemployment, urbanization, alcohol consumption, poverty, income inequality, the percentage of the population that was black, and the percentage of families headed by a single female parent. Again, states with higher rates of household firearm ownership had significantly higher homicide victimization rates for men, for women, and for children. The association was driven by gun-related homicide victimization rates; non-gun-related victimization rates were not significantly associated with rates of firearm ownership.

Individual Level Studies

Ecologic studies provide evidence about whether more guns in the community are associated with more homicides in the community. Case-control and cohort studies provide data more germane to the question of whether a gun in the home increases or reduces the risk of homicide victimization for members of the household.

Kellermann et al. examined approximately 400 homicide victims from three metropolitan areas who were killed in their homes (Kellermann et al. 1993). All died from gunshot wounds. In 83% of the homicides, the perpetrator was identified; among these cases, 95% of the time, the perpetrator was not a stranger. In only 14% of all the cases was there evidence of forced entry. After controlling for illicit drug use, fights, arrests, living alone, and whether the home was rented,

Table 1.2   NVDRS 2005–2010

	Firearm			Non-firearm		
	N	Occurred in a house/apt	Occurred at victim's residence	N	Occurred in a house/apt	Occurred at victim's residence
Homicides by age group						
0–4 yrs	81	75%	67%	1,025	90%	77%
5–14 yrs	257	72%	51%	205	78%	67%
15–24 yrs	5,679	37%	16%	1,385	47%	27%
25–34 yrs	4,906	44%	24%	1,479	56%	39%
35–64 yrs	5,003	56%	41%	3,716	62%	50%
65+ yrs	470	74%	69%	719	79%	76%
Suicides by age group						
0–4 yrs	—			—		
5–14 yrs	105	97%	88%	301	91%	88%
15–24 yrs	3,332	75%	64%	3,769	69%	65%
25–34 yrs	4,034	76%	67%	4,743	70%	65%
35–64 yrs	15,634	78%	74%	16,568	72%	70%
65+ yrs	6,019	89%	88%	2,168	80%	83%

Note: Unknowns for age (0.7%), house/apt (1.4%), home (3.6%) were set aside.

the presence of a gun in the home remained strongly associated with an increased risk for homicide in the home. Gun ownership was most strongly associated with an increased risk of homicide by a family member or intimate acquaintance.[5]

Whereas most men are murdered away from home, most children, older adults, and women are murdered at home (Table 1.2). A gun in the home is a particularly strong risk factor for female homicide victimization—with the greatest danger for women coming from their intimate partners.

The heightened risk of femicide is illustrated in a subgroup analysis of female homicide victimization from Kellermann's 1993 case-control study of homicide in the home. A spouse, a lover, or a close relative murdered most of the women decedents, and the increased risk for homicide from having a gun in the home was attributable to these homicides (Bailey, Flewelling, and Rosenbaum 1997). A case-control study by Wiebe et al. (2003) also found that the risk of homicide associated with living in a home with guns was particularly high for women (who were almost three times more likely to become homicide victims compared with women living in homes without guns). Here too, a gun in the home was a risk factor for homicide by firearm but not for homicide by other means.

Other case-control studies have also found that a gun in the home is a risk for homicide in the home, with especially heightened risk for women (Cummings et al. 1997, Dahlberg, Ikeda, and Kresnow 2004). Results from perpetrator-based case-control homicide studies also find that gun ownership is a risk for homicide perpetration. For example, a study of women murdered by intimate partners found that compared with a control group of living battered women, a gun in the house was present for 65% of perpetrators of murder versus 24% of perpetrators of nonfatal abuse. Access to a firearm by the battered woman had no protective effect (Campbell et al. 2003).

Cohort Studies

There are no studies that follow a large cohort of individuals with known characteristics, comparing homicide victimization rates of those with a gun in the home and those without.

Firearm Prevalence and Suicide

Firearm suicide rates and overall suicide rates in the United States are higher where guns are more prevalent (Miller, Hemenway, and Azrael 2007, Kubrin and Wadsworth 2009). By contrast, rates of suicide by methods other than firearms are not significantly correlated with rates of household firearm ownership (Miller, Hemenway, and Azrael 2007). This pattern has been reported in ecologic studies that have adjusted for several potential confounders, including measures of psychological distress, alcohol and illicit drug use and abuse, poverty, education, and unemployment (Miller, Azrael, and Barber 2012, Miller, Hemenway, and Azrael 2007).

Household firearm ownership has also been consistently found to be a strong predictor of suicide risk in studies that examined individual-level data. U.S. case-control studies find that the presence of a gun in the home or purchase from a licensed dealer is a risk factor for suicide (Bailey et al. 1997, Brent et al. 1993, Brent et al. 1994, Brent et al. 1991, Brent et al.1988, Conwell et al. 2002, Cummings et al. 1997, Kellermann et al. 1992, Grassel et al. 2003, Kung, Pearson, and Lui 2003, Wiebe 2003). The relative risk is large (two- to tenfold), depending on the age group and, for younger persons, how firearms in the home are stored (Miller and Hemenway 1999, Brent et al. 1991, Kellermann et al. 1992).

The only large U.S. cohort study to examine the firearm–suicide connection found that suicide rates among California residents who purchased handguns from licensed dealers were more than twice as likely to die by suicide as were age/sex matched members of the general population, not only immediately after the purchase but throughout the six-year study period (Wintemute et al. 1999). Here, too, the increase in suicide risk was attributable entirely to an excess risk of suicide with a firearm (Wintemute et al. 1999).

Drawing causal inferences about the relation between firearm availability and the risk of suicide from existing case-control and ecologic studies has been questioned on the grounds that these studies may not adequately control for the possibility that members of households with firearms are inherently more suicidal than members of households without firearms (NRC 2005). Additional cited limitations include the possibility of differential recall (by cases compared with controls) of firearm ownership and comorbid conditions, and reverse causation (whereby suicidal persons purchase firearms with the idea of committing suicide).

It is very unlikely, however, that the strong association between firearms and suicide reported consistently in U.S. studies is either spurious or substantially overstated. First, individual-level studies have often controlled for measures of psychopathology (Bailey et al. 1997, Brent et al. 1994, Brent et al. 1993, Brent et al. 1988, Conwell et al. 2002, Cummings et al. 1997, Kellermann et al. 1992, Wiebe 2003).

Second, directly answering the reverse causation critique, the risk of suicide associated with a household firearm pertains not only to gun owners but to *all* household members (Cummings et al. 1997, Kellermann et al. 1992, Wintemute et al. 1999); the relative risk is larger for adolescents than for the gun owner; and for the gun owner the risk persists for years after firearms are purchased (Cummings et al. 1997, Kellermann et al. 1992, Wintemute et al. 1999).

Third, studies that have examined whether people who live in homes with guns have higher rates of psychiatric illness, substance abuse, or other known suicide risk factors generally fail to find any indication of heightened risk (Oslin et al. 2004, Kolla, O' Connor, and Lineberry 2011). For example, four case-control studies found comparable rates of psychiatric illness and psychosocial distress among households with versus without firearms (Kellermann et al. 1992, Ilgen et al. 2008, Miller et al. 2009, Sorenson and Vittes 2008, Betz, Barber, and Miller 2011).

Fourth, there appears to be a hierarchy of suicide risk among children and young adults, depending on how securely household firearms are stored, suggesting a dose-response relationship (Grossman et al. 2005).

Finally, the consistency in magnitude, direction, and specificity of method-related risk observed in both the many individual-level and ecologic studies (the latter not being subject to recall bias or the reverse causation criticism) leads to only one conclusion: a gun in the home increases the likelihood that a family member will die from suicide.

Unintentional Firearm Deaths

Not surprisingly, ecologic and case-control studies find that where there are more guns and more guns poorly stored, there are more unintentional firearm deaths (Miller, Azrael, and Hemenway 2001, Wiebe 2003, Grossman et al. 2005). U.S. children aged 5 to 14 have eleven times the likelihood of being killed accidentally with a gun compared with similarly aged children in other developed countries (Table 1.2) (Richardson and Hemenway 2011).

Conclusion

The United States, with its many guns and highly permissive gun laws, faces a far more serious problem of lethal firearms violence than other high-income nations. The relative magnitude of our problem is illustrated in Table 1.1. This table, which compares U.S. children aged 5–14 with children of other developed countries, illustrates the stark fact that U.S. children are *thirteen* times more likely to die from a firearm homicide and *eight* times more likely to a die of a firearm suicide than children in comparable developed nations. There is no evidence that U.S. children are more careless, suicidal. or violent than children in other high-income nations. Rather, what distinguishes children in the United States from children in the rest of the developed world is the simple, devastating fact that they die—mostly by firearms—at far higher rates.

Within the United States itself, the evidence is similarly compelling: where there are more guns, there are more violent deaths—indeed, many more. The magnitude of this relationship is illustrated in Table 1.3, which compares the number of lives lost between 2001 and 2007 to homicide, suicide, and unintentional firearm accidents by sex and age groups in states with the highest compared with the lowest gun ownership rates. The consistency of findings across different populations, using different study designs, and by different researchers is striking. No credible evidence suggests otherwise.

Table 1.3   Violent deaths in states with the highest versus lowest gun ownership levels (BRFSS 2004); Mortality Data WISQARS 1999–2007

	High-gun states[a]	Low-gun states[b]	Ratio
Aggregate population of adults, 2001–2007	356 million	358 million	1.0
Proportion of households with firearms	50%	15%	3.3
Percentage of adult population reporting depression, past 12 months (NSDUH 2008–2009)	3.7%	3.7%	1.0
Percentage of adult population reporting suicidal ideation, past 12 months (NSDUH 2008–2009)	6.6%	6.5%	1.0
Number of nonlethal violent crimes in 2010 (UCR 2010)	165,739	148,287	1.1
Suicide			
Women			
Firearm suicide	4,148	563	7.4
Non-firearm suicide	4,633	4,575	1.0
Total suicide	8,781	5,138	1.7
Men			
Firearm suicide	26,314	7,163	3.7
Non-firearm suicide	11,592	12,377	0.9
Total suicide	37,906	19,540	1.9
Men ages 15–29			
Firearm suicide	5,803	1,308	4.4
Non-firearm suicide	3,192	2,671	1.2
Total suicide	8,995	3,979	2.2
5–14 year olds			
Firearm suicide	166	15	11.1
Non-firearm suicide	225	154	1.5
Total suicide	391	169	2.3
Adults 65+ years old			
Firearm suicide	6,374	1,714	3.7
Non-firearm suicide	1,182	2,270	0.5
Total suicide	7,556	3,984	1.9
Homicide			
Men			
Firearm homicide	13,755	7,799	1.8
Non-firearm homicide	5,031	3,963	1.3
Total homicide	18,786	11,762	1.6
Women			
Firearm homicide	3,165	998	3.2
Non-firearm homicide	2,855	2,132	1.3
Total homicide	6,020	3,130	1.9

Table 1.3　(Continued)

	High-gun states[a]	Low-gun states[b]	Ratio
5–14 year olds			
Firearm homicide	259	100	2.6
Non-firearm homicide	212	169	1.3
Total homicide	471	269	1.8
Men 15–29			
Firearm homicide	6,971	4,900	1.4
Non-firearm homicide	1,187	1,334	0.9
Total homicide	8,158	6,234	1.3
Adults 65+ years old			
Firearm homicide	620	139	4.5
Non-firearm homicide	794	534	1.5
Total homicide	1,414	673	2.1
Unintentional firearm deaths	109	677	6.2

Note: All data are from 1999–2007 because cell counts were suppressed beginning in 2008; terrorism-related homicides are not counted.
[a]Louisiana, Utah, Oklahoma, Iowa, Tennessee, Kentucky, Alabama, Mississippi, Idaho, North Dakota, West Virginia, Arkansas, Alaska, South Dakota, Montana, Wyoming
[b]Hawaii, New Jersey, Massachusetts, Rhode Island, Connecticut, New York

Firearm policy is often focused on guns used in crime. What is notable about the studies reviewed here, however, is the consistency of the story they tell about *all* firearms—not just those used in crime. In the United States, there are more firearm suicides than firearm homicides, and women, children, and older adults are more likely to die by gunfire from a household gun (typically, legally acquired and possessed) than from illegal guns.

The first step in ameliorating a public health problem is to identify what the problem is. For the purposes of this essay, the problem is that, year after year, many more Americans are dying by gunfire than people in any other high-income nation. Good firearm policy has the potential to reduce the toll of lethal firearm violence in the United States. Efforts to reduce this uniquely American problem will, however, be less effective than they could be if good policy is not accompanied by a shift in the kind of discussions politicians, academicians, and citizens engage in about firearms. Science can provide the content—and better science based on better data, better content. The best chance for durable and large-scale reductions in lethal violence in the United States is for all of us to commit to keeping the conversation about the costs and benefits of guns in American society civil, ongoing, and factually grounded.

ACKNOWLEDGMENTS

The text, but not the figures reported, in this essay draw in part on prior reviews written previously by the authors, often supported by the Joyce Foundation.

NOTES

1. Researchers attribute the decline in the 1990s to different causes, including reduced unemployment, increased policing, and a decline in and stabilization of illegal drug markets (Wintemute 2000). Declines in the last decade have not yet been well explained.

2. Homicide rates have been consistently higher in the southern and western regions of the United States. This is especially true for firearm homicides (CDC 2012a).

3. Measuring the availability of guns in the context of these homicides is more problematic, not least because researchers (Webster, Vernick, and Hepburn 2001, MAIG 2008) have shown that guns involved in these deaths often move across state lines from states with permissive gun laws to states with fewer guns and stronger laws.

4. Studies included in this review were those previously included in review articles by two of the authors, updated to include new articles meeting the criteria specified in these reviews which have appeared in the research literature since the time those review papers were published.

5. The study did not provide evidence about whether a gun from the home was used in any of the homicides. However, the idea that a gun in the home increased the risk of death was supported by several observations. First, the link between gun ownership and homicide was due entirely to a strong association between gun ownership and homicide by firearm; homicide by other means was not significantly linked to having a gun in the home. Second, gun ownership was most strongly associated with homicide at the hands of a family member or intimate acquaintance (i.e., guns were not significantly linked to an increased risk of homicide by non-intimate friends, unidentified persons, or strangers). Third, there was no evidence of a protective effect of keeping a gun in the home—even in the small subgroup of cases that involved forced entry.

REFERENCES

Azrael, D., J. C. Philip, and M. Miller. 2004. "State and local prevalence of firearms ownership measurement, structure, and trends." *Journal of Quantitative Criminology* 20 (1):43–62.

Bailey, S., R. Flewelling, and D. Rosenbaum. 1997. "Characteristics of students who bring weapons to school." *Journal of Adolescent Health* 20 (4):261–270.

Bailey, J. E., A. L. Kellerman, G. Somes, J. G. Banton, F. Rivara, and N. B. Rushforth. 1997. "Risk factors for violent death of women in the home." *Archives of Internal Medicine* 157 (7):777–782.

Betz, M. E., C. Barber, and M. Miller. 2011. "Suicidal behavior and firearm access: Results from the second injury control and risk survey." *Suicide and Life Threatening Behavior* 41 (4):384–391.

Blumstein, A., and J. Wallman. 2000. *The crime drop in America.* New York: Cambridge University Press.

Brent D. A. 2001. "Firearms and suicide." *Ann. N. Y. Acad. Sci.* 932:225–39.

Brent, D. A., et al. 1988. "Risk factors for adolescent suicide: A comparison of adolescent suicide victims with suicidal inpatients." *Archives of General Psychiatry* 45 (6):581–588.

Brent, D. A., J. A. Perper, C. J. Allman, G. Moritz, M. E. Wartella, and J. P. Zelenak. 1991. "The presence and accessibility of firearms in the homes of adolescent suicides: A case-control study." *JAMA* 266 (21):2989–2995.

Brent, D. A., J. A. Perper, G. Moritz, M. Baugher, J. Schweers, and C. Roth. 1994. "Suicide in affectively ill adolescents: A case-control study." *Journal of Effective Disorders* 31 (3):193–202.

Brent, D. A., J. A. Perper, G. Moritz, M. Baugher, J. Schweers, and C. Roth. 1993. "Firearms and adolescent suicide: A community case-control study." *American Journal of Diseases of Children* 147 (10):1066–1071.

Campbell, J. C., D. Webster, J. Koziol-McLain, C. Block, D. Campbell, et al. 2003. "Risk factors for femicide in abusive relationships: Results from a multisite case control study." *American Journal of Public Health* 93 (7):1089–1097.

CDC. 1997. Rates of homicide, suicide, and firearm-related death among children—26 industrialized countries. In *Morbidity and Mortality Weekly Report.* Centers for Disease Control and Prevention.

CDC. 2007. Centers for Disease Control WISQARS injury mortality report. Atlanta, GA: National Center for Injury Prevention and Control, Centers for Disease Control and Prevention.

CDC. 2012a. Centers for Disease Control and Prevention, National Center for Health Statistics: Compressed Mortality File 1999–2009. Edited by CDC. CDC WONDER Online Database, compiled from Compressed Mortality File 1999–2009

CDC. 2012b. Surveillance for violent deaths—National Violent Death Reporting System, 18 states, 2012. Centers for Disease Control and Prevention.

Conwell, Y., P. R. Duberstein, K. Connor, S. Eberly, C. Cox, and E. D. Caine. 2002. "Access to firearms and risk for suicide in middle-aged and older adults." *American Journal of Geriatric Psychiatry* 10 (4):407–416.

Cook, P. J. 1979. "The effect of gun availability on robbery and robbery murder." In *Policy studies review annual,* edited by R. H. Haveman and B. B. Zellner, 743–781. Beverly Hills, CA: Sage.

Cook, P. J., and H. L. John. 2002. "After the epidemic: Recent trends in youth violence in the United States." In *Crime and justice: A review of research,* ed. Michael Tonry, 117–153. Chicago: University of Chicago Press.

Cook, P. J., and J. Ludwig. 1997. Guns in America: National survey on private ownership and use of firearms (NCJ 1654476). Washington, DC: U.S. Department of Justice.

Cork, D. 1999. "Examining time-space interaction in city-level homicide data: Crack markets and the diffusion of guns among youth." *Journal of Quantitative Criminology* 15 (4):379–406.

Cummings, P., T. D. Koepsell, D. C. Grossman, J. Savarino, and R. S. Thompson. 1997. "The association between the purchase of a handgun and homicide or suicide." *American Journal of Public Health* 87 (6):974–978.

Dahlberg, L. L., R. M. Ikeda, and M. J. Kresnow. 2004. "Guns in the home and risk of a violent death in the home: Findings from a national study." *American Journal of Epidemiology* 160 (10):974–978.

Grassel, K. M., G. J. Wintemute, M. A. Wright, and M. P. Romero. 2003. "Association between handgun purchase and mortality from firearm injury." *Injury Prevention* 9:48–52.

Grossman, D. C., B. A. Mueller, C. Riedy, M. D. Dowd, A. Villaveces, J. Prodzinski, J. Nakagawara, J. Howard, N. Thiersch, and R. Harruff. 2005. "Gun storage practices and rise of youth suicide and unintentional firearm Injuries." *JAMA* 293 (6):707–714.

GSS. 2010. "General Social Survey."

Hemenway, D., C. Barber, and M. Miller. 2010. "Unintentional firearm deaths: A comparison of other-inflicted and self-inflicted shootings." *Accident Analysis and Prevention* 42 (2):1184–1188.

Hemenway, D., & Miller, M. (2000). "Firearm availability and homicide rates across 26 high-income countries." *Journal of Trauma, Injury, Infection, and Critical Care, 49(6), 985–988.

Hemenway, D., T. Shinoda-Tagawa, and M. Miller. 2002. "Firearm availability and female homicide victimization rates among 25 populous high-income countries." *Journal of the American Medical Women's Association* 57:1–5.

Hepburn, M., M. Miller, D. Azrael, and D. Hemenway. 2007. "The US gun stock: results from the 2004 national firearms survey." *Injury Prevention* 13:15–19.

Hepburn, L. M., and D. Hemenway. 2004. "Firearm availability and homicide: A review of the literature." *Aggression and Violent Behavior* 9:417–440.

Ilgen, M. A., K. Zivin, R. J. McCammon, and M. Valenstein. 2008. "Mental illness, previous suicidality, and access to guns in the United States." *Psychiatric Services* no. 59 (2):198–200.

Kellermann, A. L., and F. P. Rivara. 2012. "Silencing the Science on Gun Research." *JAMA* ():1–2. doi: 10.1001/jama.2012.208207.

Kellermann, A. L., F. Rivara, N. B. Rushforth, J. Banton, D. T. Reay, J. Francisco, A. B. Locci, J. Prodzinski, B. B. Hackman, and G. Somes. 1993. "Gun ownership as a risk factor for homicide in the home." *New England Journal of Medicine* 329 (15):1084–1091.

Kellermann, A. L., F. P. Rivara, G. Somes, D. T. Reay, J. Francisco, J. Banton, J. Prodzinski, C. Fligner, and B. B. Hackman. 1992. "Suicide in the home in relation to gun ownership." *New England Journal of Medicine* 327 (7):467–472.

Killias, M. 1993. "International correlations between gun ownership and rates of homicide and suicide." *Canadian Medical Association Journal* 148 (10):1721–1725.

Kolla, B. P., S. S. O' Connor, and T.W. Lineberry. 2011. "The base rates and factors associated with reported access to firearms in psychiatric inpatients." *General Hospital Psychiatry* 33 (2):191–196.

Kubrin, C. E., and T. Wadsworth. 2009. "Explaining suicide among blacks and whites: How socio-economic factors and gun availability affect race-specific suicide rates." *Social Science Quarterly* (90):1203–1227.

Kung, H. C., J. L. Pearson, and X. Lui. 2003. "Risk factors for male and female suicide decedents ages 15–64 in the United States: Results from the 1993 National Mortality Followback Survey." *Social Psychiatry and Psychiatric Epidemiology* 39 (8):419–426.

MAIG (Mayors Against Illegal Guns). 2008. The movement against illegal guns in America.

Miller, M., D. Azrael, and C. Barber. 2012. "Suicide mortality in the United States: the importance of attending to method in understanding population-level disparities in the burden of suicide." *Annual Review of Public Health* 33:393–408.

Miller, M., D. Azrael, and D. Hemenway. 2001. "Firearm availability and unintentional firearm deaths." *Accident Analysis and Prevention* 33 (4):447–484.

Miller, M., C. Barber, D. Azrael, D. Hememway, and B. E. Molnar. 2009. "Recent psychopathology, suicidal thoughts and suicide attempts in households with and without firearms: Findings from the National Comorbidity Study Replication." *Injury Prevention* 15 (3):183–187.

Miller, M., and D. Hemenway. 1999. "The relationship between firearms and suicide: A review of the literature." *Aggression and Violent Behavior* 4 (1):59–75.

Miller, M., D. Hemenway, and D. Azrael. 2007. "State-level homicide victimization rates in the US in relation to survey measures of household firearm ownership, 2001–2003." *Social Science & Medicine* 64 (3):656–664.

Miller, M., S. J. Lippmann, D. Azrael, and D. Hemenway. 2007. "Household firearm ownership and rates of suicide across the 50 states." *Journal of Trauma Injury, Infection and Critical Care* 62 (4):1029–1035.

Nock, M. K., G. Borges, E. J. Bromet, C. B. Cha, R. C. Kessler, and S. Lee. 2008. "Suicide and suicidal behavior." *Epidemiology Reviews* 30 (1):133–154.

NRC. 2005. National Research Council: Firearms and violence: A critical review. Washington, DC: National Academies Press.

Oslin, D.W., C. Zubritsky, G. Brown, M. Mullahy, and A. Puliafico. 2004. "Managing suicide in late life: Access to firearms as a public health risk." *American Journal of Geriatric Psychiatry* 12 (1):30–36.

Pickett, W., F, J. Elgar, F. Brooks, M. de Looze, and K. Rathman. 2013. "Trends and socioeconomic correlates of adolescent physical fighting in 30 countries." *Pediatrics* 131 (1):18–26.

Richardson, E. G., and D. Hemenway. 2011. "Homicide, suicide, and unintentional firearm fatality: Comparing the United States with other high-income countries, 2003." *Journal of Trauma Injury, Infection and Critical Care* 70 (1):238–243.

SAS. 2007. "Completing the count: Civilian firearms: Annexe 1: Seventy-nine countries with comprehensive civilian ownership data." In *The small arms survey: Guns in the city*, ed. Small Arms Survey Geneva. Cambridge, UK: Cambridge University Press.

Shaffer, D., M. S. Gould, P. Fisher, P. Trautman, and D. Moreau. 1996. "Psychiatric diagnosis in child and adolescent suicide." *Archives of General Psychiatry* 53 (4):339–348.

Smith, T. W. 2000. 1999 National gun policy survey of the National Opinion Research Center: Research findings. Chicago, IL: National Opinion Research Center, University of Chicago.

Sorenson, S. B., and K. A. Vittes. 2008. "Mental health and firearms in community-based surveys: Implications for suicide prevention." *Evaluation Review* 32 (3):239–256.

van Kesteren, J., P. Mayhew, and P. Nieuwbeerta. 2001. Criminal victimization in seventeen industrialized countries: Key findings from the 2000 international crime victims survey. In *Netherlands Ministry of Justice: Research and Documentation Centre Netherlands.*

Webster, D., J. Vernick, and L. Hepburn. 2001. "Relationship between licensing, registration, and other gun sales laws and the source state of crime guns." *Injury Prevention* 7 (3):184–189. doi: 10.1136/ip.7.3.184.

Wiebe, D. J. 2003. "Homicide and suicide risks associated with firearms in the home: A national case-control study." *Annals of Emergency Medicine* 41 (6):771–782.

Wintemute, G. J. 2000. "Guns and gun violence." In *The crime drop in America*, ed. A. Blumstein and J. Wallman. Cambridge: Cambridge University Press.

Wintemute, G. J., C. A. Parham, J. J. Beaumont, M. Wright, and C. Drake. 1999. "Mortality among recent purchasers of handguns." *New England Journal of Medicine* 341 (21):1583–1589.

The Limited Impact of the Brady Act

Evaluation and Implications

Philip J. Cook and Jens Ludwig

Federal firearms law divides the population into two groups: those prohibited from legally possessing a firearm due to their criminal record or certain other disqualifying conditions and everyone else. The vast majority of the adult public is allowed to acquire and possess all the firearms they want, thus preserving the personal right to "keep and bear arms" that has been established by recent U.S. Supreme Court rulings.[1] But that right, like all rights, has limits. People with serious criminal records or severe mental illness may reasonably be deemed at such high risk of misusing firearms that public-safety concerns take precedence over gun rights. While in practice it is impossible to keep all members of high-risk groups disarmed in a gun-rich environment, a selective prohibition may cause some reduction in gun misuse and save enough lives to be worthwhile.

Philip J. Cook, PhD, is the ITT/Terry Sanford Professor of Public Policy and professor of economics and sociology at Duke University, and he is the co-director of the National Bureau of Economic Research working group on the economics of crime. Jens Ludwig, PhD, MA, is the McCormick Foundation Professor of Social Service Administration, Law and Public Policy at the University of Chicago, director of the University of Chicago Crime Lab, and co-director of the National Bureau of Economic Research working group on the economics of crime.

The effectiveness of this selective-prohibition approach may depend on how it is enforced. The two mechanisms in use to discourage disqualified people from obtaining guns are deterrence through the threat of criminal prosecution ("felon in possession" cases) and regulation of firearms transactions. The current regulatory framework was created by the Gun Control Act of 1968 (GCA), which required that those in the business of selling guns obtain a federal firearms license (FFL) and that interstate shipments of guns be limited to licensees. Anyone purchasing a gun from an FFL is required by the GCA to fill out a form 4473 stating that he or she did not have a felony conviction or other disqualifying condition, although under federal law dealers were not required to verify the information reported by the prospective buyer.

The GCA's requirement was greatly strengthened by subsequent legislation, the Brady Handgun Violence Prevention Act, implemented in 1994. The Brady Act required that FFLs conduct a background check on would-be buyers—the buyer's signature on a 4473 was no longer enough. This new regulation was enacted with high hopes of reducing gun violence, despite its limitations. Most gun crimes are committed with weapons that were not purchased from dealers, but rather acquired through off-the-books transactions. Such transactions are generally permitted and not regulated by the Brady Act. However, some disqualified individuals do attempt to buy guns from FFLs, and the *Brady* background checks have blocked over 2 million sales since the law was implemented (Bowling et al. 2010).

On March 2, 2000, President Bill Clinton declared at a news conference that "the Brady Bill is saving people's lives and keeping guns out of the wrong hands," a claim justified in part by the substantial number of people who had been denied handguns as a result of the law.[2] During the first five years of the Brady Act, 312,000 applications to purchase handguns from dealers (2.4% of the total) were denied due to a felony record or other disqualifying characteristic (Bowling et al. 2010). Other would-be buyers with criminal records may have been deterred from even attempting to buy a firearm. The logic is clear: Since guns are more lethal than knives and other likely substitutes, any reduction in criminal gun use due to *Brady* would likely translate into a net reduction in homicides (Zimring 1968, 1972).

The same year that President Clinton claimed success we published an evaluation of the Brady Act in the *Journal of the American Medical Association* (Ludwig and Cook 2000). Our conclusion was less positive—we found no evidence of a reduction in the homicide rate that could be attributed to

Brady. We also considered the possibility that *Brady* reduced the overall suicide rate, but found no discernible impact on that outcome either. In presenting these findings, we cautioned that our statistical method rested on certain untested (though in our judgment, reasonable) assumptions, and that our null results still left some room for the possibility that *Brady* had an effect, albeit small, and either positive or negative. Further, even if our null results are correct for the early years of *Brady*, they do not preclude the possibility that a different regulatory scheme might be more effective in achieving the purpose. Indeed, the Brady Act itself incorporated potentially important changes that were implemented in December 1998. While the initial "interim" phase, from 1994 to 1998, was limited to handgun purchases, the second "permanent" phase expanded the background check requirement to include purchasers of rifles and shotguns. Perhaps more importantly, the interim phase required a five-day waiting period from application to delivery of the handgun, while the permanent phase replaced the waiting period with a new system, known as the National Instant Criminal Background Check System (NICS). Our evaluation focused entirely on the interim phase.

In this essay we provide a summary of our evaluation, discussing its strengths and limitations, and then go on to consider two questions that are vital to the current debate: (1) What are the most important limitations of the current selective prohibition system?; and (2) How could this general approach be strengthened?

Background and Findings

James Brady, press secretary to President Reagan, was shot during an assassination attempt against the president in March 1981. Together with his wife, Sarah, Brady became a leader of the gun control movement, and through Handgun Control, Inc. worked for seven years to achieve passage of what became known as the Brady Handgun Violence Prevention Act. The first set of provisions was implemented in February 1994, requiring that FFLs conduct a background check and wait for five business days before transferring a handgun to a customer. Only 32 states were directly affected by these provisions, because the other 18 states and the District of Columbia already met the minimum requirements of the Act. In effect these provisions created a sort of natural experiment, with 32 states in the "change" or "treatment" condition, and the 18 no-change states serving as "controls." Our evaluation took advantage of this experiment-like setting to estimate the causal effect of the Brady Act on certain outcomes.

Our main outcome measure was the homicide rate from the Vital Statistics records. While other types of crime are also of interest, the data on homicides are more detailed and far more accurate than for the other violent crimes, such as robbery and assault. (The main limitation of the Vital Statistics data for our purposes is the lack of information on perpetrators.) We also analyzed the effects of the *Brady* regulations on suicide. The focus of our analysis for both homicide and suicide was on adult victims, and in particular for those 21 years of age and older. The primary rationale for this age limitation is that the Brady Act would logically have little or no effect on access to guns by those under 21; federal law sets 21 as the minimum age to purchase a handgun from an FFL, and the age of the customer was subject to check even before *Brady* by a requirement that he or she show identification. Of course, limiting the homicide outcome to adult victims does not provide exactly what we would like to have, namely rates of homicide *committed* by those age 21 or over; *Brady* regulations are aimed at the potential perpetrators rather than the victims. But in practice teenage killers select teenage victims, and few homicide victims aged 21 years or over are shot by perpetrators under 21 years of age (Cook and Laub 1998). It turns out that limiting the analysis to adults is not only logical given the nature of the intervention, it also enhances the validity of our evaluation method, since it helps avoid potential biases introduced by the volatility of juvenile homicides during our sample period that was associated with the rise and fall in crack-market activity (Blumstein 1995; Cork 1999).

The importance of having a control group for evaluating the effect of *Brady* on the "treatment" states' homicide rates is that other factors were at play, and homicide rates were dropping nationwide in the 1990s. In particular, the national homicide rate dropped by 34% from 1990 to 1998. Most of the crime drop during the 1990s (which was by no means limited to homicide) has been attributed to causes that are unrelated to changes in firearm regulations. Among the factors that have been suggested to explain the crime drop of the 1990s are increased imprisonment and spending on police, the waning of the crack cocaine "epidemic" that began in the mid-1980s, and, more controversially, the legalization of abortion in the early 1970s (Blumstein and Wallman 2000; Levitt 2004; Cook and Laub 2002). In any event, an evaluation of the Brady Act based only on the trend in homicide rates in the *Brady* treatment states would mistakenly attribute to the Brady Act the effects of all of the other forces that were driving crime rates down over the 1990s.

Our assumption that the 18 states that were not directly affected by the Brady Act provide a valid control group is supported by the remarkable similarity in pre-*Brady* trends in adult homicide rates. Evidently other causal factors did exert similar impacts on the *Brady* treatment and control states. Thus if the trends in homicide rates (and especially gun homicide rates) had diverged between the two groups after *Brady*, then it would be plausible to attribute that divergence to the new regulations introduced by the Act. Our evaluation approach is further supported by the fact that the law in question was exogenous to the individual states—there is no "self-selection" problem here, as might arise if we were evaluating laws that were changed by the act of individual state legislatures (perhaps in response to state-specific changes in crime).

A distinct concern in evaluating the effects of the Brady Act is that the new law may have reduced gun running from the treatment to control states, in which case comparing the two groups of states might understate the overall effects of the law (Weil 1997). The concern here is that homicide rates in the "control" states were in fact affected by the intervention. Some support for this concern comes from ATF trace data in Chicago showing that the fraction of crime guns in the city that could be traced to the *Brady* treatment states declined dramatically following implementation of the law (Cook and Braga 2001). However, the proportion of homicides in Chicago committed with guns did not change over this period, despite the substantial changes in gun-trafficking patterns (Cook and Ludwig 2003). One explanation of these results is that traffickers were able to substitute in-state sources for out-of-state sources at little extra cost. If correct, they suggest that while *Brady* did affect trafficking to the control states, the effect was not of much consequence for gun availability to those at risk of violence in those states.

Here are the specifics of our quantitative evaluation. We utilize a "difference in difference" approach that compares the pre- and post-*Brady* changes for the treatment and control groups. The econometric technique is panel regression analysis utilizing specification (1) below, where Y_{it} represents a mortality measure for state (i) in period (t), and X_{it} represents a set of control variables.[3] The model includes separate dichotomous indicator variables for each state, d_i, to capture unmeasured state-specific "fixed effects" that cause the level of violence to differ across states, a set of year indicator variables, g_t, that capture changes in the overall rate of violence in the U.S. conditional on the observed covariates, and the indicator variable T_{it} that is equal to 1 in the treatment states following implementation of the Brady Act and equal to 0 otherwise. From Vital Statistics data, we had available four years of post-*Brady* data (1994 to 1997). For comparability, we define the pre-*Brady* period as the four years prior to the law's implementation (1990 to 1993).

$$Y_{it} = b_0 + b_1 X_{it} + b_2 T_{it} + d_i + g_t + e_{it} \qquad (1)$$

Since state-specific fixed effects are included in the model, the key coefficient of interest (b_2) reflects the difference between the treatment and control states in the change in violence rates from the pre- to post-*Brady* periods. The coefficient b_2 captures any one-time shift in the rate of gun violence in the treatment versus control states around the time of the Brady Act, and should be negative if *Brady* reduced gun violence.

Equation (1) was estimated via weighted least squares, a technique that corrects for heteroskedasticity in the stochastic term by pre-multiplying the dependent and explanatory variables by the square root of the state's population. We calculated Huber-White standard errors to adjust for the non-independence of observations from the same state.

The findings from this regression analysis are summarized in Table 2.1. We find no statistically discernible difference in homicide trends between the *Brady* (treatment) and non-*Brady* (control) states among people aged 21 and older. While our point estimates are negative, they are even more negative for non-gun homicide than for gun homicide (and in every case statistically insignificant). In this pattern of results we see no case for a causal effect of *Brady*. The 95% confidence interval for one version of our estimates ranges from an increase of 8% to a reduction of 13%.[4]

Of course the Brady Act may have affected outcomes other than homicide. In particular, the waiting period required during phase one of *Brady* may have slowed handgun acquisition by some people experiencing a suicidal impulse. As shown in Table 2.1, our analysis of suicide rates found some evidence that *Brady* may have reduced gun suicide rates among people aged 55 and older. However, these gains were at least partially offset by an increase in non-gun suicides (perhaps due to weapon substitution), so whether waiting periods reduced overall suicides among this age group is unclear.

Table 2.1 Effects of the Brady Act on homicide and suicide changes from
pre- to post-Brady period in treatment relative to control states
(Standard-error estimates in parentheses)

	Victims aged 21 and older	Victims aged 55 and older
Homicide (rate per 100,000)	−0.36 (0.64)	−0.09 (0.27)
Gun homicide rate	−0.14 (0.52)	0.05 (0.10)
Non-gun homicide rate	−0.22 (0.15)	−0.14 (0.20)
% homicides committed with gun	1.1 (1.0)	3.3 (2.4)
Suicide (rate per 100,000)	−0.12 (0.27)	−0.54 (0.37)
Gun suicide rate	−0.21 (0.19)	−0.92** (0.25)
Non-gun suicide rate	0.09 (0.13)	0.38* (0.20)
% suicides committed with gun	−0.3 (0.5)	−2.2** (0.9)

Source: Cook and Ludwig (2003). The original results reported in Ludwig and Cook
(2000) were based on a data set with several minor errors which we subsequently
corrected.
Note: The pre-Brady period is defined as 1990 to 1993 and post-Brady period as 1994
to 1997. Regressions are calculated by estimating equation (2) in text using state
population as weights to adjust for heteroskedasticity.
   **Statistically different from zero at the 5% p-value
   *Statistically different from zero at the 10% p-value

How do we reconcile our findings of no detectable impacts on homicide
with administrative records on the numbers of people denied handguns as a
result of Brady background check requirements? About 2.4% of potential
handgun buyers were denied handguns during the interim phase of the Brady
Act as a result of background checks (Bowling et al. 2010). One explanation is
that the type of person who is disqualified from legally buying a gun but shops
at an FFL anyway tends to be at relatively low risk for misusing a gun (compared with other disqualified individuals). Data from California show that
individuals who were denied purchase of a handgun due to a felony record have
23% fewer violent-crime arrests than those who have been arrested but not convicted for a felony, and thus were able to successfully purchase a handgun from
an FFL (Wright, Wintemute and Rivara 1999). Yet the follow-up arrest rates
for both groups are fairly low, and only around 3% of violent-crime arrests are
for homicide (Wright and Wintemute 1999). Projecting the California data to
the nation suggests that those 312,000 convicted felons who were denied a
handgun in Brady states in the interim phase (from 1994 to 1998) would have
committed about 60 fewer homicides as a result.

Discussion

Suppose that our null findings are correct and that the first phase of the Brady Act had little or no impact on homicide or suicide rates. What are the likely explanations, and what can we conclude about the possibility of saving lives through the Gun Control Act's ban on gun possession by certain high-risk groups?

The most prominent of the likely explanations is simply that by limiting the background-check requirement to sales by FFLs, the Brady Act's background-check requirement had no direct effect on the vast majority of transactions that provide criminals with guns. Surveys of prisoners in the 1980s show that only one-fifth obtained their guns directly from a licensed gun dealer (Wright & Rossi, 1994), even though at that time dealers in most states were not required to conduct background checks to verify the buyer's eligibility.[5] Most crime guns are obtained from people who are not licensed FFLs through private transactions that are largely unregulated under existing federal law—that is, these crime guns are obtained in the off-the-books secondary gun market.

While this "private sale loophole" is the most compelling explanation for limited impact of the Brady Act, there are several other considerations that should be taken into account. First, a majority of adults who end up using a gun in crime are not disqualified from possessing a gun. Cook, Ludwig and Braga (2005) find that nearly three in five homicide offenders in Illinois in 2001 did not have a felony conviction within the 10 years prior to the homicide. Not that they had spotless records—only one-quarter of homicide offenders had not been arrested at least once during the 10 years prior to the homicide. Expanding the crime-related disqualification criteria to include, say, conviction of any violent misdemeanor (rather than the current disqualification, which is limited to felonies and misdemeanor domestic violence) could help in this respect.

Second, even if a disqualified person did seek to buy guns from an FFL after *Brady*, there is a good chance of success, simply because the relevant records are often incomplete or difficult to access. In recognition of this problem Congress established the National Criminal History Improvement Program (NCHIP) to provide grants and technical assistance to the states to improve the quality and immediate accessibility of criminal history records and related information. This federal investment resulted in an 83% increase in the criminal records accessible for background checks by 2003 (Ramker 2006), thereby increasing the chance that a disqualified person would be identified as such through the NICS process. NCHIP has continued to provide modest funding for improving records and was supplemented in 2007 by a new program focused on assisting states to incorporate mental health records in the NICS system. A few states have made large gains in this respect, but most do not yet have a reliable system in place for submitting relevant records on severe mental illness or drug abuse (Mayors Against Illegal Guns 2011).

In sum, the limitations of the current system for screening firearms buyers to prevent gun crimes include, in order of importance, the private sales loophole, the fact that a large share of gun criminals are not disqualified, and the incomplete coverage of the databases utilized in the NICS. The same limitations apply if the screening system is intended to prevent gun suicides, although for suicides the relative importance of these three changes differs: those at risk of suicide may be more likely to obtain guns from FFLs (in which case the private-sales loophole would be less important) but much less likely to be disqualified under current standards.[6]

There has been considerable interest in closing the private-sales loophole by simply requiring that all gun sales, whether in the primary or secondary market, be subject to background checks. California has instituted such a system for firearms transactions, which must go through an FFL who then charges a fee for conducting the background check. Such a system, were it to be enforceable, would make it more difficult for disqualified people to obtain a gun. The fundamental question is how to enforce such a system. California requires that handguns be registered to their owner, which is useful in holding owners accountable for the disposition of their handguns. Even without a registration requirement, a universal background check system could be enforced in a variety of ways, including law-enforcement oversight of gun shows and undercover "buy and bust" operations by the police. Whether the California system is successful in reducing gun violence has not been established (but see Webster, Vernick, and Bulzacchelli 2009).

While the prospects are dim for decisive victories against gun violence through modest improvements in the regulation of gun transfers, the stakes are very high. Even just a one percent reduction in gun homicides and suicides would amount to over 300 lives saved—enough to justify a billion-dollar program by the usual reckoning of the value of life. The findings from our evaluation of the Brady Act certainly do not rule out the possibility that it saved several times that many lives during each of the early years, and hence was worthwhile. Neither our evaluation method nor any other that we know of would be precise enough to detect such a proportionally small effect.

ACKNOWLEDGMENTS

The original research reported in this essay was supported by a grant from the Joyce Foundation. The authors thank Bob Malme, Chris Clark, Heath Einstein, Meghan McNally, and Esperanza Ross for valuable research assistance, and Roseanna Ander, Steve Hargarten, David Hemenway, Arthur Kellermann, Debby Leff, Willard Manning, James Mercy, John Mullahy, William Schwab, Daniel Webster, Garen Wintemute, and Mona Wright for useful comments. All opinions and any errors are the authors'.

NOTES

1. *District of Columbia v. Heller* (554 US 570 (2008)) established a personal right to keep a handgun in the home for self-defense purposes. *McDonald v. Chicago* (561 US 3025 (2010)) extended this right beyond federal jurisdiction to encompass state and local governments.

2. Brady Campaign to Prevent Gun Violence, 'Saving Lives by Taking Guns Out of Crime: The Drop in Gun-Related Crime Deaths Since Enactment of the Brady Law,' Executive Summary, downloaded from http://www.bradycenter.org/xshare /Facts/brady-law-drop-in-crime.pdf

3. In our reported specification, we controlled for state-level changes in the following factors that may influence rates of crime and violence: consumption of alcohol per capita (measured in gallons of ethanol), percentage of the population living in metropolitan areas, percentage of the population living below the official poverty line and income level per worker (in 1998 constant dollars) percentage who are African American, and the percentage of the population falling into 7 different age groups.

4. In this version we used the log form of the dependent variable in each of the regressions. The results using other specifications are similar.

5. For a more recent estimate of the percent of crime guns obtained directly from an FFL, see the essay by Webster, Vernick, McGinty, and Alcorn (in this volume).

6. In a personal communication dated January 14, 2013, Mallory O'Brien, Director of the Milwaukee Homicide Review Commission, reports evidence that suicides, unlike violent criminals, are quite likely to obtain their guns directly from an FFL. "From January 1, 2010 to December 31, 2012, firearms were recovered from 59 suicide victims in the City of Milwaukee. ATF eTrace data was used to determine: first purchaser, time to event and firearm type. ATF was able to successfully trace firearms

for 52 of the victims. In 31 (60%) cases the suicide victim purchased the firearm from a licensed firearm dealer. Ten of these victims who purchased the firearm from an FFL used the weapon within a year of the event."

REFERENCES

Blumstein, Alfred. 1995. "Youth Gun Violence, Guns, and the Illicit-Drug Industry," *Journal of Criminal Law and Criminology* 86: 10–36.

Blumstein, Alfred and Joel Wallman, eds. 2000. *The Crime Drop in America.* New York: Cambridge University Press.

Bowling, Michael, Ronald J. Frandsen, Gene A. Lauver, Allina D. Boutilier, Devon B. Adams. 2010. *Background Checks for Firearms: Statistical Tables.* Bureau of Justice Statistics Bulletin NCJ 231679.

Brady Campaign to Prevent Gun Violence. 2002. "Saving Lives by Taking Guns Out of Crime: The Drop in Gun-Related Crime Deaths Since Enactment of the Brady Law," Executive Summary, downloaded from www.bradycampaign.org/facts /research/savinglives.asp, accessed on April 17.

Cook, Philip J. and Anthony A. Braga. 2001. "A Comprehensive Firearms Tracing: Strategic and Investigative Uses of New Data on Firearms Markets," *Arizona Law Review* 43(2): 277–310.

Cook, Philip J. and John H. Laub. 1998. "The Unprecedented Epidemic of Youth Violence" in *Crime and Justice: An Annual Review of Research.* Michael H. Moore and Michael Tonry, Editors (Chicago: University of Chicago Press), 26–64.

Cook, Philip J. and John H. Laub. 2002. "After the Epidemic: Recent Trends in Youth Violence in the United States" in *Crime and Justice: A Review of Research,* edited by Michael Tonry. Chicago: University of Chicago Press, 117–153.

Cook, Philip J. and Jens Ludwig. 2003. "The Effects of the Brady Act on Gun Violence" in Bernard E. Harcourt (ed.) *Guns, Crime, and Punishment in America.* New York: NYU Press: 283–298.

Cook, Philip J., Stephanie Molliconi, and Thomas B. Cole. 1995. "Regulating Gun Markets." *The Journal of Criminal Law and Criminology* 86(1): 59–92.

Cork, Daniel. 1999. "Examining Time-Space Interaction in City-Level Homicide Data: Crack Markets and the Diffusion of Guns Among Youth." *Journal of Quantitative Criminology* 15 (4): 379–406.

Levitt, Steven D. 2004. "Understanding Why Crime Fell in the 1990s: Four Factors that Explain the Decline and Six that Do Not." *Journal of Economic Perspectives,* 18(1): 163–190.

Ludwig, Jens and Philip J. Cook. 2000. "Homicide and suicide rates associated with the implementation of the Brady Handgun Violence Prevention Act." *Journal of the American Medical Association* 284(5): 585–591.

Mayors Against Illegal Guns. 2011. *Fatal Gaps: How missing records in the federal background check system put guns in the hands of killers.* http://mayorsagainstille galguns.org/downloads/pdf/maig_mimeo_revb.pdf

Ramker, Gerard F. 2006. *Improving Criminal History Records for Background Checks, 2005.* Bureau of Justice Statistics Program Report NCJ 211485.

Webster Daniel W, Jon S Vernick, and MT Bulzacchelli. 2009. "Effects of state-level firearm seller accountability policies on firearms trafficking." *Journal of Urban Health*; 86:525–537.

Weil, Douglas S. 1997. *Traffic Stop: How the Brady Act Disrupts Interstate Gun Trafficking*. Washington, DC: Center to Prevent Handgun Violence.

Wright, James D. and Peter H. Rossi. 1986. *Armed and Considered Dangerous: A Survey of Felons and Their Firearms*, New York: Aldine de Gruyter.

Wright, Mona A., Garen J. Wintemute, and Frederick P. Rivara. 1999. "Effectiveness of Denial of Handgun Purchase to Persons Believed to Be at High Risk for Firearm Violence." *American Journal of Public Health* 89(1): 88–90.

Wright, Mona A. and Garen J. Wintemute. 1999. Unpublished calculations. Davis, CA: Violence Prevention Research Program, University of California at Davis Medical Center.

Zimring, Franklin E. 1968. "Is Gun Control Likely to Reduce Violent Killings?" *The University of Chicago Law Review* 35: 721–737.

Zimring, Franklin E. 1972. "The Medium is the Message: Firearm Calibre as a Determinant of Death from Assault," *Journal of Legal Studies*. 1: 97–124.

3

Preventing Gun Violence Involving People with Serious Mental Illness

Jeffrey W. Swanson, Allison Gilbert Robertson, Linda K. Frisman, Michael A. Norko, Hsiu-Ju Lin, Marvin S. Swartz, and Philip J. Cook

The December 2012 tragedy at Newtown may soon settle in the collective memory of senseless rampages by unstable young men. But in the immediate aftermath, the question of what might have been done to prevent those 28 untimely deaths may galvanize the attention of policymakers desperate to respond. Shall we now hold mental health systems more accountable for failing

Jeffrey W. Swanson, PhD, is a professor in the Department of Psychiatry and Behavioral Sciences at Duke University School of Medicine. Allison Gilbert Robertson, PhD, MPH, is an assistant professor in the Department of Psychiatry and Behavioral Sciences at Duke University School of Medicine. Linda K. Frisman, PhD, is a research professor with the University of Connecticut School of Social Work and a senior research scientist with the Connecticut Department of Mental Health and Addiction Services. Michael A. Norko, MD, MAR, is an associate professor of psychiatry in the Law and Psychiatry Division at Yale University School of Medicine and director of Forensic Services for the Connecticut Department of Mental Health and Addiction Services. Hsiu-Ju Lin, PhD, is an associate research professor in the School of Social Work at the University of Connecticut and the principal data analyst for the Research Division at the Connecticut Department of Mental Health and Addiction Services. Marvin S. Swartz, MD, is a professor and head of the Division of Social and Community Psychiatry and director of Behavioral Health for the Duke University Health System. Philip J. Cook, PhD, is the ITT/Terry Sanford Professor of Public Policy and professor of economics and sociology at Duke University, and he is the codirector of the National Bureau of Economic Research working group on the economics of crime.

to find, treat, or confine people who incline to violence? Should we fault the loose enforcement of federal firearms restrictions, and a loophole-ridden system of background-checks, for failing to keep guns out of the hands of dangerous people? Does the problem lie with the laws themselves, with their blunt and archaic definitions that leave risky people untouched while sweeping up legions of the harmless?

Cogent answers to these questions—and any guidance for the reforms they might imply—must first acknowledge that a multiple-casualty shooting by a disturbed individual is a statistically rare and virtually unpredictable event (Nielssen et al. 2009; Swanson 2011). As such, a singular horrific incident plays an important but ambiguous role in the national conversation on gun violence and in the emergent policy discussion on what to do about it. On the one hand, gun policy scholars hope that the tragedy will focus public consciousness on the pervasive problem of firearms-related injury and mortality. On the other hand, mental health stakeholders and advocates reasonably worry that viewing the public health epidemic of firearm violence through the lens of a massacre of schoolchildren—an act nobody can imagine a sane person committing—is to misplace emphasis on an atypical and presumed psychopathology while ignoring the larger, complex, and more salient causes of a broad societal scourge (Appelbaum and Swanson 2010).

In this essay, we take as a starting place the inherent tension between public safety and civil rights in considering mental illness as a significant concern for firearms policy and law. This means grappling with the full range of social benefits and costs that may accrue in casting a wide net with a broad mesh to find a few dangerous people among the many with largely non-dangerous disorders of thought, mood, and behavior. Whatever the evidence suggests about people with mental illness and violence—and for most there is no linkage—they are often portrayed as dangerous in the mass media and perceived as such by the general public (Pescosolido et al. 1999). Fear stokes avoidance and social rejection, which in turn beget discrimination. And if they are no longer "one of us," coercion, loss of privacy, and unwarranted deprivation of liberty become easy to justify. Ironically, this alienates people with serious but treatable mental health conditions and encumbers their desire to seek help with worry about what that might entail. A public policy of categorical exclusion based on the presumed dangerousness of one group may serve the public interest but not without overreaching and not without social cost.

We acknowledge that the exigencies of policymaking must sometimes outpace the evidence for what works. But it is also true that crisis-driven law is not always carefully deliberated and that the results can make things worse and be difficult to undo. Prudence, then, makes it crucial that available empirical research contribute as much as possible to the policymaking process, even if the existing research is messy, incomplete, and not wholly generalizable. In that spirit, we present new findings from an empirical study of the effectiveness of federal gun prohibitions in reducing the risk of violent crime in a Connecticut sample of more than 23,000 people with serious mental illness. Using merged administrative records from the state's public mental health and criminal justice systems for the years 2002 through 2009, our quasi-experimental analysis spans the periods before and after Connecticut began reporting mental health records to the National Instant Criminal Background Check System (NICS) in 2007. We consider implications of our research results for possible (and perhaps newly feasible) policy reforms to reduce gun violence.

In 1968, Congress passed the Gun Control Act, which categorically prohibited people from buying firearms if they had ever been involuntarily committed to a mental hospital or "adjudicated as a mental defective" (Simpson 2007). (The latter term is gratuitous and should be amended. It has almost no clinical meaning today, and many mental health stakeholders find the language stigmatizing and offensive.) As defined more specifically in the regulations, the exclusion covers people who have been determined by an authoritative legal process to be dangerous or incompetent to manage their own affairs due to a mental illness. It also covers individuals found incompetent to stand trial or acquitted by reason of insanity.

The legacy of the 1968 Gun Control Act prohibitions remains with us today, long after civil commitment reforms and deinstitutionalization have run their course, radically reducing and reshaping the ranks of the involuntarily committed (Appelbaum 1994; Fisher and Grisso 2010). The categories of exclusion were encoded in federal regulations and retained in the 1994 Brady Violence Prevention Act, which instituted background checks—now increasingly conducted through the NICS—to screen out prohibited persons who may attempt to buy guns from a licensed gun dealer. The mental health prohibitions, in particular, are based on a set of assumptions that may have sounded reasonable 45 years ago, but today invite careful scrutiny in light of voluminous research evidence that has accumulated over the ensuing decades.

The suspect assumptions are these: that serious mental illnesses—of the sort that landed people in mental hospitals against their will—were strongly and causally associated with risk of violent behavior; that people with these dangerous mental health conditions will inevitably come to the attention of psychiatrists, who could then reliably discern the risk of violence and confine the appropriate patients to a mental hospital; that, once discharged, involuntarily treated psychiatric patients will always carry with them some risk of relapse to their dangerous mental health conditions and, thus, should be categorically prohibited from obtaining firearms; and, finally, that the law could effectively deter prohibited individuals from purchasing firearms from a licensed gun dealer—either because they would not try to buy a gun or because they would truthfully disclose their gun-disqualifying mental health histories in the attempt and, thus, be stopped. In order for the logic of the law to work effectively, *all* of these assumptions had to hold true; they were links in a chain of prevention. As it turned out, all of the assumptions were flawed.

Subsequent epidemiological research showed that mental illness contributes little to population violence over all (Fazel and Grann 2006; Swanson 1994; Van Dorn, Volavka, and Johnson 2012). The very small proportion of people with mental illnesses who are inclined to be dangerous often do not seek treatment before they do something harmful; they therefore do not acquire a gun-disqualifying record of mental health adjudication (or a criminal record, either) that would show up in a background check. Psychiatrists, using clinical judgment, cannot accurately foresee which patients will be violent (Lidz, Mulvey, and Gardner 1993) and commit many patients for reasons unrelated to violence risk. States vary widely in commitment criteria and the dangerousness standards that underlie them (Fisher and Grisso 2010). The federal background checks only affect persons who buy guns through a federally licensed gun dealer, while a substantial proportion of firearms transfers are private transactions (Cook and Ludwig 1997). And many people have access to guns in the home, even if they would not legally be able to purchase a gun (North Carolina State Center for Health Statistics 2001).

Some advocates believe the answer to preventing gun rampages by disturbed individuals lies in extending the reach of states' reporting to the NICS (Mayors Against Illegal Guns 2011). Unfortunately, there is no evidence to suggest that merely filling the NICS with more records of people with gun-disqualifying mental health histories would have any measurable impact on reducing firearm violence in the population or, for that matter, on preventing mass shootings. Indeed, there would seem to be plenty of circumstantial evidence to the contrary. Still, what has been missing is a direct empirical evaluation of the law and policy in a single state, using longitudinal individual-level outcome data that would enable us to compare results for people with serious psychiatric disorders who have been subjected to the law's strictures and exposed to the NICS-reporting policy with those who have not. What follows is a report of the findings of such a study in Connecticut.

Effectiveness of Firearms Prohibitions in Reducing Violence among People with Serious Mental Illness in Connecticut, 2002–2009: Findings from a New Research Study

Connecticut began reporting mental health records to the NICS in early 2007. The Department of Public Safety is responsible for forwarding to the NICS all data regarding gun-prohibited persons. This now occurs by automatic transfer of gun-disqualifying mental health records through a "black box" system, so that confidential psychiatric records are not released to anyone outside of the state mental health authority. The state uploaded 3,062 mental health records to NICS in its first year of reporting, and by 2013 nearly 14,000 records had accumulated in the database. Presumably, the persons whose records were newly made available to the gun background check system had subsequently diminished access to new guns; insofar as they might otherwise have acquired and used guns to commit violent crimes, their risk of committing a violent crime should also have diminished. What has been the impact, if any, in reduced violent crime by gun-disqualified persons with serious mental illness in the state? Our study addressed that question.

Data

Administrative records for adults with serious mental illness spanning 8 years were assembled and merged from Connecticut's public mental health and criminal justice agencies. All research activities involving the use of private health information for this study were reviewed and approved by the relevant jurisdictional Institutional Review Boards (IRBs). Merged records from January 2002 through December 2009 were assembled for 23,292 adults meeting the following criteria: (1) diagnosis of schizophrenia, bipolar disorder, or major depressive disorder and (2) hospitalization in a state psychiatric hospital—either voluntarily or involuntarily—during the study period. Two study cohorts were constructed for comparison: persons with at least one of the four types of mental health adjudications reported to NICS (involuntary commitment, incompetent to stand trial, insanity acquittals, and conservatorships); and persons with at least one voluntary psychiatric hospitalization but no mental health adjudications. Data were structured in person-month format.

The sample is representative of the population of persons diagnosed with a serious mental illness who use services in the public mental health care system and who either have a history of mental health adjudication or have been hospitalized voluntarily in a state-operated facility for a mental health or co-occurring substance abuse disorder. As such, the sample would not generalize well to the population of all persons in the community who meet criteria for a mental illness or those who have less severe conditions not requiring inpatient treatment or who have private health insurance. The study sample is likely to have more severe and disabling psychiatric conditions, higher rates of substance abuse comorbidity, and a higher proportion who are involved with the criminal justice system. The base rate of violent crime in the sample is much higher than estimates of crime in community samples of persons with mental illness. Records of arrest include all available information but may not have captured lifetime arrests, especially for crime events occurring remotely in the individual's past.

Measures

The primary outcome variable was arrest for any violent crime (firearms-related or otherwise) within a given month. Violent crimes included murder, manslaughter, arson, kidnapping, sexual assault, other assault, robbery, and burglary. Ideally, we would have employed firearms charges as our primary outcome, but only arrests that resulted in conviction were available for analysis. Independent analysis from the Office of Legislative Research in Connecticut has shown that about 92% of firearms violations (e.g., illegal possession, transfer, use of a firearm in a crime, etc.) in the state do not result in convictions, due to plea bargaining and consolidation of charges (Reinhart 2007). Firearms conviction per se is thus an insensitive measure of gun-related crime. Instead, we used violent crime conviction as a proxy for gun use in crime. Violent crime is an important public health and safety outcome—arguably the distal goal of reducing the illegal use of guns—and the two variables are correlated.

Categorical variables were constructed to indicate whether a gun-disqualifying mental health record was present in a given month, whether a criminal disqualifier was in effect (record of felony conviction, misdemeanor drug crime, or misdemeanor domestic violence offense), and whether the observation month occurred before or after NICS reporting began in Connecticut. Age, sex, race, primary psychiatric diagnosis, and co-occurring substance use diagnoses were included as covariates.

Analysis

We used multivariable categorical regression with repeated measures to estimate effects on violent crime events. The dependent variable was lagged to ensure proper temporal ordering and to avoid confounding the occurrence of gun-disqualifying events with outcome events. We tested the change in risk of violent offending from before to after NICS reporting began. We also tested, in separate regressions not shown, the differences in violent crime risk in people who were disqualified versus not disqualified, for the pre- and post-NICS periods. We controlled for covarying effects of individuals' coincident criminal disqualification and clinical and demographic characteristics as described above. We adjusted the analysis for time at risk by removing observations when individuals were hospitalized or incarcerated. We adjusted for the non-independence of intraperson observations over time.

Results

The mean age of participants was 36 years, and a majority were male (62.5%). The racial-ethnic composition of the sample was 62.7% non-Hispanic white, 18.4% African American, 16.6% Hispanic, and 2.3% other racial-ethnic groups. Regarding primary psychiatric diagnosis, 28.1% had schizophrenia, 30.6% had bipolar disorder, and 41.2% had depression. Across diagnostic groups, 85.9% had a co-occurring alcohol or illicit drug abuse problem at some time during the study period. The prevalence of substance abuse comorbidity is higher in this sample than would be found in a community-representative sample, due in part to the inclusion criterion of hospitalization in a state facility, which would tend to select individuals who have had more complex and severe psychiatric problems.

Table 1 shows the numbers of individuals and proportions of the sample that were disqualified from purchasing a firearm during any time in the study period by type of disqualification. About 40% of the sample was disqualified either for mental health adjudication or a criminal record. Disqualification due to a criminal record was far more common than losing gun rights due to a mental health record (34.9% vs. 7.0%). Of the 1,634 individuals in the study with a

Table 1. Prevalence of gun-disqualifying mental health and criminal records in sample of people with seroius mental illness

Type of gun-disqualifying record	N	Percent
Involuntary civil commitment	1,086	(4.7%)
Incompetent to stand trial	464	(2.0%)
Not guilty by reason of insanity	29	(0.1%)
Conservatorship	152	(0.7%)
Any mental health disqualification	1,634	(7.0%)
Criminal disqualification	8,129	(34.9%)
Any criminal or mental health disqualification	9,246	(39.7%)
Both criminal and mental health disqualification	512	(2.2%)
Not disqualified	14,046	(60.3%)

mental health disqualification, 512 (31.3%) were dually disqualified on the basis of a criminal record. The large majority (93.7%) of the participants who were convicted of a gun-disqualifying crime during the study period were never involuntarily committed or otherwise disqualified due to a mental health record.

A substantial proportion of the sample (39.0%) was convicted of a violent crime at some time during the 8-year study period. The proportion of these crimes that involved use of guns is unknown, but 4% of the sample received a conviction specifically on a gun charge, such as illegal possession of a firearm. Table 2 shows the unadjusted frequencies of violent crime events as a proportion of the person-month observations available for analysis, by status of disqualification from firearms, for observations before and after NICS reporting began. In the full sample, there was a small decline in the estimated annualized rate of violent crime associated with NICS reporting in those with a mental health disqualification—from 7.8% to 6.5%, a proportional decline of 17%. In the subgroup of observations without any criminal disqualifications, the corresponding decline was greater—from 6.7% before NICS to 3.2% after NICS, a proportional decline of 53%. These unadjusted results are consistent with a NICS reporting effect, although they do not prove a causal relationship. An appropriate quasi-experimental test of statistical significance requires a robust multivariable analysis.

Table 3 displays the multivariable regression analysis for the full sample. Having a gun-disqualifying criminal record did not reduce the likelihood of

Table 2. Unadjusted frequencies of violent crime by gun-disqualifying mental health status and NICS policy exposure (person-month level of analysis)

	N person-months	Number of violent crime months	Percent of person-months with violent crime	Estimated annualized percent of group with violent crime
FULL SAMPLE [1]				
Gun-disqualifying mental health record and NICS policy exposure				
Legally disqualified, before NICS reporting began	44,345	289	0.65	7.8
Legally disqualified, after NICS reporting began	51,254	278	0.54	6.5
Not legally disqualified, before NICS reporting began	1,314,007	7,066	0.54	6.5
Not legally disqualified, after NICS reporting began	778,678	3,776	0.48	5.8
Total	*2,188,284*	*11,409*	*0.52*	*6.3*
NOT-CRIMINALLY-DISQUALIFIED SUBSAMPLE [2]				
Gun-disqualifying mental health record and NICS policy exposure				
Legally disqualified, before NICS reporting began	34,842	194	0.56	6.7
Legally disqualified, after NICS reporting began	35,248	93	0.26	3.2
Not legally disqualified, before NICS reporting began	1,128,574	5,552	0.49	5.9
Not legally disqualified, after NICS reporting began	537,325	1,753	0.33	3.9
Total	*1,735,989*	*7,592*	*0.44*	*5.2*

[1] Includes all person-months with community tenure; months spent hospitalized or incarcerated were removed from analysis.

[2] N=452,292 person-month observations were removed for the subsample analysis due to a gun-disqualifying criminal history.

Table 3. Adjusted odds ratios for monthly violent crime associated with legal restrictions on firearms access for people with serious mental illness in Connecticut from 2002-2009, before and after initation of state policy of reporting gun-disqualifying mental health records to the National Instant Check System

	Adusted Odds Ratio	95% Confidence Interval	Statistical Significance
Gun-disqualifying criminal record			
No criminal disqualification [reference category]	[1.00]		
Criminal disqualification	1.60	(1.52 - 1.68)	***
Gun-disqualifying mental health record and NICS policy exposure			
Legally disqualified, before NICS reporting began [reference category]	[1.00]		
Legally disqualified,after NICS reporting began	0.92	(0.76 - 1.13)	ns
Not legally disqualified, before NICS reporting began	0.76	(0.65 - 0.88)	***
Not legally disqualified, after NICS reporting began	0.78	(0.67 - 0.91)	***
Primary psychiatric diagnosis			
Major depression [reference category]	[1.00]		
Schizophrenia	0.90	(0.84 - 0.96)	***
Bipolar disorder	1.13	(1.07 - 1.20)	**

Substance abuse

No co-occurring alcohol or illicit drug use disorder [reference category]	[1.00]	
Any co-occurring alcohol or illicit drug use disorder	2.93	(2.57 - 3.34) ***
Demographic characteristics		
Age in years	0.98	(0.97 - 0.98) ***
Sex		
Female [reference category]	[1.00]	
Male	2.00	(1.90 - 2.14) ***
Race/ethnicity		
Non-hispanic white [reference category]	[1.00]	
Black	1.77	(1.67 - 1.88) ***
Hispanic	1.20	(1.11 - 1.26) ***
Other race/ethnicity	0.41	(0.29 - 0.58) ***

Analytic model specifications: General estimating equations (GEE) logistic regression for repeated measures with a lagged dependent variable, controlling for time and adjusting for non-independence of intra-person observations.

N=2,187,732 person-months observations

Statistical significance: ns - not significant; ***p<0.001;

future violent crime but rather increased the likelihood of a future violent offense by a factor of 1.6. The odds ratios for violent crime were significantly lower for people with no mental health adjudications, compared with those were disqualified in the pre-NICS period. Among all those who were disqualified, the odds of violent crime did not significantly decline after NICS reporting began. The model also shows that violent crime was associated with having a substance use disorder, being younger, male, of African American or Hispanic background, and having bipolar disorder versus depression. These tend to be factors associated with crime in the population without mental disorders, assuming that racial-ethnic minority status is functioning here as a proxy indicator of social and economic disadvantage, which we did not measure directly. Bipolar disorder was positively associated with violent crime compared with depression. Schizophrenia was negatively associated with violent crime compared with depression (a finding also reported in the MacArthur Violence Risk Study; Monahan et al. 2001.)

Table 4 shows the same analysis for the sample that was uniquely susceptible to the mental-health-related strictures in the federal law and the corresponding NICS reporting policy in Connecticut, without the potentially confounding effect of criminal history on violent crime recidivism. In this analysis, all of the observations were removed for any person-months in which an individual had a criminal disqualification in effect. This model shows a significant result of reduced violent offending among those with a disqualifying mental health record after NICS reporting began. The likelihood of violent crime was lower by a factor of 0.69 among those disqualified in the post-NICS-reporting period compared with those in the pre-NICS period. Indeed, the likelihood of violent crime in disqualified individuals whose records were reported to NICS was reduced to about the same level as seen in people who had never been disqualified. However, in groups who were never disqualified, the odds ratios for violent crime were approximately the same before and after the NICS policy was implemented—0.65 versus 0.62—suggesting, as would be expected, that NICS reporting did not affect people with no record to report to NICS.

Discussion and Implications for Policy

Considering our study population as a whole, we find little evidence that that Brady Act prohibitions serve to reduce the risk of violent crime. Indeed, having a gun-disqualifying criminal record serves as marker for significantly *in-*

creased risk of committing a future violent crime. To the extent that guns were involved in the commission of these crimes by people who could not legally buy a gun, it is clear that the perpetrators did not need to patronize a federally licensed gun dealer and undergo a background check; other ways, means, and suppliers abound for those willing to exploit them.

However, considering separately the subgroup of people with serious mental illness who do not have criminal records, our data seem to suggest that the Brady Law background checks can have some positive effect, if enforced. In those with a gun-disqualifying mental health record, risk of violent criminal offending declined significantly after Connecticut began reporting gun-disqualifying mental health records to the NICS.

These findings do not prove a causal relationship between the background check system and reduced violent crime. There may be other explanations, for example, that post-2007 improvements in the mental health and criminal justice system specifically affected people with gun-disqualifying mental health adjudications, resulting in improved treatment outcomes and a concomitant lower risk of criminal offending. The study has other limitations. We used violent crime as a proxy measure for gun use in crime. The research was conducted in a single state, and the findings may not generalize well to other states.

We conclude that the existing federal criteria for mental health prohibitions on firearms are far from perfect—they tend to be both overinclusive and underinclusive—but they are indeed correlated with increased risk of violent crime in this study. And here is at least some evidence, from one state, that having a mental health adjudication record archived in the NICS can significantly reduce risk of a first violent crime. Achieving comprehensive state reporting of mental health records to NICS may thus help reduce violent crime that is facilitated by guns and, thus, improve public safety.

However, this measured step will not prevent gun violence by dangerous individuals who today can easily skirt the background check system to obtain a firearm. It does nothing to prevent disqualified persons from using the guns they may already have. And even where it appears to work, the policy can affect only a small proportion of the population of persons with serious mental illness, because the base rate of mental health adjudication in Connecticut (as many states) is very low. Only about 7% of the sample had any disqualifying mental health adjudication, and an even smaller proportion—5%—were uniquely disqualified on the basis of a mental health history without also being

Table 4. Adjusted odds ratios for first violent crime associated with legal restrictions on firearms access for people with serious mental illness in Connecticut from 2002-2009, before and after initation of state policy of reporting gun-disqualifying mental health records to the National Instant Check System: SUBSAMPLE WITH NO PRE-EXISTING FELONY CONVICTION OR OTHER GUN DISQUALIFYING CRIMINAL RECORD

	Adusted Odds Ratio	95% Confidence Interval	Statistical Significance
Gun-disqualifying mental health record and NICS policy exposure			
Legally disqualified, before NICS reporting began [reference category]	[1.00]		
Legally disqualified,after NICS reporting began	0.69	(0.57 - 0.82)	***
Not legally disqualified, before NICS reporting began	0.65	(0.54 - 0.79)	**
Not legally disqualified, after NICS reporting began	0.62	(0.46 - 0.83)	***
Primary psychiatric diagnosis			
Major depression [reference category]	[1.00]		
Schizophrenia	0.80	(0.74 - 0.86)	***
Bipolar disorder	1.05	(0.98 - 1.13)	ns
Substance abuse			
No co-occurring alcohol or illicit drug use disorder [reference category]	[1.00]		
Any co-occurring alcohol or illicit drug use disorder	3.08	(2.68 - 3.54)	***

Demographic characteristics

Age in years	0.98	(0.97 - 0.98) ***
Sex		
Female [reference category]	[1.00]	
Male	2.18	(2.04 - 2.34) ***
Race/ethnicity		
Non-hispanic white [reference category]	[1.00]	
Black	1.89	(1.76 - 2.03) ***
Hispanic	1.30	(1.21 - 1.41) ***
Other race/ethnicity	1.26	(0.24 - 0.54) ***

Analytic model specifications: General estimating equations (GEE) logistic regression for repeated measures with a lagged dependent variable, controlling for time and adjusting for non-independence of intra-person observations.

N=1,735,437 person-months observations

Statistical significance: ns - not significant; ** p<0.01; =**p<0.001;

disqualified on the basis of a criminal history. In the non-criminally-disqualified subsample, those with a mental health disqualifier accounted for 3.0% of the sample and 3.4% of the violent crime. In the post-NICS period, they accounted for 6.2% of the sample and 5.0% of the violent crime. In contrast, 96% percent the crimes were committed by individuals who did not have a mental health disqualifier in effect, at least not at the time of the offense. These proportions suggest that background checks to enforce the federal mental health prohibitions—even if they are completely effective—will have a very small impact on overall violent crime in persons with serious mental illness; most of those at risk are unaffected by the law.

Revisions to the outdated federal criteria for mental health prohibitions on guns are needed. Minimum standards should be both *efficient* in prohibiting dangerous people from accessing guns and *fair* in preserving the rights of those who are not dangerous. Ideally, a balancing of safety and rights should inform more practical and less onerous rules for denying firearms rights to persons with mental illness who are dangerous, and the same balancing should inform parallel criteria for timely restoration of rights to persons with the mental illness who are no longer dangerous. Most important, then, changes to the prohibited category standards should focus on individual dangerousness, rather than relying on a presumed correlation between violence risk and membership in a category of persons with a mental health adjudication record, irrespective of its remoteness or the circumstances besides dangerousness that might have required it.

Innovative models of gun disqualification exist at the state level and could provide some guidance, at least in principle, for a more rational federal minimal standard. Indiana's "dangerous persons" law (Parker 2010), for example, is not tied to involuntarily commitment or even necessarily to having a diagnosis of mental illness but rather to a determination of dangerousness. In addition, the law focuses on removing current access to guns rather than merely foreclosing the future purchase of a new gun. The Indiana law allows clinicians or the police to take steps to have firearms removed without a warrant from individuals who are assessed to pose a danger to themselves or others (Parker 2010). Another promising approach worthy of consideration is California's law that allows seizure of guns from individuals with mental illness who are detained for dangerousness in a 72-hour hold, pending a judicial hearing in 14 days (Simpson 2007). The point of the law, in both cases, is to take a public health and safety approach to more accurately identify people who pose an appreciable risk of harming themselves or others instead of apply a broad categorical exclusion that is both insensitive and nonspecific as a practical index of gun violence risk.

Our study results suggest that, among people with mental illness who have a history of criminal offending and involvement with the justice system, existing law and policy designed to prevent access to firearms through federally licensed gun dealers is likely to be of limited effectiveness. Efforts to prevent gun violence in known criminal offenders with mental illness should also focus on reducing socially determined criminogenic risk factors; improving community-based mental health outcomes; and decreasing criminal recidivism in mentally ill offenders through targeted programs such as mental health courts, jail diversion, and community reintegration services for persons with mental illness who have been incarcerated (Monahan and Steadman 2012; Swanson 2010). Added to those measures, we should surely advocate for a range of population-based, gun-safety reforms that remain possible within constitutional limits.

Finally, a word about what might be considered the "elephant in the room" for a serious discussion of mental illness and firearm mortality: it is not homicide but suicide. When we bring suicide into the picture of gun violence, mental illness legitimately becomes a strong vector of concern; it should become an important component of effective policy to prevent firearm violence. Suicides account for 61% of all firearm fatalities in the United States—19,393 of the 31,672 gun deaths recorded in 2010 (Centers for Disease Control and Prevention 2013). Suicide is the third leading cause of death in Americans aged 15 to 24, perhaps not coincidentally the age group when young people go off to college, join the military, and experience a first episode of major mental illness. The majority of suicide victims had identified mental health problems and a history of some treatment. "How did they get a gun?" is an important question to answer. "Where was the treatment, and why did it fail?" may be even more important.

Depression is the particular psychiatric illness most strongly associated with suicide. Social disadvantage plays a role both in the etiology of depressive illness and disparities in its treatment. Depression is not, however, a disorder that gets most individuals a gun-disqualifying record of involuntarily commitment. In other words, people suffering from the one mental health condition that is most closely and frequently linked to suicidality are unlikely to show up in a gun background check. Even if every state were to report all of its records of mental health adjudications to the NICS, this "gap" would not close. But reporting to the authorities everyone who makes a suicide threat is probably not a good idea, either; it could merely drive people away from the treatment they need. Arguably, though, better access to evidence-based treatment for depression—particularly for low-income people, the elderly, and the unemployed (not to mention college students and returning veterans)—might prevent more firearm fatalities than would relying solely on improved NICS reporting to keep guns out of the hands of dangerous people.

ACKNOWLEDGMENT

Funding for the research presented in this essay was provided by a grant from the National Science Foundation, with additional support from the Robert Wood Johnson Foundation Program on Public Health Law Research.

REFERENCES

Appelbaum, Paul. 1994. Almost a Revolution: Mental Health Law and the Limits of Change. New York: Oxford University Press.

Appelbaum, Paul S., and Jeffrey W. Swanson. 2010. "Gun laws and mental illness: How sensible are the current restrictions?" Psychiatric Services 61: 652–654.

Bonnie, Richard J., James S. Reinhard, Phillip Hamilton, and Elizabeth L. McGarvey. 2009. Mental Health System Transformation After The Virginia Tech Tragedy. Health Affairs 28: 793–804.

Centers for Disease Control and Prevention. 2013. Injury Prevention & Control: Data & Statistics Web-based Injury Statistics Query and Reporting System (WISQA-RSTM). Fatal Injury Data and Nonfatal Injury Data. http://www.cdc.gov/injury/wisqars/index.html

Cook, Philip J., and Jens Ludwig. 1997. "Guns in America: National Survey on Private Ownership and Use of Firearms." National Institute of Justice, Research in Brief, Washington, DC: Department of Justice. http://www.ncjrs.gov/pdffiles/165476.pdf

Fazel, Seena, and Martin Grann. 2006. "The Population Impact of Severe Mental Illness on Violent Crime." The American Journal of Psychiatry 163: 1397–1403.

FBI. 2013. http://www.fbi.gov/about-us/cjis/nics

Fisher, William, and Thomas Grisso. 2010. "Commentary: Civil Commitment Statutes—40 Years of Circumvention." The Journal of the American Academy of Psychiatry Law 38(3): 365–368.

Lidz, Charles W., Edward P. Mulvey, and William Gardner. 1993. "The Accuracy of Predictions of Violence to Others." The Journal of American Medical Association 269: 1007–1011.

Mayors Against Illegal Guns. 2011. "Fatal Gaps: How Missing Records in the Federal Background Check System Put Guns in the Hands of Killers." http://www.mayors againstillegalguns.org/downloads/pdf/maig_mimeo_revb.pdf

Monahan, John, and Henry J. Steadman. 2012. "Extending Violence Reduction Principles to Justice-Involved Persons with Mental Illness." In Applying Social Science to Reduce Violent Offending, edited by Joel A. Dvoskin, Jennifer L. Skeem, Raymond W. Novaco, and Kevin S. Douglas, 245–261. New York: Oxford University Press.

Monahan, John, Henry J. Steadman, Eric Silver, et al. 2001. Rethinking Risk Assessment: The MacArthur Study of Mental Disorder and Violence. New York: Oxford University Press.

Nielssen, Olav, Dominique Bourget, Taina Laajasalo, et al. 2009. "Homicide of Strangers by People with a Psychotic Illness." Schizophrenia Bulletin 35: 1012–1021.

Norko, Michael A., and Victoria M. Dreisbach. 2008. Letter to the Editor. Journal of the American Academy of Psychiatry and the Law 36: 269.

North Carolina State Center for Health Statistics Behavioral Risk Factor Surveillance System. 2001. http://www.schs.state.nc.us/schs/brfss/2001/us/firearm3.html

Parker, George. 2010. "Application of a Firearm Seizure Law Aimed at Dangerous Persons: Outcomes from the First Two Years." Psychiatric Services 61: 478–482.

Pescosolido, Bernice A., John Monahan, and Bruce G. Link, et al. 1999. "The Public's View of the Competence, Dangerousness, and Need for Legal Coercion of Persons with Mental Health Problems." American Journal of Public Health 89: 1339–1345.

Price, M., and D. M. Norris. 2008. "National Instant Criminal Background Check Improvement Act: Implications for Persons with Mental Illness." Journal of the American Academy of Psychiatry and the Law 36: 123–130.

Reinhart, Christopher. 2007. "Case Statistics for Firearms Violations." OLR Research Report, 2007-R-0442, Connecticut Office of Fiscal Analysis Database. http:// worldcat.org/arcviewer/1/CZL/2007/08/02/0000070154/viewer/file1.html26782.75

Simpson, Joseph R. 2007. "Bad Risk? An Overview of Laws Prohibiting Possession of Firearms by Individuals with a History of Treatment for Mental Illness." Journal of the American Academy of Psychiatry and the Law 35: 330–338.

Skeem, Jennifer, and John Monahan. 2011. "Current Directions in Violence Risk Assessment." Current Directions in Psychological Science 20: 38–42.

Swanson, Jeffrey W. 1994. "Mental Disorder, Substance Abuse, and Community Violence: An Epidemiological Approach." In Violence and Mental Disorder, edited by J. Monahan and H. Steadman, 101–136. Chicago: University of Chicago Press.

Swanson, Jeffrey W. 2010. "Explaining Rare Acts of Violence: The Limits of Population Research Evidence." Psychiatric Services 62: 1369–1371.

Swanson, Jeffrey W. 2011. "Preventing the Unpredicted: Managing Violence Risk in Mental Health Care." Psychiatric Services 59: 191–193.

Van Dorn, Richard A., Jan Volavka, and Norman Johnson. 2012. "Mental Disorder and Violence: Is There a Relationship beyond Substance Use?" Social Psychiatry and Psychiatric Epidemiology 47(3): 487–503.

4

Evidence for Optimism

Policies to Limit Batterers' Access to Guns

April M. Zeoli and Shannon Frattaroli

In 2010, at least 1,082 women and 267 men were killed by their intimate partners. Fifty-four percent of these victims were killed with guns (United States Department of Justice 2012). For at least the past twenty-five years, more intimate partner homicides (IPHs) have been committed with guns than with all other weapons combined (Fox and Zawitz 2009). Furthermore, women are more likely to be killed by an intimate partner than by any other offender group (Fox and Zawitz 2009; Moracco, Runyan, and Butts 1998). The evidence is clear: when a woman is killed, it is most likely to be at the hands of an intimate partner with a gun.

In this essay, we focus on policies to limit batterers' access to guns, the evidence that supports these policies, and evidence for improvement in their implementation and expansion. We begin with an overview of the evidence about gun usage in domestic violence and how batterers become known to

April M. Zeoli, PhD, MPH, is an assistant professor in the School of Criminal Justice at Michigan State University. Shannon Frattaroli, PhD, MPH, is an associate professor at the Johns Hopkins Bloomberg School of Public Health.

the justice system. Second, we discuss existing legislation to remove guns from batterers. We then present promising evidence about policies to limit batterers' access to guns and their relationship to IPH, and we discuss implementation and enforcement of those laws. We conclude with federal gun policy recommendations to prevent IPH.

Domestic Violence and Guns: A Brief Overview

Guns are the weapons of choice for IPH perpetrators. Domestic violence involving a gun is more likely to result in homicide than domestic violence that involves a knife, other weapon, or bodily force (Saltzman et al. 1992). Indeed, the risk of homicide increases when a violent intimate has access to a gun (Bailey et al. 1997; Kellerman et al. 1993), with one study estimating a fivefold increased risk (Campbell et al. 2003). Intimate partners are more likely to use guns to kill their female victims than are non-intimate partners who kill women (Arbuckle et al. 1996; Moracco et al. 1998). Moreover, there is growing evidence documenting the role of guns in nonfatal domestic violence perpetrated by men against women (Moracco et al. 2006; Rothman et al. 2005; Sorenson and Wiebe 2004; Tjaden and Thoennes 2000). These nonfatal uses of guns may warn of future fatal violence: batterers' use of weapons to threaten has been associated with a fourfold increased risk of homicide (Campbell et al. 2003).

There is a history of male-to-female domestic violence in the relationships of most women and men killed by their intimate partners (Bailey et al. 1997; Campbell et al. 2003; McFarlane et al. 1999; Smith, Moracco, and Butts 1998), making domestic violence against the female partner the leading risk factor for IPH (Campbell et al. 2007). Stalking may also be an important risk factor for IPH (Campbell et al. 2003), with one study reporting that 76% of homicide victims and 85% of attempted homicide victims were stalked by their abusers prior to the incident (McFarlane et al. 1999). Often this abuse is known to the authorities. Roughly half of women killed by their intimate partners had contact with the justice system to report violence and stalking within the year preceding their murders. These women reported domestic violence/stalking to the police, had their assailants arrested, filed criminal charges, and obtained domestic violence restraining orders (DVROs) against their batterers (McFarlane et al. 1999; Moracco, Runyan, and Butts 1998).

When women seek assistance from the justice system, they create opportunities for intervention that may prevent future violence and homicide. If equipped with a comprehensive set of domestic violence laws, law enforcement may be better positioned to safeguard victims and save more lives. Laws that restrict batterers' access to guns are an essential component of any comprehensive approach to address domestic violence.

Current Federal Law: Responding to the Risks

Two provisions under federal law address the dangerous combination of batterers and guns. In 1994, Congress amended the Gun Control Act to prohibit individuals who are under qualifying DVROs from purchasing or possessing guns (18 U.S.C. § 922(g)(8)). To qualify, a DVRO must be issued after a court hearing about which the respondent was notified and in which he had the opportunity to participate. This type of DVRO is often referred to as *permanent.* Eligible DVRO respondents include the petitioner's current or former spouse, someone the petitioner shares a child with, or a current or former cohabitant (18 U.S.C. § 921(a)(32)).

In 1996, Congress amended the Gun Control Act to prohibit those convicted of domestic violence misdemeanors from purchasing or possessing guns (18 U.S.C. § 922(g)(9)). This expansion is a lifetime ban and includes any misdemeanor that "has, as an element, the use or attempted use of physical force, or the threatened use of a deadly weapon" and was committed by an intimate partner (18 U.S.C. § 921(a)(33)). The list of those included as intimate partners under the misdemeanor law is more expansive than the DVRO gun prohibition and includes parents or guardians as well as those "similarly situated to a spouse, parent or guardian" (18 U.S.C. § 921(a)(33)). Importantly, this law applies to law enforcement and the military and includes qualifying offenses that pre-date the law.

State-Level Domestic Violence Gun Legislation

Many states have laws limiting DVRO respondents' access to guns. State laws are often more inclusive than federal laws and some, for example, expand the definition of qualifying DVROs to include temporary DVROs. Courts usually consider and grant temporary DVROs before respondents have been notified of petitioners' requests for protection from abuse. This decision in the absence of the respondent is unusual in the U.S. justice system, but it is a direct response to the danger that DVRO petitioners face. Respondents to

DVROs have high rates of criminal justice system involvement (Klein 1996; Moracco et al. 2010; Vittes and Sorenson 2006) and often have committed severe domestic violence (Holt et al. 2003; Logan, Shannon, and Walker 2005; Sorenson and Shen 2005). Furthermore, women who seek DVROs often do so in the context of separation from their batterer (Logan et al. 2008), a time of heightened homicide risk (Campbell et al. 2007; Wilson and Daly 1993). Temporary DVROs allow victims to gain the protection a DVRO provides without requiring them to wait for a hearing.

Some states limit domestic violence misdemeanants' access to guns. These laws may also be more expansive than the federal legislation. One way in which both state DVRO and domestic violence misdemeanor gun restrictions increase coverage is by expanding the categories of intimate partners covered by the law, for example by including current or former dating partners. Current dating partners were responsible for 35 percent of IPHs committed between 1976 and 2005, but the share of IPHs committed annually by current dating partners has been increasing (Fox and Zawitz 2009). Additionally, one study found that more than half of DVRO applications were against current or former dating partners or fiancés and that applications against this group were more likely to mention guns than applications against current and former spouses combined (Vittes and Sorenson 2006).

There is great variation in state DVRO and domestic violence misdemeanant gun laws, including whether purchase of a gun is prohibited or only possession is prohibited. Not all states provide more coverage than the federal legislation, and many do not have these types of gun prohibitions. Because some states have only the federal law to rely on and because federal restrictions may be stronger than state restrictions, federal law is crucial.

Evidence

Federal legislative strategies to address the risks associated with armed batterers rely on the existing system of identifying and prosecuting violent intimates through the criminal justice system and the DVRO system in place in courts in all fifty states. This approach is consistent with the evidence: past abuse in a relationship is the best predictor of future abuse and is the leading risk factor associated with IPH. It is also consistent with our current approach to regulating access to guns. Prohibitions on purchase and possession are largely based on disqualifying behaviors, with criminal

nondomestic violence convictions constituting the largest category of prohibited purchasers denied through background checks (Federal Bureau of
Investigation 2011).

Evaluating Impacts

Three studies have examined how state laws limiting access to guns for
DVRO respondents and domestic violence misdemeanants affect IPH (Vigdor and Mercy 2003, 2006; Zeoli and Webster 2010). Vigdor and Mercy examined the effects of state DVRO and domestic violence misdemeanant gun
restrictions on state-level IPH from 1982 to 1998 (2003), and again from 1982
to 2002 (2006). In both studies, DVRO laws were significantly associated with
reductions in IPH risk, both for IPHs committed with guns and total IPHs.
Further investigation uncovered that these reductions rested on the capacity
of states to support background checks on would-be gun purchasers (Vigdor
and Mercy 2003, 2006). This finding highlights the importance of ensuring
that systems for implementing these laws are in place and supported: the prohibition against purchasing a gun can be effective only if background checks
yield current, comprehensive, and accurate disqualifying information.

There was also a measurable difference in the effect of laws prohibiting
gun purchases compared to laws prohibiting possession only (Vigdor and
Mercy 2006). In states prohibiting purchase, total and gun IPH had an associated reduction of 10% to 12%; there was no measurable impact of possession-
only laws. Purchase may be the more effective prohibited action because the
restriction on possession relies on respondents to voluntarily surrender their
guns or law enforcement to collect guns from newly prohibited respondents
(Vigdor and Mercy 2006).

A later analysis of state domestic violence gun laws and IPH in 46 U.S. cities from 1979 to 2003 provides further evidence of the state DVRO laws' impact (Zeoli and Webster 2010). The 46 cities were in 27 states, 15 of which have
DVRO gun prohibitions and 9 of which have domestic violence misdemeanant gun prohibitions. Cities in states with DVRO gun restrictions had 19%
fewer IPHs and 25% fewer IPHs committed with guns compared to cities
without those state laws (Zeoli and Webster 2010).

Taken together, these three studies provide compelling evidence that DVRO
gun restrictions reduce IPH. Importantly, the results of all three studies show
that those reductions are not limited to IPHs committed with guns, suggesting
that there is no discernible substitution effect. Would-be killers do not replace

guns with other weapons to affect the same number of killings. Or, put another way, the evidence suggests that state DVRO gun prohibitions save lives.

Unlike the beneficial effects associated with DVRO laws, the three studies found no measurable impact on IPH of state laws restricting domestic violence misdemeanants' access to guns. This may be for a number of reasons. Misdemeanor convictions for domestic violence may be too few for researchers to detect an associated reduction in homicide (Vigdor and Mercy 2006). In addition, the statute under which a batterer is charged also may determine whether he is identified through a background check as prohibited or not, and many states do not have a specific domestic violence misdemeanor crime to charge (Vigdor and Mercy 2006). Finally, a lack of implementation and enforcement of the law may impact its effectiveness.

Implementation and Enforcement

With the evidence concerning laws that address the risks associated with guns and violent intimates came attention to the implementation and enforcement of these laws. DVRO policies have been a focus of this research, which offers empirical insight into why DVRO laws prohibiting purchase fare better than policies that only prohibit possession and provides strategies for strengthening the possession prohibition. We are unaware of any research examining how domestic violence misdemeanor prohibitions are implemented and enforced. However, we suspect there are similarities in the processes involved because both laws require that information about the prohibiting offense be included in the background check system and that processes for retrieving guns from newly disqualified individuals be in place.

One evaluation of North Carolina's DVRO gun law found no measurable reduction in intimate partner gun violence among petitioners post-law but also documented no change in DVROs requiring respondents to surrender their guns or cases where guns were recovered from respondents (Moracco et al. 2006). The conclusion from this study is not that the law is flawed but rather that the implementation of the law did not allow for a real test of its merits. The implementation failure is likely not unique to North Carolina. Indeed, several reports offer anecdotal evidence of neglected implementation (Attorney General's Task Force on Local Criminal Justice Response to Domestic Violence 2005; Frattaroli and Teret 2006; Gwinn 2006; Webster et al. 2010).

Behind the failures to implement the gun possession prohibition are opportunities to better ensure the prohibition is realized (Frattaroli and Teret

2006; Wintemute et al. 2012). It is essential to know whether a respondent possesses guns and, if so, how many. Such information can be obtained from state registries and gun sale databases (where they exist), DVRO petitions, and petitioners. One evaluation of an initiative to implement the California DVRO law concluded that while each source provides some unique data about respondents' guns, the information is still incomplete (Wintemute et al. 2012). Facilitating disclosure of information about guns by petitioners through the DVRO application and hearing processes is critical (Frattaroli and Teret 2006; Webster et al. 2010; Wintemute et al. 2012), and the value of complete registry or record-of-sales databases that capture all gun transactions (long guns and handguns; private sales and dealer sales) cannot be overstated for any effort to fully enforce DVRO possession prohibitions (Wintemute et al. 2012). Knowledge of which respondents may have firearms allows law enforcement to better prepare for interacting with the respondent safely, and it may increase the likelihood that guns are recovered (Wintemute et al. 2012).

Even with information about the presence of guns, that information does not always translate into DVROs issued with instructions to surrender guns (Frattaroli and Teret 2006; Sorenson and Shen 2005; Webster et al. 2010). Still, there is evidence that oversight may reduce underuse of the DVRO gun law. Following an examination of the state's DVRO database, the California Department of Justice sent letters to relevant local agencies that called attention to the low utilization of the gun prohibition on DVROs in the database (Seave 2006). A review of the data following this exchange revealed a reduction in the percentage of orders without a gun prohibition (Seave 2006).

Service of issued DVROs is also a major barrier to realizing a DVRO gun prohibition. For those orders that are served by law enforcement, the act of service offers a chance for officers to facilitate removal of guns to ensure compliance with the DVRO. The value of law enforcement access to record-of-sale databases and to information provided by the petitioner to the recovery of guns has been documented, as has the importance of trained officers tasked with handling these exchanges (Wintemute et al. 2012).

Given the findings from the above studies, we hypothesize that the documented effects associated with DVRO gun restrictions likely reflect an effect of the purchase prohibitions and not the possession prohibitions. While the implementation of this law is complex and involves participation from different agencies, these barriers are not insurmountable, as the California initiative demonstrates (Wintemute et al. 2012). Additionally, a recent report suggests that a small number of localities are engaging in innovative strategies to ensure that DVRO laws are being used to improve public safety (Klein 2006). Between the emerging initiatives at the local level and the literature that is developing on this topic, the time is right for federal action to organize and encourage the efforts needed to reduce the documented risks that result when violent intimates have access to guns.

Policy Implications

There are many ways to strengthen federal law to reduce the violence documented at the start of this essay. Following is a list of recommendations that are evidence-informed and actionable—although not exhaustive.

Goal: Prevent DVRO respondents and DV misdemeanants from purchasing or possessing guns.

Policy: Require all gun purchasers to submit to a background check.

• Rationale: Under federal law, background checks are not required for sales from private sellers, providing prohibited batterers with easy access to guns. Requiring background checks for all gun sales will eliminate an important source of guns for prohibited batterers.

Policy: Incentivize states to automate DVRO and domestic violence misdemeanor records for reporting to background check systems.

• Rationale: Background check systems must be automated and updated regularly so that disqualifying information is included in the system and immediately available to gun sellers.

Policy: Incentivize states to create gun registries or gun purchase databases.

• Rationale: A mechanism to allow law enforcement to quickly learn whether a DVRO respondent or a person convicted of a domestic violence misdemeanor owns a gun would aid efforts to enforce existing prohibitions on gun possession among this group of people known to be violent.

Goal: Expand federal law to prohibit other categories of violent intimates from purchasing and possessing guns.

Policy: Extend the DVRO prohibition to include those covered by temporary DVROs.

• Rationale: The initial period after filing for a DVRO, during which a temporary DVRO is in place, is a dangerous time for petitioners. Federal law should recognize and reduce this danger by extending the prohibition to include temporary DVROs.

Policy: Expand the definition of intimate partners.

- Rationale: Current and former dating partners should be included in federal law so all victims of violent intimate partners receive equal protection.

Policy: Extend federal gun prohibitions to cover those convicted of misdemeanor stalking.

- Rationale: Stalking is an important risk factor for intimate partner homicide. However, because misdemeanor stalking laws often do not include "the use or attempted use of physical force, or the threatened use of a deadly weapon," the domestic violence misdemeanor gun prohibition does not apply.

Policy: Extend federal gun prohibitions to cover persons who have violated a DVRO (permanent and temporary) because of threatened or actual violence.

- Rationale: Those who violate court-issued DVROs because of violence may be especially dangerous and should be subject to the lifetime ban on gun purchase and possession to which domestic violence misdemeanants are subject.

Goal: Provide the resources and support needed for state and local systems to implement and enforce domestic violence gun prohibitions.

Policy: Establish and fund a center that will provide the training and technical assistance needed to realize full implementation of laws that prohibit DVRO respondents and misdemeanants from possessing guns.

- Rationale: Federal law enforcement authorities, with the help of model state programs such as the California Armed and Prohibited Persons System, are well-positioned to assist state and local law enforcement in developing their infrastructures to ensure these laws are realized for the benefit of public safety.

REFERENCES

Arbuckle, J., L. Olson, M. Howard, J. Brillman, C. Anctil, and D. Sklar. 1996. Safe at home? Domestic violence and other homicides among women in New Mexico. *Ann Emerg Med* 27: 210–15.

Attorney General's Task Force on Local Criminal Justice Response to Domestic Violence. 2005. Keeping the promise: Victims' safety and batterer accountability. Sacramento, CA: California Department of Justice.

Bailey, J., A. Kellerman, G. Somes, J. Banton, F. Rivara, and N. Rushforth. 1997. Risk factors for violent death of women in the home. *Arch Intern Med* 157: 777–82.

Campbell, J.C., N. Glass, P.W. Sharps, K. Laughon, and T. Bloom. 2007. Intimate partner homicide: Review and implications of research and policy. *Trauma, Violence & Abuse* 8: 246–60.

Campbell, J.C., D.W. Webster, J. Koziol-Mclain, C. Block, D. Campbell, M.A. Curry, F. Gary, N. Glass, J. Mcfarlane, C. Sachs, P. Sharps, Y. Ulrich, S.A. Wilt, J. Manganello, X. Xu, J. Schollenberger, V. Frye, and K. Laughon. 2003. Risk factors for femicide in abusive relationships: Results from a multisite case control study. *American Journal of Public Health* 93: 1069–97.

Federal Bureau of Investigation. 2011. National Instant Criminal Background Check System (NICS) operations. Washington, D.C.: U.S. Department of Justice.

Fleury, R.E., C. Sullivan, and D. Bybee. 2000. When ending the relationship does not end the violence: Women's experiences of violence by former partners. *Violence Against Women* 6: 1363–83.

Fox, J.A., and M.W. Zawitz. 2009. Homicide trends in the United States: Bureau of Justice Statistics. http://bjs.ojp.usdoj.gov/content/homicide/homtrnd.cfm.

Frattaroli, S., and S.P. Teret. 2006. Understanding and informing policy implementation: A case study of the domestic violence provisions of the Maryland Gun Violence Act. *Evaluation Review* 30: 347–60.

Gwinn, C. 2006. Domestic violence and firearms: Reflections of a prosecutor. *Evaluation Review* 30: 237–44.

Holt, V.L., M.A. Kernic, M.E. Wolf, and F. Rivara. 2003. Do protection orders affect the likelihood of future partner violence and injury? *American Journal of Preventive Medicine* 24: 16–21.

Kellerman, A., F. Rivara, N. Rushforth, J. Banton, D. Reay, J. Francisco, A. Locci, J. Prodzinski, B. Hackman, and G. Somes. 1993. Gun ownership as a risk factor for homicide in the home. *New England Journal of Medicine* 329: 1084–91.

Klein, A.R. 1996. Re-abuse in a population of court-restrained male batterers: Why restraining orders don't work. In *Do arrests and restraining orders work?*, 192–213. Thousand Oaks, CA: Sage.

———. 2006. Enforcing domestic violence firearm prohibitions: A report on promising practices. Washington, D.C.: Office on Violence Against Women. http://www.bwjp.org/files/bwjp/articles/Enforcing_Firearms_Prohibitions.pdf.

Kurz, D. 1996. Separation, divorce, and woman abuse. *Violence Against Women* 2: 63–81.

Logan, T.K., L. Shannon, and R. Walker. 2005. Protective orders in rural and urban areas: A multiple perspective study. *Violence Against Women* 11: 876–911.

Logan, T.K., R. Walker, L. Shannon, and J. Cole. 2008. Factors associated with separation and ongoing violence among women with civil protective orders. *Journal of Family Violence* 23: 377–85.

McFarlane, J., J.C. Campbell, S.A. Wilt, C. Sachs, Y. Ulrich, and X. Xu. 1999. Stalking and intimate partner femicide. *Homicide Studies* 3: 300–16.

Moracco, K.E., K. Andersen, R.M. Buchanan, C. Espersen, J.M. Bowling, and C. Duffy. 2010. Who are the defendants in domestic violence protection order cases? *Violence Against Women* 16: 1201–23.

Moracco, K.E., K.A. Clark, C. Espersen, and J.M. Bowling. 2006. Preventing firearms violence among victims of intimate partner violence: An evaluation of a new North Carolina law: U.S. Department of Justice.

Moracco, K.E., C.W. Runyan, and J.D. Butts. 1998. Femicide in North Carolina, 1991–1993: A statewide study of patterns and precursors. *Homicide Studies* 2: 422–46.

Rothman, E.F., D. Hemenway, M. Miller, and D. Azrael. 2005. Batterers' use of guns to threaten intimate partners. *Journal of the American Medical Women's Association* 60: 62–68.

Saltzman, L.E., J.A. Mercy, P. Ocarroll, M. Rosenberg, and P. Rhodes. 1992. Weapon involvement and injury outcomes in family and intimate assaults. *Journal of the American Medical Association* 267: 3043–47.

Seave, P.L. 2006. Disarming batterers through restraining orders: The promise and the reality in California. *Evaluation Review* 30: 245–65.

Smith, P.H., K.E. Moracco, and J.D. Butts. 1998. Partner homicide in context: A population-based perspective. *Homicide Studies* 2: 400–421.

Sorenson, S.B., and H. Shen. 2005. Restraining orders in California: A look at state-wide data. *Violence Against Women* 11: 912–33.

Sorenson, S.B., and D.J. Wiebe. 2004. Weapons in the lives of battered women. *American Journal of Public Health* 94: 1412–17.

Tjaden, P., and N. Thoennes. 2000. Extent, nature, and consequences of intimate partner violence. Washington, DC: U.S. Department of Justice.

United States Department of Justice. 2012. Uniform crime reporting program data: Supplementary homicide reports, 2010. Icpsr33527-v1. Ann Arbor, MI: Inter-university Consortium for Political and Social Research [distributor].

Vigdor, E.R., and J.A. Mercy. 2003. Disarming batterers: The impact of domestic violence firearm laws. In *Evaluating gun policy*, 157–214. Washington, DC: The Brookings Institution.

———. 2006. Do laws restricting access to firearms by domestic violence offenders prevent intimate partner homicide? *Evaluation Review* 30: 313–46.

Vittes, K.A., and S.B. Sorenson. 2006. Are temporary restraining orders more likely to be issued when applications mention firearms? *Evaluation Review* 30: 266–82.

Webster, D.W., S. Frattaroli, J.S. Vernick, C. O'Sullivan, J. Roehl, and J.C. Campbell. 2010. Women with protective orders report failure to remove firearms from their abusive partners: Results from an exploratory study. *Journal of Women's Health* 19: 93–98.

Wilson, M.I., and M. Daly. 1993. Spousal homicide risk and estrangement. *Violence and Victims* 8: 3–16.

Wintemute, G., S. Frattaroli, K.A. Vittes, B. Claire, M. Wright, and D.W. Webster. 2012. Firearms and domestic violence education and intervention project: Final report of process and outcome evaluations. Sacramento, CA: Violence Prevention Research Program, University of California, Davis.

Zeoli, A.M., and D.W. Webster. 2010. Effects of domestic violence policies, alcohol taxes and police staffing levels on intimate partner homicide in large us cities. *Injury Prevention* 16: 90–95.

5

Reconsidering the Adequacy of Current Conditions on Legal Firearm Ownership

Katherine A. Vittes, Daniel W. Webster, and Jon S. Vernick

An important objective of successful gun violence prevention policy is to keep guns from high-risk individuals without infringing on the rights of law-abiding citizens to use firearms for protection or recreation. Given the potential of laws designed to keep guns from dangerous individuals to save lives, the categories of individuals to be prohibited from possessing firearms merits careful consideration. The goals of this chapter are to (1) briefly review the current federal prohibitory criteria for firearm possession and the rationale for these prohibitions, (2) make the case for broadening these criteria to limit access to firearms among additional categories of individuals, and (3) put forth specific policy recommendations based on the available research evidence. This chapter does not address prohibitory criteria related to mental

Katherine A. Vittes, PhD, MPH, is a research associate at the Johns Hopkins Center for Gun Policy and Research. Daniel W. Webster, ScD, MPH, is a professor in the Department of Health Policy and Management at the Johns Hopkins Bloomberg School of Public Health. Jon S. Vernick, JD, MPH, is an associate professor and associate chair in the Department of Health Policy and Management at the Johns Hopkins Bloomberg School of Public Health.

health status and only touches on prohibitions for violent misdemeanants, because these are covered elsewhere in this volume.

Rationale for Current Conditions that Prohibit Firearm Possession

Recognizing that certain categories of individuals are at high risk for committing violence, federal law prohibits firearm possession by the following groups: felons; fugitives; persons convicted of a misdemeanor crime for domestic violence; those who are subject to certain restraining orders for domestic violence; unlawful users of or those addicted to controlled substances; those who have been found by a judge to be mentally incompetent, a danger to themselves or others as a result of mental illness, or have been involuntarily committed to a mental institution; those who have been dishonorably discharged from the military; illegal aliens; and persons who have renounced their U.S. citizenship. In addition, federal law sets 21 years as the minimum age at which a person can lawfully purchase a handgun from a federally licensed firearms dealer but sets 18 as the minimum legal age for handgun possession and for transfers of handguns from anyone who is not a licensed gun dealer (*18 U.S.C. §922 (d) (2012)*). No minimum possession age applies to long guns (rifles and shotguns) under federal law.

Research provides justification for restricting firearm possession for many of these groups. Convicted felons are much more likely to commit subsequent violent crimes—including homicide—than are nonfelons (Cook, Ludwig, and Braga 2005). Similarly, persons with a history of committing intimate partner violence are at increased risk for killing an intimate partner (Campbell et al. 2003) and for committing violence against nonfamily members (Etter and Birzer 2007; Fagan, Stewart, and Hansen 1983; Gayford 1975; Hotaling, Straus, and Lincoln 1989).

Research also supports restricting firearm possession for drug abusers. Illicit drug use and abuse is strongly associated with violent and criminal behavior (Afifi et al. 2012; Friedman 1998; Kelleher et al. 1994; Parker and Auerhahn 1998; Rivara et al. 1997; Walton-Moss et al. 2005) and suicide (Borges, Walters, and Kessler 2000; Borowsky, Ireland, and Resnick 2001; Rivara et al. 1997). For example, homicide offenders are nearly five times more likely to abuse drugs than are nonoffenders, and the use of illicit drugs is associated with a seven times higher risk of suicide (Rivara et al. 1997).

There also is strong evidence for restricting access to firearms by young people. Involvement in violent crime, either as a perpetrator or victim, increases dramatically during adolescence and in early adulthood (Fabio et al. 2006; Fox and Zawitz 2010). Brain structures related to risk taking and impulse control are developing throughout adolescence, and this may contribute to heightened risk of violent behavior among this age group (Johnson, Blum, and Giedd 2009; Steinberg 2004).

The Case for Broadening Firearm Prohibitions for High-Risk Persons

Federal law sets the minimum standards for legal firearm ownership, but many states have laws that disqualify additional categories of high-risk individuals. The differences across states are significant. For example, New Jersey prohibits firearm possession by anyone who has been convicted of a crime for which the penalty can be 6 months or more of imprisonment and sets the minimum legal age for handgun possession at 21 years. (Federal law sets age 18 as the minimum legal age to *possess* a handgun.) In contrast, 13 states have standards for legal firearm possession that either mirror or are weaker than federal standards. In these 13 states, individuals who are likely at high risk for committing violence against themselves or others can legally possess firearms.

A recent study, using data from a survey of inmates in state prisons, examined the criminal history and ages of 253 persons incarcerated for committing gun-related crimes in the 13 U.S. states with the least stringent criteria for legal firearm possession.[1] Sixty percent ($n = 151$) of the offenders in the study were legally permitted to possess firearms prior to committing the gun crime that led to their incarceration, including 4% who had prior misdemeanor convictions involving violence or firearms, 6% convicted of other misdemeanors, 5% convicted of a serious offense as a juvenile, and 13% who had prior arrests but no convictions. It is important to note that, if these 13 states had laws prohibiting firearm possession for these additional high-risk groups, nearly half of the 151 offenders ($n = 73$) who were legally in possession of firearms would have been prohibited when they committed the gun offense for which they were incarcerated (Vittes, Vernick, and Webster 2012). Some portion of these gun crimes might have been prevented if these offenders had been prohibited from possessing firearms when they committed the offenses for which they were incarcerated.

Few rigorous scientific studies directly examine whether laws prohibiting individuals in specific high-risk groups from purchasing or possessing firearms reduce criminal offending by prohibited individuals (Hahn et al. 2005; Welford, Pepper, and Petrie 2004). However, studies that examine the effects of prohibiting access to firearms by perpetrators of domestic violence suggest that these laws can effectively reduce violence. For example, Wintemute and colleagues (2001) examined a California law that expanded firearm prohibitions to include persons convicted of violent misdemeanors. The study found that misdemeanants who were denied purchase of a handgun due to a change in the law were less likely than handgun purchasers to commit subsequent violent and gun-related crime. Studies also have found that state laws prohibiting firearm possession by those subject to certain types of domestic violence restraining orders are associated with lower rates of intimate partner homicide (Vigdor and Mercy 2003, 2006; Zeoli and Webster 2010).

Despite the lack of specific evaluations of prohibitory criteria for firearm possession for some categories of individuals, ample evidence shows that certain categories of individuals are at increased risk for violent and criminal behavior. We draw upon this literature to make the case for broadening prohibitions for firearm possession to include alcohol abusers, persons less than 21 years of age, and adults convicted of serious crimes as juveniles.

Alcohol Abusers

Unlike illicit drug abusers, alcohol abusers are not prohibited from purchasing or possessing firearms under federal law. Yet, alcohol abuse is at least as strongly associated with the perpetration and victimization of violence (Afifi et al. 2012; Friedman 1998; Kelleher et al. 1994; Parker and Auerhahn 1998; Rivara et al. 1997; Sharps et al. 2001; Walton-Moss et al. 2005) and suicide (Borges, Walters, and Kessler 2000; Borowsky et al. 2001; Rivara et al. 1997). For example, a case-control study that examined risk factors for homicide and suicide in three large urban areas in the United Sates found that subjects who drank alcohol, had ever been in trouble at work for drinking, or were ever hospitalized for alcohol abuse were at increased risk for homicide and suicide compared with controls (Rivara et al. 1997). Another multicity case-control study found that victim and perpetrator alcohol abuse was strongly associated with nonfatal and fatal intimate partner violence (Sharps et al. 2001).

Several studies suggest that firearm owners may be at increased risk for abusing alcohol (Diener and Kerber 1979; Miller, Hemenway, and Wechsler 1999, 2002; Nelson et al. 1996; Wintemute 2011). This is especially concerning, given that alcohol has been shown to hamper shooting accuracy and impair judgment about when it might be appropriate to use a gun (Carr et al. 2009). A recent study that analyzed population-based survey data from eight U.S. states found that respondents who owned firearms were more likely than those who did not live in a home with a firearm to engage in binge drinking, drive under the influence of alcohol, and have at least 60 drinks per month. Heavy drinking was also more common among firearm owners who carried a gun for protection and stored a gun loaded and unlocked (Wintemute 2011). College students who own firearms are more likely than their unarmed counterparts to binge drink (Miller, Hemenway, and Wechsler 1999, 2002), to drive after binge drinking (Miller et al. 1999, 2002), to be arrested for driving under the influence of alcohol (Miller et al. 1999), and to damage property after drinking alcohol (Miller et al. 1999).

State laws vary with regard to firearm purchase and possession prohibitions for alcohol users or problem drinkers (Carr et al. 2010; Webster and Vernick 2009). Unfortunately, the state laws that do exist may be ineffective because they fail to provide precise definitions of who is disqualified, making them impossible to enforce (Webster and Vernick 2009). Pennsylvania is an exception in that it prohibits firearm purchase by persons who have been convicted of three or more drunk driving offenses within a five-year period. Webster and Vernick (2009) point out that Pennsylvania's law is particularly useful because it provides a definition of alcohol abuser that is sufficiently specific to allow for the identification of prohibited persons. It is also highly justifiable given the abundant evidence that repeat drunk driving offenders are a high-risk group. Not only have they demonstrated reckless behavior, people who drive under the influence are also more likely to abuse illicit drugs or alcohol and to have concurrent psychiatric disorders (Freeman, Maxwell, and Davey 2011; Lapham et al. 2001, 2006; Laplante et al. 2008), have lower self-control (Keane, Maxim, and Teevan 1993), and have higher rates of repeated arrests (Lucker et al. 1991).

Youth under Age 21

Under federal law, a person must be 18 years of age to purchase a long gun and 21 years of age to purchase a handgun from a federally licensed firearms dealer. But persons 18 years of age and older may purchase a handgun from a private seller and may possess a handgun. And there is no minimum age to possess a long gun or to purchase one from a private seller. Yet, research shows that risk for violent perpetration and victimization continues into young adulthood. Young people between the ages of 18 and 20 have some of the highest rates of homicide offending, and age-specific homicide offending rates rise sharply in the late teens and peak at age 20 (*Homicide Trends in the U.S.* 2012).

Laws that set 21 years as the minimum legal age for alcoholic beverage consumption were enacted in all 50 states in response to the recognition that heightened risk-taking behavior by individuals in this age group was a public safety concern. These laws led to significant reductions in deaths from motor vehicle crashes involving drivers between the ages of 18 and 20 (O'Malley and Wagenaar 1991).

The few studies that have evaluated laws banning juvenile gun purchase or possession have found no effect on juvenile homicide *victimization* or suicide (Marvell 2001; Rosengart et al. 2005; Webster et al. 2004). However, there has yet to be a study on the effect of these types of laws on the *commission* of violent crimes or homicide. Violent crime and homicide perpetration may be particularly relevant outcomes. Access to firearms by juveniles increases their risk for violent offending and victimization into early adulthood (Ruback, Shaffer, and Clark 2011). In addition, a recent study of gun-using offenders incarcerated in state correctional facilities in the 13 states with the weakest standards for legal gun possession found that the largest segment of offenders who would have been prohibited in states with stricter standards were those between 18 and 20 years of age (Vittes et al. 2012).

Another type of age-based firearm restriction warrants mention. Recognizing that children and adolescents lack the requisite maturity and self-control to be trusted with firearms (Hardy 2003), child access prevention (CAP) laws hold adult gun owners criminally responsible if a child gains access to and uses a gun that is not securely stored. Eighteen states and the District of Columbia currently have some form of CAP laws (Legal Community Against Violence 2008). Studies have found that CAP laws—particularly those that carry felony rather than misdemeanor penalties—are effective in reducing accidental shootings of children (Cummings et al. 1997; Hepburn et al. 2006). Research also shows that enacting CAP laws is associated with lower rates of adolescent suicides (Webster et al. 2004).

Persons Convicted of Serious Juvenile Offenses

A sizeable body of research suggests that the commission of crimes at a young age is a robust predictor of subsequent criminal activity and violent offending (Berk et al. 2009; Brame, Bushway, and Paternoster 2003; Farrington 1987; Ou and Reynolds 2010). For example, a study analyzing data from a cohort of low-income minority youth in Chicago found that men who were arrested before age 18 had a 38% higher likelihood of a subsequent felony conviction by age 26 compared with those who had not been arrested (Ou and Reynolds 2010). A study of probationers and parolees in Philadelphia found that serious criminal offending at a young age strongly predicted the subsequent commission of homicide or attempted homicide (Berk et al. 2009).

There is also a sizable literature suggesting that criminal recidivism is inversely associated with time since criminal conviction and with age (Blumstein and Nakamura 2009; Kurlychek, Brame, and Bushway 2005, 2007; Kurlychek, Bushway, and Brame 2012; Soothill and Francis 2009). Many of the states that have laws that restrict firearm possession from these offenders take this into account by making the restriction effective for a specified period of time or until the offender reaches a certain age. For example, Massachusetts bans firearm possession for five years after conviction for a serious juvenile offense, and California and Pennsylvania prohibit firearm possession until age 30 for juveniles adjudicated of certain felonies and misdemeanors.

Policy Recommendations

Despite the contentious debate among policymakers and others in the United States about policies governing the ownership and use of firearms, there is wide agreement that access ought to be restricted for individuals deemed to be at high risk for using guns to inflict harm on themselves or others. There also is a growing research literature that supports prohibiting firearm access among such dangerous persons. Nonetheless, some may argue that expanding prohibitory criteria for firearm possession is unfairly discriminatory or too difficult to achieve.

Persons who are barred from firearm possession, however, do have some legal recourse under the relief from federal firearms disabilities program. Under the provisions of the Gun Control Act of 1968, felons and other persons who have been prohibited under federal law from possessing firearms can apply to the attorney general to have this prohibition lifted. The U.S. Bureau of Alcohol, Tobacco, Firearms and Explosives (ATF) is responsible for reviewing and responding to requests for relief from firearms disability submitted by individual applicants. In recent years, however, appropriations have not been provided for this program (ATF 2013). Providing adequate appropriations for the relief from firearms disabilities program could make policies that broaden denial criteria for legal firearm possession more politically palatable.

Although many of the federal prohibitory criteria for firearm possession were established decades ago by the Gun Control Act of 1968, it is not the case that the categories of persons that are prohibited under federal law are unchangeable or even that they have not been changed recently. In fact, persons convicted of a domestic violence misdemeanor and those subject to certain types of domestic violence restraining orders were added to the list of prohibited firearm possessors as recently as 1996 and 1994, respectively (Vernick and Hepburn 2003).

The following recommendations are based on the evidence presented in the previous sections:

1. Prohibit firearm purchase for persons convicted of two or more crimes involving drugs or alcohol within any three-year period for a period of 10 years.
2. Raise the federal minimum age requirement for handgun purchase or possession to 21 years of age.
3. Prohibit firearm purchase for persons who have committed one or more serious juvenile offenses until age 30.

The research presented in this chapter indicates that alcohol abusers, young people, and persons who have been convicted of serious crimes as juveniles are at increased risk for violence. Access to firearms by individuals in these groups increases their own and the public's risk for injury and death. Firearm prohibitions for individuals in other high-risk groups such as domestic violence misdemeanants and respondents to domestic violence restraining orders are effective injury prevention policies. Evaluations of policies that can isolate the effect of firearm restrictions on high-risk groups are needed. Universal background checks, discussed elsewhere in this volume, would aid in the implementation and enforcement of these policies. Meanwhile, broadening these prohibitions has the potential to save additional lives.

NOTES

1. The 13 U.S. states with the least stringent criteria for legal firearm possession are Arkansas, Georgia, Idaho, Louisiana, Maine, Michigan, Mississippi, Montana, New Hampshire, New Mexico, Vermont, Wisconsin, and Wyoming.

REFERENCES

18 U.S.C. §922 (d) (2012).

Afifi, T. O., C. A. Henriksen, G. J. G. Asmundson, and J. Sareen. 2012. "Victimization and perpetration of intimate partner violence and substance use disorders in a nationally representative sample." *Journal of Nervous and Mental Disease* 200(8): 684–691. doi: 10.1097/NMD.0b013e3182613f64.

ATF. 2013. *General Questions.* Bureau of Alcohol, Tobacco, Firearms, and Explosives. Available from http: //www.atf.gov/firearms/faq/general.html.

Berk, R., L. Sherman, G. Barnes, E. Kurtz, and L. Ahlman. 2009. "Forecasting murder within a population of probationers and parolees: A high stakes application of statistical learning." *Journal of the Royal Statistical Society* 172(1): 191–211.

Blumstein, A., and K. Nakamura. 2009. "Redemption in the presence of widespread criminal background checks." *Criminology* 47(2): 327–359.

Borges, G., E. E. Walters, and R. C. Kessler. 2000. "Associations of substance use, abuse, and dependence with subsequent suicidal behavior." *American Journal of Epidemiology* 151(8): 781–789.

Borowsky, I. W., M. Ireland, and M. D. Resnick. 2001. "Adolescent suicide attempts: Risks and protectors." *Pediatrics* 107(3): 485–493.

Brame, R., S. D. Bushway, and R. Paternoster. 2003. "Examining the prevalence of criminal desistance." *Criminology* 41(2): 23–448.

Campbell, J. C., D. W. Webster, J. Koziol-McLain, et al. 2003. "Risk factors for femicide in abusive relationships: Results from a multisite case control study." *American Journal of Public Health* 93(7): 1089–1097.

Carr, B. G., G. Porat, D. J. Wiebe, and C. C. Branas. 2010. "A review of legislation restricting the intersection of firearms and alcohol in the US." *Public Health Reports* 125(5) : 674–679.

Carr, B. G., D. J. Wiebe, T. S. Richmond, R. Cheney, and C. C. Branas. 2009. "A randomised controlled feasibility trial of alcohol consumption and the ability to appropriately use a firearm." *Injury Prevention* 15(6): 409–412.

Cook, P. J., J. Ludwig, and A. A. Braga. 2005. "Criminal records of homicide offenders." *Journal of the American Medical Association* 294(5): 598–601.

Cummings, P., D. C. Grossman, F. P. Rivara, and T. D. Koepsell. 1997. "State gun safe storage laws and child mortality due to firearms." *Journal of the American Medical Association* 278(13) : 1084–1086.

Diener, E., and K. W. Kerber. 1979. "Personality characteristics of American gun-owners." *Journal of Social Psychology* 107(2): 227–238.

Etter, G. W., and M. L. Birzer. 2007. "Domestic violence abusers: A descriptive study of the characteristics of defenders in protection from abuse orders in Sedgwick County, Kansas." *Journal of Family Violence* 22(3): 113–119.

Fabio, A., R. Loeber, G. K. Balasubramani, J. Roth, W. Fu, and D. P. Farrington. 2006. "Why some generations are more violent than others: Assessment of age, period, and cohort effects." *American Journal of Epidemiology* 164(2): 151–160.

Fagan, J. A., D. K. Stewart, and K. V. Hansen. 1983. "Violent men or violent husbands? Background factors and situational correlates." In *The Dark Side of Families: Current Family Violence Research*, edited by D. Finkelhor, R. Gelles, G. Hotaling, and M.A. Straus, 49–68. Beverly Hills, CA: Sage Publications.

Farrington, D. P. 1987. "Predicting individual crime rates." *Crime and Justice: A Review of Research* 9: 53–101. doi: 10.1086/449132.

Fox, J. A. , and M. W. Zawitz. 2010. Homicide trends in the US: Age, gender, and race trends. Washington, DC: Bureau of Justice Statistics, U.S. Department of Justice.

Freeman, J., J. C. Maxwell, and J. Davey. 2011. "Unraveling the complexity of driving while intoxicated: A study into the prevalence of psychiatric and substance abuse comorbidity." *Accident Analysis and Prevention* 43(1): 34–39. doi: 10.1016 /j.aap.2010.06.004.

Friedman, A. S. 1998. "Substance use/abuse as a predictor to illegal and violent behavior: A review of the relevant literature." *Aggression and Violent Behavior* 3(4): 339–355. doi: 10.1016/s1359-1789(97)00012-8.

Gayford, J. J. 1975. "Wife battering: A preliminary study of 100 cases." *British Medical Journal* 1(5951): 194–197.

Hahn, R. A., O. Bilukha, A. Crosby, et al. 2005. "Firearms laws and the reduction of violence: A systematic review." *American Journal of Preventive Medicine* 28(2, Supp 1): 40–71.

Hardy, M. S. 2003. "Effects of gun admonitions on the behaviors and attitudes of school-aged boys." *Journal of Developmental & Behavioral Pediatrics* 24(5): 352–358.

Hepburn, L., D. Azrael, M. Miller, and D. Hemenway. 2006. "The effects of child access prevention laws on unintentional child firearm fatalities, 1979–2000." *Journal of Trauma* 61(2): 423–428.

Homicide Trends in the U.S. Bureau of Justice Statistics, March 20, 2012 2012. Available from http: //bjs.ojp.usdoj.gov/content/homicide/teens.cfm.

Hotaling, G. T., M. A. Straus, and A. J. Lincoln. 1989. "Intrafamily violence, and crime and violence outside the family." In *Family Violence*, edited by L. Ohlin and M. Tonry, 315–375. Chicago: University of Chicago Press.

Johnson, S. B., R. W. Blum, and J. N. Giedd. 2009. "Adolescent maturity and the brain: The promise and pitfalls of neuroscience research in adolescent health policy." *Journal of Adolescent Health* 45(3): 216–221.

Keane, C., P. S. Maxim, and J. J. Teevan. 1993. "Drinking and driving, self-control, and gender: Testing a general-theory of crime." *Journal of Research in Crime and Delinquency* 30(1): 30–46.

Kelleher, K., Chaffin M., J. Hollenberg, and E. Fischer. 1994. "Alcohol and drug disorders among physically abusive and neglectful parents in a community-based sample." *American Journal of Public Health* 84(10): 1586–1590.

Kurlychek, M. C., R. Brame, and S. D. Bushway. 2005. "Scarlet letters and recidivism: Does an old criminal record predict future offending?" *Criminology & Public Policy* 5(3): 483–504.

———. 2007. "Enduring risk? Old criminal records and predictions of future criminal involvement." *Crime & Delinquency* 53(1): 64–83.

Kurlychek, M. C., S. D. Bushway, and R. Brame. 2012. "Long-tern crime desistance and recidivism patterns: Evidence from the Essex County convicted felon study." *Criminology* 50(1): 71–103. doi: 10.1111/j.1745-9125.2011.00259.x.

Lapham, S. C., J. C. Baca, G. P. McMillan, and J. Lapidus. 2006. "Psychiatric disorders in a sample of repeat impaired-driving offenders." *Journal of Studies on Alcohol* 67: 707–713.

Lapham, S. C., E. Smith, J. C. Baca, I. Y. Chang, B. J. Skipper, G. Baum, and W. C. Hunt. 2001. "Prevalence of psychiatric disorders among persons convicted of driving while impaired." *Archives of General Psychiatry* 58: 943–949.

Laplante, D. A., S. E. Nelson, S. S. Odegaard, R. A. Labrie, and H. J. Shaffer. 2008. "Substance and psychiatric disorders among men and women repeat driving under the influence offenders who accept a treatment-sentencing option." *Journal of Studies on Alcohol and Drugs* 69(2): 209–217.

Legal Community Against Violence. 2008. Regulating guns in America: An evaluation and comparative analysis of federal, state, and selected local gun laws. San Francisco, CA.

Lucker, G. W., V. L. Holt, D. J. Kruzich, and J. D. Gold. 1991. "The prevalence of antisocial behavior among U.S. Army DWI offenders." *Journal of Studies on Alcohol* 52(4): 318–320.

Marvell, T. B. 2001. "The impact of banning juvenile gun possession." *Journal of Law & Economics* 44(2): 691–713.

Miller, M., D. Hemenway, and H. Wechsler. 1999. "Guns at College." *Journal of American College Health* 48 (1): 7–12.

———. 2002. "Guns and gun threats at college." *Journal of American College Health* 51(2): 57–65.

Nelson, D. E., J. A. Grant-Worley, K. Powell, J. Mercy, and D. Holtzman. 1996. "Population estimates of household firearm storage practices and firearm carrying in Oregon." *Journal of the American Medical Association* 275(22): 1744–1748. doi: 10.1001/jama.275.22.1744.

O'Malley, P. M., and A. C. Wagenaar. 1991. "Effects of minimum drinking age laws on alcohol use, related behaviors and traffic crash involvement among American youth: 1976–1987." *Journal of Studies on Alcohol* 52(5): 478–491.

Ou, S. R., and A. J. Reynolds. 2010. "Childhood predictors of male adult crime." *Children and Youth Services Review* 32(8): SI 1097–1107.

Parker, R. N., and K. Auerhahn. 1998. "Drugs, alcohol, and homicide: Issues in research and theory." In *Homicide: A Sourcebook of Social Research*, edited by M. D. Smith and M. A. Zahn. Thousand Oaks, CA: Sage.

Rivara, F. P., B. A. Mueller, G. Somes, C. T. Mendoza, N. B. Rushforth, and A. L. Kellermann. 1997. "Alcohol and illicit drug abuse and the risk of violent death in the home." *Journal of the American Medical Association* 278(7): 569–575.

Rosengart, M., P. Cummings, A. Nathens, P. Heagerty, R. Maier, and F. Rivara. 2005. "An evaluation of state firearm regulations and homicide and suicide death rates." *Injury Prevention* 11(2): 77–83.

Ruback, R. B., J. N. Shaffer, and V. A. Clark. 2011. "Easy access to firearms: Juveniles' risks for violent offending and violent victimization." *Journal of Interpersonal Violence* 26(10): 2111–2138. doi: 10.1177/0886260510372948.

Sharps, P.W., J. Campbell, D. Campbell, F. Gary, and D. Webster. 2001. "The role of alcohol in intimate partner femicide." *American Journal of Addictions* 10(2): 122–135.

Soothill, K., and B. Francis. 2009. "When do ex-offenders become like non-offenders?" *The Howard Journal* 48(4): 373–387.

Steinberg, L. 2004. "Risk taking in adolescence: what changes, and why?" *Annals of the New York Academy of Science* 1021: 51–58.

Vernick, J. S, and L. M. Hepburn. 2003. "Examining state and federal gun laws: Trends for 1970–1999." In *Evaluating Gun Policy*, edited by Jens Ludwig and Philip J. Cook, 345–411. Washington, DC: Brookings Institution Press.

Vigdor, E. R., and J. A. Mercy. 2003. "Disarming batterers: The impact of domestic violence firearm laws." In *Evaluating Gun Policy*, edited by Jens Ludwig and Philip J. Cook, 157–201. Washintgon, DC: Brookings Institution Press.

———. 2006. "Do laws restricting access to firearms by domestic violence offenders prevent intimate partner homicide?" *Evaluation Review* 30(3): 313–346.

Vittes, K. A., J. S. Vernick, and D. W. Webster. 2012. "Legal status and source of offenders' firearms in states with the least stringent criteria for gun ownership." *Injury Prevention* epub. doi: 10.1136/injuryprev-2011-040290.

Walton-Moss, B.J., J. Manganello, V. Frye, and J. C. Campbell. 2005. "Risk factors for intimate partner violence and associated injury among urban women." *Journal of Community Health* 30(5): 377–389.

Webster, D. W., and J. S. Vernick. 2009. "Keeping firearms from drug and alcohol abusers." *Injury Prevention* 15(6): 425–427.

Webster, D. W., J. S. Vernick, A. M. Zeoli, and J. A. Manganello. 2004. "Association between youth-focused firearm laws and youth suicides." *Journal of the American Medical Association* 292(5): 594–601.

Welford, C. F., J. V. Pepper, and C. V. Petrie. 2004. *Firearms and Violence: A Critical Review*. Edited by Division of Behavioral and Social Science and Education Committee on Law and Justice, National Research Council of the National Academies. Washington, DC: The National Academies Press.

Wintemute, G. J. 2011. "Association between firearm ownership, firearm-related risk and risk reduction behaviours and alcohol-related risk behaviours." *Injury Prevention* 17(6): 422–427.

Wintemute, G. J., M. A. Wright, C. M. Drake, and J. J. Beaumont. 2001. "Subsequent criminal activity among violent misdemeanants who seek to purchase handguns: Risk factors and effectiveness of denying handgun purchase." *Journal of the American Medical Association* 285(8): 1019–1026.

Zeoli, A. M., and D. W. Webster. 2010. "Effects of domestic violence policies, alcohol taxes and police staffing levels on intimate partner homicide in large US cities." *Injury Prevention* 16(2): 90–95.

6

Broadening Denial Criteria for the Purchase and Possession of Firearms

Need, Feasibility, and Effectiveness

Garen J. Wintemute

This essay presents the findings of research relating to criminal activity among legal purchasers of firearms—those who have passed their background checks—and the evidence that extending the denial criteria to additional high risk populations is feasible and effective. Its primary subject is persons convicted of violent misdemeanor crimes, a group sometimes referred to as not-so-law-abiding gun owners. It will briefly consider persons who abuse alcohol, which is discussed more fully in the essay by Katherine A. Vittes (in this volume).

Background

Federal statute prohibits the purchase and possession of firearms by persons convicted of any felony or a misdemeanor domestic violence offense, anyone

Garen J. Wintemute, MD, MPH, is the Susan P. Baker–Stephen P. Teret Chair in Violence Prevention and a professor of emergency medicine in the University of California, Davis, School of Medicine.

who is "an unlawful user of or addicted to any controlled substance," and others (U.S. Code). From the inception of the Brady Act in 1994 through 2009, the most recent year for which data are available, 107,845,000 background checks were performed; 1,925,000 (1.8%) firearm purchases were denied (Bowling et al. 2010). In 2009 alone, 10,764,000 background checks were performed, and 150,000 (1.4%) denials resulted. Well over 90% of denials result from the would-be purchaser's prior criminal activity.

While recent Supreme Court decisions have affirmed that any individual right to possess firearms is subject to restriction (*District of Columbia v. Heller* 2008, *McDonald v. City of Chicago* 2010), there is no agreement on what those restrictions should be.

The existing federal denial criteria do not extend to all persons who are at increased risk for committing crimes. This problem of incomplete coverage has been noted at least since 1981, when Cook and Blose noted that a "considerable fraction of people who commit violent crimes are legally entitled to own guns" (Cook and Blose 1981). One notable gap concerns prior convictions for violent misdemeanors. While persons convicted of misdemeanor assault on their intimate partners are prohibited persons, those convicted of misdemeanor assault on anyone else, or of misdemeanor violence of other kinds, are not. Another important omission concerns persons who abuse alcohol. Alcohol is specifically excluded from the list of controlled substances referred to in statutes regulating firearm purchase and possession.

Two recent studies highlight the importance of such gaps in coverage. Among individuals arrested for homicide in Illinois in 2001, 42.6% had prior felony convictions. Many of the remaining 57.4% were likely not prohibited from purchasing firearms at the time of their arrests (Cook, Ludwig, and Braga 2005). The second study concerned inmates incarcerated for firearm-related felonies in 13 states where denial criteria reflected those in federal statutes. This study considered all denial criteria related to criminal activity. Of 253 inmates, 102 (40.3%) were prohibited persons at the time of their arrests (Vittes, Vernick, and Webster 2012).

This evidence suggests that most of those who commit firearm-related violent crimes are eligible to purchase firearms, under federal standards at least, at the time the crimes are committed. In fact, the narrow scope of the current federal denial criteria has been proposed as one of the reasons that the Brady Handgun Violence Prevention Act did not measurably reduce homicide rates (Ludwig and Cook 2000, Wintemute 2000).

Given the important gaps in federal regulation, many states have enacted additional prohibitions on firearm purchase and possession. Twenty-six states include at least some misdemeanor crimes, and 20 include persons with a history of alcohol abuse (Bureau of Justice Statistics 2006). The specifics vary from state to state.

Since 1991, California has denied firearm purchases to persons convicted of essentially all violent misdemeanors, including crimes such as assault and battery and brandishing a firearm, since 1991. The prohibition lasts for 10 years. Criminal convictions account for 80% to 90% of denials in California, and convictions for violent crimes account for 40% to 55% (Wintemute et al. 1999, Wright, Wintemute, and Claire 2005). Denials for felony convictions and violent misdemeanor convictions are about equal in number. Approximately 25% of denials for misdemeanor assault are for domestic violence offenses (Wright, Wintemute, and Claire 2005).

Such extensions can substantially expand the size of the population that is denied purchase and possession of firearms. Of the 253 felons in the 13-state study discussed, an additional 28.9% would have been prohibited persons under stricter criteria that are now in effect in other states (Vittes, Vernick, and Webster 2012).

Evidence

Two important empirical questions should be addressed when considering expansions of the denial criteria. First, are there subgroups of persons who purchase firearms legally, at least under federal statute, who are demonstrably at increased risk for committing violent crimes? Second, does denial *work*—does it decrease risk for firearm-related and violent crimes among the individuals who are directly affected? There is good evidence on both questions for persons convicted of violent misdemeanors, and on the first for alcohol abusers.

Misdemeanor Violence

The research on misdemeanor violence comes from California. The first study concerned 5,923 authorized purchasers of handguns ages 21 to 49 in 1977 (Wintemute et al. 1998). Of these handgun purchasers, 3,128 had at least one prior misdemeanor conviction (not necessarily for a violent offense), and 2,795 had no prior criminal history. Over 15 years of follow-up, 50.4% of purchasers with prior convictions, but only 9.8% of those with no prior criminal history, were arrested for a new offense (Table 6.1). Approximately one in six purchasers with a prior misdemeanor conviction (15.4%) was arrested for a violent Crime Index offense: murder, rape, robbery, or aggravated assault.

There was a strong dose-response relationship among men; risk of arrest increased with the number of prior convictions (Table 6.1). There also appeared to be some specificity of association, in that prior convictions for offenses involv-

Table 6.1   Incidence of and relative risk for new criminal activity, by type of offense, among authorized purchasers of handguns in California

Type and number of prior conviction(s)	Nature of new offense			
Study group	Any offense n (%)	Nonviolent firearm offense n (%)	Violent offense n (%)	Violent Crime Index offense n (%)
Prior misdemeanor conviction (*n*=2,735)	1379 (50.4)	361 (13.2)	682 (24.9)	421 (15.4)
No prior criminal history (*n*=2,442)	239 (9.8)	50 (2.0)	108 (4.4)	60 (2.5)
Males[a]	RR (95% CI)	RR (95% CI)	RR (95% CI)	RR (95% CI)
Any conviction(s)				
1	5.9 (5.1–6.9)	5.0 (3.6–7.0)	5.0 (4.0–6.2)	5.1 (3.8–6.9)
≥2	8.4 (7.2–9.8)	7.7 (5.6–10.5)	7.3 (5.9–9.1)	7.6 (5.7–10.2)
Conviction(s), none involving firearms or violence				
1	5.9 (5.0–6.9)	4.8 (3.4–6.7)	4.8 (3.8–6.0)	5.0 (3.7–6.8)
≥2	7.8 (6.7–9.2)	6.5 (4.7–9.1)	6.8 (5.4–8.6)	6.4 (4.7–8.7)
Conviction(s) involving firearms, but none involving violence				
1	6.4 (4.9–8.2)	7.7 (4.8–12.3)	4.4 (3.0–6.6)	5.2 (3.1–8.5)
≥2	10.9 (6.0–20.0)	14.7 (5.8–36.9)	13.0 (6.3–26.7)	12.4 (5.0–31.0)
Conviction(s) involving violence				
1	9.3 (7.7–11.3)	8.7 (6.0–12.6)	8.9 (6.8–11.6)	9.4 (6.6–13.3)
≥2	11.3 (8.3–15.3)	11.7 (6.8–20.0)	10.4 (6.9–15.8)	15.1 (9.4–24.3)

Source: Wintemute GJ, Drake CM, Beaumont JJ, Wright MA, Parham CA. Prior Misdemeanor Convictions as a Risk Factor for Later Violent and Firearm-Related Criminal Activity among Authorized Purchasers of Handguns. *JAMA* 1998;280:2083–2087.

RR=relative risk; CI=confidence interval

[a]Comparison is to subjects with no prior criminal history. Results are adjusted for age and time elapsed since handgun purchase.

ing firearms or violence were associated with the greatest risk of subsequent arrests for violent or firearm-related offenses. Handgun purchasers with two or more prior convictions for violent crimes were at substantially increased risk of arrest for violent crimes generally (relative risk 10.4), and the violent Crime Index offenses (relative risk 15.1). But even purchasers with only a single prior misdemeanor conviction, and that for an offense involving neither firearms nor violence, were still approximately five times as likely as those with no prior criminal history to be arrested subsequently for firearm-related or violent crimes.

At the time these handgun purchases were made, California still relied on the criminal history criteria in federal statute, as many states do today. On that parameter, this study population is generally comparable to persons who purchase handguns now from licensed retailers across the United States.

More recent research measured the incidence of criminal activity serious enough to prohibit firearm ownership among people who had previously, and legally, purchased handguns (Wright and Wintemute 2010). This study was conducted after California began prohibiting violent misdemeanants from purchasing firearms, and such persons are not part of the study population. A cohort of 7,256 handgun purchasers in 1991, 2,761 with a non-prohibiting criminal history and 4,495 with no criminal record at the time of purchase, were followed for up to five years. During that time, 21.0% of purchasers with convictions for non-violent misdemeanors were arrested, and 4.5% were convicted of a crime that prohibited firearm ownership under federal law. The incidence of criminal activity among those with no criminal history was much lower; 3.7% were arrested for any reason, and 0.9% became prohibited persons. Prior conviction for a non-violent misdemeanor was associated with a five-fold increase in risk of conviction for a prohibiting offense (hazard ratio 5.1), as in the prior study.

Risk was related inversely to age and, as before, was related directly to the extent of the prior criminal history (Table 6.2). Compared to handgun purchasers with no criminal history, and after adjustment for age and sex, those with three or more prior convictions for nonviolent misdemeanors had a hazard ratio of 13.6 for conviction for any prohibiting offense and a hazard ratio of 11.0 for a conviction for a violent Crime Index offense (Table 6.2).

Age and prior criminal history acted synergistically as risk factors. As compared to purchasers aged 35 to 49 with no prior criminal history, those aged 21 to 24 with three or more prior misdemeanor convictions had arrest rates for all types of offenses that were increased by a factor of approximately 200.

Table 6.2   Risk of arrest and new prohibition among legal purchasers of handguns in California[a]

Characteristic	Arrest for any crime	Conviction for prohibiting offense	Conviction for violent Crime Index crime[b]
Misdemeanor conviction(s)	HR (95% CI)	HR (95% CI)	HR (95% CI)
No criminal history	Referent	Referent	Referent
1	5.6 (4.5–6.9)	4.2 (2.5–6.8)	4.9 (2.2–11.1)
2	9.0 (6.7–12.2)	10.4 (5.7–18.8)	9.2 (3.1–26.8)
≥3	11.4 (8.3–15.7)	13.6 (7.2–25.6)	11.0 (3.4–35.6)
Sex			
Male	1.0 (0.7–1.3)	0.6 (0.3–1.1)	0.9 (0.3–3.1)
Female	Referent	Referent	Referent
Age, yr			
21–24	4.9 (3.7–6.4)	6.1 (3.5–10.8)	7.7 (2.8–20.9)
25–34	2.4 (1.9–3.1)	2.4 (1.4–4.1)	2.6 (1.0–6.9)
35–49	Referent	Referent	Referent

Adapted from Wright MA, Wintemute GJ. Felonious or Violent Criminal Activity That Prohibits Gun Ownership among Prior Purchasers of Handguns: Incidence and Risk Factors. *J Trauma* 2010;69:948–955.
HR=hazard ratio; CI=confidence interval.
[a]Adjusted for all variables in the table.
[b]Murder, forcible rape, robbery, aggravated assault.

Alcohol Abuse

Alcohol abuse is a major risk factor for firearm-related violence of all types (Kellermann et al. 1992, Kellermann et al. 1993, Rivara et al. 1997, Conner et al. 2001, Karch, Dahlberg, and Patel 2010). Moreover, several studies have identified an association between personal firearm ownership and heavy or abusive alcohol consumption (Diener and Kerber 1979, Schwaner et al. 1999, Miller, Hemenway, and Wechsler 1999, 2002, Nelson et al. 1996, Smith 2001, Casiano et al. 2008).

A recent study of data from the 1996 and 1997 Behavioral Risk Factor Surveillance System surveys examined this association more closely (Wintemute 2011). After adjustment for demographics and state of residence, firearm owners were more likely than persons who had no firearms at home to have five or more drinks on one occasion (odds ratio 1.3), to drink and drive (odds ratio 1.8), and to have 60 or more drinks per month (odds ratio 1.5) (Table 6.3).

Of particular interest—and perhaps not surprisingly—firearm owners who engaged in risk behaviors with firearms were also more likely than other firearm owners to drink excessively. For example, as compared with persons who had no firearms at home, firearm owners who also drove or rode in a vehicle with a loaded firearm were at greatest risk for drinking and driving (odds ratio 4.3). Firearm owners who did not travel in a vehicle with a loaded firearm available, were still at increased risk for drinking and driving (odds ratio 2.1), but less so.

Table 6.3   Alcohol use and alcohol-related risk behaviors among firearm owners by presence or absence of specific firearms-related behavior[a]

Characteristic or behavior	Any alcohol OR (95% CI)	≥5 Drinks/ occasion OR (95% CI)	Drink and drive OR (95% CI)	≥60 Drinks/ month OR (95% CI)
Exposure to firearms				
Firearm owner	1.3 (1.2–1.5)	1.3 (1.2–1.5)	1.8 (1.3–2.4)	1.5 (1.1–1.8)
Household	1.2 (1.1–1.3)	1.0 (0.9–1.3)	1.3 (0.8–1.9)	1.3 (0.8–2.0)
No firearms	Referent	Referent	Referent	Referent
Loaded unlocked firearm at home				
Firearm owner, 'yes'	1.4 (1.2–1.7)	1.8 (1.5–2.3)	3.5 (2.3–5.4)	2.3 (1.6–3.3)
Firearm owner, 'no'	1.3 (1.2–1.4)	1.2 (1.1–1.4)	1.5 (1.9–2.0)	1.3 (1.0–1.7)
No firearms	Referent	Referent	Referent	Referent
Drive/ride in vehicle with loaded firearm				
Firearm owner, 'yes'	1.5 (1.3–1.9)	1.7 (1.4–2.2)	3.0 (1.9–4.7)	2.2 (1.4–3.3)
Firearm owner, 'no'	1.3 (1.2–1.4)	1.2 (1.1–1.4)	1.6 (1.2–2.2)	1.3 (1.0–1.7)
No firearms	Referent	Referent	Referent	Referent
Carry firearm for protection against people				
Firearm owner, 'yes'	1.3 (0.9–1.8)	1.5 (1.0–2.1)	2.1 (1.0–4.6)	1.6 (0.8–3.1)
Firearm owner, 'no'	1.3 (1.2–1.5)	1.3 (1.1–1.5)	1.7 (1.3–2.3)	1.4 (1.1–1.8)
No firearms	Referent	Referent	Referent	Referent

Source: Wintemute GJ. Association between firearm ownership, firearm-related risk and risk reduction behaviors and alcohol-related risk behaviors. *Injury Prevention* 2011;17(6):422–427.

OR=odds ratio; CI=confidence interval

[a]Adjusted for state of residence, age, sex, and race.

The limited data available suggest that firearm ownership itself is associated with an increased risk of arrest (Cook and Ludwig 1996, Diener and Kerber 1979) or, among college students, "trouble with the police" (Miller, Hemenway, and Wechsler 2002). Carrying a firearm in public has also been linked to arrest for a non-traffic offense (Cook and Ludwig 1996, Smith 2001) and aggressive or hostile driving behavior (Miller et al. 2002, Hemenway, Vriniotis, and Miller 2006). Given the findings just presented, it is plausible that alcohol abuse among firearm owners is partly responsible for the association between firearm ownership and involvement with the criminal justice system.

Does Denial Work?

If denying firearm purchases reduces risk for future criminal activity, it most likely does so through incapacitation. To the extent that denial deprives high-risk persons of access to firearms, it reduces their capacity for committing firearm-related and violent crimes.

Some argue that denial simply prevents ineligible persons from acquiring firearms from licensed retailers and note that firearms can easily be obtained from private parties. Jacobs and Potter, partly on this basis, have labeled background checks and denial as nothing more than "a sop to the widespread fear of crime" (Jacobs and Potter 1995). The evidence is, however, that criminal firearm markets do not function smoothly; firearms are not always easily obtained through them (Cook et al. 2005). We have no data on how frequently firearm acquisitions are merely redirected by purchase denials and not prevented.

Background check and recordkeeping requirements do divert prohibited persons away from licensed retailers. Observational research at gun shows, where licensed retailers and private party sellers operate side by side, has documented cases in which individuals who are unable to purchase firearms from licensees do so from private parties instead (Wintemute 2009). In the 1991 Survey of State Prison Inmates, half of those who purchased their most recent firearm from an illegal source said that they had not bought their weapon from a licensee because of concerns about the background check (Bureau of Justice Statistics 1994). Vittes and colleagues reported that just 3.9% of the prohibited persons in their inmate sample had gotten those weapons from a licensed retailer (Vittes, Vernick, and Webster 2012).

Comprehensive background check requirements, which subject private party sales to the same safeguards that are applied to sales by licensed retailers, interfere with the operations of criminal firearms markets (Webster,

Vernick, and Bulzacchelli 2009, Pierce et al. 2012, Mayors Against Illegal Guns 2010). These studies are reviewed in the essay by Webster (in this volume).

Most importantly, denial appears to reduce risk for new criminal activity among those persons who are denied. The strongest evidence for this comes from a quasi-experimental evaluation of California's decision to extend its prohibitions to persons convicted of violent misdemeanors (Wintemute et al. 2001). The prohibition lasts for 10 years following their convictions. Study subjects were aged 21 to 34; all had prior convictions for violent misdemeanors. The intervention group comprised 927 persons who sought to purchase handguns in 1991 and were denied under the terms of the new policy. The control group included 727 persons who sought to purchase handguns in 1989 or 1990, just before the policy changed, and whose purchases were approved. Subjects were followed for up to three years.

Overall, 33.0% of subjects were arrested during follow-up: 21.8% for a firearm-related or violent offense and 22.1% for offenses of other types (Table 6.4). Persons whose purchases were approved were more likely than those who were denied to be arrested for a firearm-related or violent offense (relative hazard 1.2) but not for other offenses (relative hazard 0.9). In both groups, as always, risk of arrest was strongly related to age and the number of prior misdemeanor convictions (Table 6.4).

Denial was associated with a significant decrease in risk of arrest, both overall and for subjects stratified by age or number of prior convictions. These findings persisted in multivariate analysis (Table 6.5). Purchasers were more likely than denied persons to be arrested for new firearm-related or violent crimes (relative hazard 1.3), but not for other crimes (relative hazard 1.0). Similar results were seen in subgroups stratified by age, number of prior convictions for any crime, and number of prior convictions for a firearm-related or violent crime. The only exception was for subjects with three or more prior convictions for firearm-related or violent crimes. In this group with an established pattern of such activity, denial of handgun purchase may have no effect.

The authors called attention to the fact that there was a decrease in arrest rates only for the types of crimes the new policy might be thought to affect. They interpreted this specificity of effect as consistent with the hypothesis that the observed effect was related to the new policy.

A second study with a similar design estimated the effectiveness of denial of purchase based on a prior felony conviction (Wright, Wintemute, and Rivara 1999). As this policy has been enforced for decades in California, no

Table 6.4   Incidence and relative hazard of first arrest for new crimes among violent misdemeanants who applied to purchase handguns

Characteristic	Subjects, n	Firearm-related and/or violent crime		Non-firearm, nonviolent crime	
		Persons arrested n (%)	RH (95% CI)	Persons arrested n (%)	RH (95% CI)
All subjects	1654	360 (21.8)		366 (22.1)	
Purchase status					
Denied	927	186 (20.1)	Referent	211 (22.8)	Referent
Approved	727	174 (23.9)	1.2 (1.0–1.5)	155 (21.3)	0.9 (0.8–1.1)
Sex					
Female	65	11 (16.9)	Referent	15 (23.1)	Referent
Male	1589	349 (22.0)	1.3 (0.7–2.5)	351 (22.1)	0.9 (0.6–1.6)
Age, yr					
21–24	377	108 (28.6)	Referent	117 (31.0)	Referent
25–29	719	152 (21.1)	0.7 (0.6–0.9)	152 (21.1)	0.7 (0.5–0.8)
30–34	558	100 (17.9)	0.6 (0.4–0.8)	97 (17.4)	0.5 (0.4–0.7)
Prior convictions					
Any crime					
1	815	144 (17.7)	Referent	126 (15.5)	Referent
2	429	90 (21.0)	1.2 (0.9–1.6)	104 (24.2)	1.7 (1.3–2.1)
3	200	57 (28.5)	1.7 (1.3–2.3)	58 (29.0)	2.0 (1.5–2.8)
≥4	198	63 (31.8)	2.0 (1.5–2.7)	73 (36.9)	2.8 (2.1–3.7)
Firearm-related and/or violent crime					
1	1217	230 (18.9)	Referent	241 (19.8)	Referent
2	302	86 (28.5)	1.6 (1.3–2.1)	81 (26.8)	1.4 (1.1–1.8)
≥3	115	37 (32.2)	1.8 (1.3–2.6)	36 (31.3)	1.7 (1.2–2.5)

Source: Wintemute GJ, Wright MA, Drake CM, Beaumont JJ. Subsequent Criminal Activity among Violent Misdemeanants Who Seek to Purchase Handguns. *JAMA* 2001;285(8):1019–1026.
    RH = relative hazard; CI = confidence interval

non-intervention group was available. Instead, 177 individuals who sought to purchase handguns in 1977 but were denied as a result of a prior felony conviction were compared to 2,470 persons who purchased handguns in 1977 and at that time had records of felony arrests. (Members of this group might have been convicted of those offenses, but at the misdemeanor level.) Subjects

Table 6.5   Risk of arrest for new crimes for handgun purchasers compared with denied persons among violent misdemeanants who applied to purchase handguns[a]

Characteristic	Firearm-related and/or violent crime RH (95% CI)	Non-firearm, nonviolent crime RH (95% CI)
Age, yr		
21–24	1.4 (0.9–2.0)	1.0 (0.7–1.5)
25–29	1.1 (0.8–1.5)	0.9 (0.7–1.3)
30–34	1.6 (1.1–2.5)	1.0 (0.6–1.5)
Prior convictions		
Any crime		
1	1.3 (0.9–1.8)	1.0 (0.7–1.4)
2	1.2 (0.8–1.8)	0.9 (0.6–1.3)
3	1.1 (0.7–1.9)	1.3 (0.8–2.3)
≥4	1.8 (1.1–3.1)	0.9 (0.6–1.5)
Firearm-related and/or violent crime		
1	1.4 (1.1–1.8)	1.0 (0.7–1.3)
2	1.3 (0.8–2.0)	1.1 (0.7–1.8)
>3	0.9 (0.5–1.8)	0.8 (0.4–1.7)

Source: Wintemute GJ, Wright MA, Drake CM, Beaumont JJ. Subsequent Criminal Activity among Violent Misdemeanants Who Seek to Purchase Handguns, Risk Factors and Effectiveness of Denying Handgun Purchase. *JAMA* 2001;285:1019–1026.
RH = relative hazard; CI = confidence interval
[a]The comparison is to persons whose handgun purchases were denied. Adjusted for sex and all variables in the table.

were followed for up to three years following their attempted or completed purchases. The small size of the study population precluded multivariate adjustment. In separate analyses adjusting for age and for the nature and extent of the prior criminal history, the felony arrestees whose purchases were approved had statistically significant increases in risk of arrest for offenses involving firearms or violence (relative risk of 1.1 to 1.3) as compared to the felons whose purchases were denied.

Studies evaluating prohibitions on firearm ownership at the population level have yielded mixed findings. State-level firearm prohibitions for persons subject to domestic violence restraining orders were associated with 7% to 20% declines in the female intimate partner homicide rate (Vigdor and Mercy 2003, 2006, Zeoli and Webster 2010). The Brady Handgun Violence Prevention Act, however, was found to have no effect on rates of firearm homicide (Ludwig and Cook 2000). Specific reasons for this other than a lack of effect of denial on the persons directly affected have been proposed, including effects on interstate trafficking and the fact that private party transfers are not regulated by the Brady Act. These studies are discussed elsewhere.

Recommendations

Federal and state governments should broaden their criteria for denial of firearm purchase and possession to include persons convicted of violent misdemeanors. An unknown, but possibly substantial, proportion of such persons were arrested on felony charges but convicted at the misdemeanor level in plea bargain arrangements. Among those who purchase firearms, persons convicted of violent misdemeanors are at substantially increased risk for violent crime in the future. Denial of firearm purchase can reduce that risk by an amount that is of real-world importance. The list of offenses now in use in California provides a reasonable model. At the federal level, this could perhaps be accomplished by deleting the word "domestic" from the phrase "misdemeanor crime of domestic violence" in 18 USC §922(d) and reworking the definition of the phrase as appropriate.

Federal and state governments should also deny the purchase and possession of firearms to persons who abuse alcohol. Multiple definitions of alcohol abuse are in use, and it might be reasonable to consider the second instance of any alcohol-related offense (DUI, drunk and disorderly, etc.) as the criterion for denial. This can be explored further and refined as needed. We do not have specific evidence that denial is effective in such cases, but there is good evidence that alcohol abuse is a risk factor for crime, that its prevalence is increased among firearm owners, and that it and other behaviors that increase risk for violence co-occur among firearm owners.

The question of how long these prohibitions should last has not been definitively answered. Risk of recidivism following an index arrest declines over time. Among 18-year-olds arrested for violent or property crimes, risk of arrest returned to the level seen for the never-arrested after approximately 20 years (Blumstein and Nakamura 2009). Other studies, again of juveniles and young adults, have seen risk return to baseline after less than 10 years (Kurlychek,

Brame, and Bushway 2007, 2006). In the United Kingdom, the time required is between 10 and 15 years (Soothill and Francis 2009). There appears to be no parallel research on older offenders or firearm owners. California's 10-year policy is consistent with the available evidence.

Background checks that extend to misdemeanor convictions and alcohol-related offenses will be more complex and take longer to complete. ATF encountered 3,166 cases in 2011 in which a firearm was acquired by a prohibited person because the three-day waiting period ended before the background check could be completed (Federal Bureau of Investigation 2012). In such cases, ATF agents must contact the purchasers and recover or arrange other dispositions for the firearms (Frandsen 2010). To avoid a massive increase in delayed denials, as such cases are known, the waiting period should be extended in individual cases until the background check is completed.

Support for Broadened Denial Criteria

Survey research in the late 1990s found high levels of support among the general population and firearm owners for denial criteria that included violent and firearm-related misdemeanors and alcohol abuse (Table 6.6) (Teret et al. 1998). Results for the general population were confirmed in the 2001 General Social Survey (Smith 2007).

In a 2012 survey of firearm owners, 75% of members of the National Rifle Association (NRA) felt that persons with a history of misdemeanor violence

Table 6.6   Support overall and among firearm owners for denial of firearm purchases by persons convicted of specific misdemeanor offenses

Offense	Overall %	Firearm owners %
Public display of a firearm in a threatening manner	95	91
Possession of equipment for illegal drug use	92	89
Domestic violence	89	80
Assault and battery without a lethal weapon or serious injury	85	75
Drunk and disorderly conduct	74	73
Carrying a concealed weapon without a permit	83	70
Driving under the influence of alcohol	71	59

Source: Teret SP, Webster DW, Vernick JS, et al. Support for new policies to regulate firearms. *N Engl J Med.* 1998;339:813–818.

should not receive concealed weapon permits. Many states provide such permits to anyone who is legally eligible to possess firearms. Therefore, a judgment that a class of persons should not receive concealed weapon permits suggests a judgment that they should not possess firearms (Luntz Global 2012).

Drawbacks and Costs

Background checks are useful only to the extent that the databases on which they are performed are accurate and complete. There will be costs, which may be substantial, to compile the data for background checks that include these offenses. There will also be costs associated with the increasing number of denials and, presumably, appeals of those denials. Personnel, facility, and other resource requirements will all increase. No estimates of cost, or of offsetting financial benefit in crimes and injuries prevented, have been developed.

Compiling additional data on violent misdemeanors and alcohol-related offenses will take some time. Estimates of how long, and exploration of ways to shorten the time to implementation, will be needed.

These hurdles notwithstanding, California's experience with misdemeanor denials shows that such policies can be implemented and sustained over time and that a robust firearms market can operate with such regulation in place. More than 601,000 firearms were sold in California in 2011 (California Department of Justice), and the industry describes the state's market as "lucrative" (Anonymous 2007).

REFERENCES

Anonymous. "California Market Still Lucrative." 2007. *The New Firearms Business*, 15 March, 5.
Blumstein, Alfred, and Kiminori Nakamura. 2009. "Redemption in the Presence of Widespread Criminal Background Checks." *Criminology*, no. 47: 327–359.
Bowling, Michael, et al. 2010. Background Checks for Firearms Transfers, 2009— Statistical Tables. Washington, DC: Bureau of Justice Statistics.
Bureau of Justice Statistics. 1994. Firearms and Crimes of Violence. Washington, DC: Department of Justice.
Bureau of Justice Statistics. 2006. Survey of State Procedures Related to Firearm Sales, 2005. Washington, DC: Bureau of Justice Statistics.
California Department of Justice. 2012. Dealers Record of Sale Transactions.
Casiano, Hygiea, et al. 2008. "Mental Disorder and Threats Made by Noninstitutionalized People with Weapons in the National Comorbidity Survey Replication." *Journal of Nervous and Mental Disease*, no. 196: 437–445.

Conner, Kenneth R, et al. 2001. "Violence, Alcohol, and Completed Suicide: A Case-Control Study." *American Journal of Psychiatry*, no. 158: 1701–1705.

Cook, Philip J, et al. 2005. Underground Gun Markets. Cambridge, MA: National Bureau of Economic Research.

Cook, Philip J, and J Blose. 1981. "State Programs for Screening Handgun Buyers." *The Annals of the American Academy of Political and Social Science*, no. 445: 80–91.

Cook, Philip J, and Jens Ludwig. 1996. *Guns in America: Results of a Comprehensive National Survey on Firearms Ownership and Use*. Washington, DC: The Police Foundation.

Cook, Philip J, Jens Ludwig, and Anthony A Braga. 2005. "Criminal Records of Homicide Offenders." *Journal of the American Medical Association*, no. 294: 598–601.

Diener, Edward, and Kenneth W Kerber. 1979. "Personality Characteristics of American Gun-Owners." *Journal of Social Psychology*, no. 107: 227–238.

District of Columbia v. Heller, 128 S.Ct. 2783 (2008).

Federal Bureau of Investigation. 2012. National Instant Criminal Background Check System (NICS) Operation 2011. Washington, DC: Federal Bureau of Investigation.

Frandsen, Ronald J. 2010. Enforcement of the Brady Act, 2008: Federal and State Investigations and Prosecutions of Firearm Applicants Denied by a NICS Check in 2008. Final Report to the U.S. Department of Justice. Document Number: 231052.

Hemenway, David, M Vriniotis, and Matthew Miller. 2006. "Is an Armed Society a Polite Society?" *Accident Analysis and Prevention*, no. 38: 687–695.

Jacobs, James B, and Kimberly A Potter. 1995. "Keeping Guns out of the 'Wrong' Hands: The Brady Law and the Limits of Regulation." *Journal of Criminal Law and Criminology*, no. 86: 93–120.

Karch, Debra L, Linda L Dahlberg, and Nimesh Patel. 2010. "Surveillance for Violent Deaths - National Violent Death Reporting System, 16 States, 2007." *Morbidity and Mortality Weekly Report (MMWR)*, no. 59: 1–50.

Kellermann, Arthur L, et al. 1992. "Suicide in the Home in Relation to Gun Ownership." *New England Journal of Medicine*, no. 327: 467–472.

Kellermann, Arthur L, et al. 1993. "Gun Ownership as a Risk Factor for Homicide in the Home." *New England Journal of Medicine*, no. 329: 1084–1091.

Kurlychek, Megan C, Robert Brame, and Shawn D Bushway. 2006. "Scarlet Letters and Recidivism: Does an Old Criminal Record Predict Future Offending?" *Criminology & Public Policy*, no. 5: 483–504.

Kurlychek, Megan C, Robert Brame, and Shawn D Bushway. 2007. "Enduring Risk? Old Criminal Records and Predictions of Future Criminal Involvement." *Crime & Delinquency*, no. 53: 64–83.

Ludwig, Jens A, and Philip J Cook. 2000. "Homicide and Suicide Rates Associated with Implementation of the Brady Handgun Violence Prevention Act." *Journal of the American Medical Association*, no. 284: 585–591.

Luntz Global. 2012. Gun Owners Poll. New York, NY: Mayors Against Illegal Guns.

Mayors Against Illegal Guns. 2010. "Trace the Guns: The Link between Gun Laws and Interstate Gun Trafficking," www.MayorsAgainstIllegalGuns.org, www.TraceTheGuns.org.

Mcdonald v. City of Chicago, 130 S.Ct. 3020 (2010).

Miller, Matthew, et al. 2002. "'Road Rage' in Arizona: Armed and Dangerous." *Accident Analysis and Prevention*, no. 34: 807–814.

Miller, Matthew, David Hemenway, and Henry Wechsler. 1999. "Guns at College." *Journal of American College Health,* no. 48: 7–12.

Miller, Matthew, David Hemenway, and Henry Wechsler. 2002. "Guns and Gun Threats at College." *Journal of American College Health,* no. 51: 57–65.

Nelson, David E, et al. 1996. "Population Estimates of Household Firearm Storage Practices and Firearm Carrying in Oregon." *Journal of the American Medical Association,* no. 275: 1744–1748.

Pierce, Glenn L, et al. 2012. New Approaches to Understanding and Regulating Primary and Secondary Illegal Firearms. Washington, DC: National Institute of Justice.

Rivara, Frederick P, et al. 1997. "Alcohol and Illicit Drug Abuse and the Risk of Violent Death in the Home." *Journal of the American Medical Association,* no. 278: 569–575.

Schwaner, Shawn L, et al. 1999. "Who Wants a Gun License?" *Journal of Criminal Justice,* no. 27: 1–10.

Smith, Tom W. 2001. National Gun Policy Survey of the National Opinion Research Center: Research Findings. Chicago, IL: National Opinion Research Center, University of Chicago.

Smith, Tom W. 2007. Public Attitudes Towards the Regulation of Firearms. Chicago, IL: National Opinion Research Center, University of Chicago.

Soothill, Keith, and Brian Francis. 2009. "When Do Ex-Offenders Become Like Non-Offenders?" *The Howard Journal,* no. 48: 373–387.

Teret, Stephen P, et al. 1998. "Support for New Policies to Regulate Firearms: Results of Two National Surveys." *New England Journal of Medicine,* no. 339: 813–818.

Title 18, *U.S. Code,* Part 1, Chapter 44, Section 922(d).

Vigdor, Elizabeth Richardson, and James A Mercy. 2003. "Disarming Batterers: The Impact of Domestic Violence Firearm Laws" In *Evaluating Gun Policy: Effects on Crime and Violence,* ed. Jens A Ludwig and Philip J Cook. Washington, DC: Brookings Institution Press, 157–213.

Vigdor, Elizabeth Richardson, and James A Mercy. 2006. "Do Laws Restricting Access to Firearms by Domestic Violence Offenders Prevent Intimate Partner Homicide?" *Evaluation Review,* no. 30: 313–346.

Vittes, Katherine A, Jon S Vernick, and Daniel W Webster. 2012. "Legal Status and Source of Offenders' Firearms in States with the Least Stringent Criteria for Gun Ownership." [Published Online Ahead of Print June 23, 2012] *Injury Prevention,* DOI: 10.1136/injuryprev-2011-040290.

Webster, Daniel W, Jon S Vernick, and Maria T Bulzacchelli. 2009. "Effects of State-Level Firearm Seller Accountability Policies on Firearm Trafficking." *Journal of Urban Health,* no. 86: 525–537.

Wintemute, Garen J. 2000. "Impact of the Brady Act on Homicide and Suicide Rates." (Letter) *Journal of the American Medical Association,* no. 284: 2719–2720.

Wintemute, Garen J. 2009. *Inside Gun Shows: What Goes on When Everybody Thinks Nobody's Watching.* Sacramento, CA: Violence Prevention Research Program.

Wintemute, Garen J. 2011. "Association between Firearm Ownership, Firearm-Related Risk and Risk Reduction Behaviours and Alcohol-Related Risk Behaviours." *Injury Prevention,* no. 17: 422–427.

Wintemute, Garen J, et al. 1998. "Prior Misdemeanor Convictions as a Risk Factor for Later Violent and Firearm-Related Criminal Activity among Authorized

Purchasers of Handguns." *Journal of the American Medical Association,* no. 280: 2083–2087.

Wintemute, Garen J, et al. 1999. "Denial of Handgun Purchase: A Description of the Affected Population and a Controlled Study of Their Handgun Preferences." *Journal of Criminal Justice,* no. 27: 21–31.

Wintemute, Garen J, et al. 2001. "Subsequent Criminal Activity among Violent Misdemeanants Who Seek to Purchase Handguns: Risk Factors and Effectiveness of Denying Handgun Purchase." *Journal of the American Medical Association,* no. 285: 1019–1026.

Wright, Mona A, and Garen J Wintemute. 2010. "Felonious or Violent Criminal Activity That Prohibits Gun Ownership among Prior Purchasers of Handguns: Incidence and Risk Factors." *Journal of Trauma,* no. 69: 948–955.

Wright, Mona A, Garen J Wintemute, and Barbara E Claire. 2005. "People and Guns Involved in Denied and Completed Handgun Sales." *Injury Prevention,* no. 11: 247–250.

Wright, Mona A, Garen J Wintemute, and Frederick A Rivara. 1999. "Effectiveness of Denial of Handgun Purchase to Persons Believed to Be at High Risk for Firearm Violence." *American Journal of Public Health,* no. 89: 88–90.

Zeoli, April M, and Daniel W Webster. 2010. "Effects of Domestic Violence Policies, Alcohol Taxes and Police Staffing Levels on Intimate Partner Homicide in Large Us Cities." *Injury Prevention,* no. 16: 90–95.

7

Comprehensive Background Checks for Firearm Sales

Evidence from Gun Shows

Garen J. Wintemute

Many lines of evidence bear on whether to institute a comprehensive background check policy that would extend the current background check and recordkeeping requirements for sales by licensed retailers to sales by private parties. This essay presents evidence from observational and other research related to gun shows and makes recommendations based on that evidence. For simplicity's sake, "sales" will be used to refer to transfers of all types.

Background

In 1995, Philip Cook and colleagues defined buying and selling by licensed retailers as the primary market for firearms; both new and used firearms are involved (Cook, Molliconi, and Cole 1995). The secondary market consists of

Garen J. Wintemute, MD, MPH, is the Susan P. Baker–Stephen P. Teret Chair in Violence Prevention and a professor of emergency medicine in the University of California, Davis, School of Medicine.
Portions of this chapter are based on prior work by the author.

transfers by unlicensed private parties such as the individual attendees at gun shows (Cook, Molliconi, and Cole 1995, Braga et al. 2002).

The secondary market is quite large. According to the National Survey of Private Ownership of Firearms, approximately 40% of all firearms transactions occur directly between private parties (Cook and Ludwig 1996). Other estimates concur. In the 2004 National Firearms Survey, for example, 55% of 566 firearm owners reported that their most recent acquisition had been from a store (Hepburn et al. 2007). Another 8% reported purchasing their firearm from a licensed retailer at a gun show (unpublished data, National Firearms Survey).

The Federal Double Standard

In order to sell a firearm, a federally licensed retailer must see the buyer's identification. The buyer must complete a lengthy Firearms Transaction Record and certify, under penalty of perjury, that he is buying the firearm for himself and is not a member of any prohibited class. The National Instant Criminal Background Check System (NICS), administered by the Federal Bureau of Investigation (FBI), must perform a background check. In over 90% of cases this background check is completed within minutes, but if important information is missing the buyer may have to wait up to three business days to acquire the firearm (Federal Bureau of Investigation 2012b).

The retailer must keep a permanent record of each purchase that includes specific identifying information for both the buyer and the firearm. If the same person buys more than one handgun from him within five business days, the retailer must file a special report with the U.S. Bureau of Alcohol, Tobacco, Firearms and Explosives (ATF).

These procedural safeguards are intended to ensure that the buyer is who he says he is, that he and not someone else will be the actual owner of the firearm, and that he is not prohibited from owning it. They help prevent the large-volume purchasing that otherwise might fuel trafficking operations. They establish a chain of ownership that will help law enforcement authorities link the firearm to its buyer if it is used in a future crime.

But a private party can sell that same firearm—or many firearms—and none of these federal safeguards will be in place. Private-party sellers are not required to ask for identification. They *cannot* initiate a background check, except in Delaware, Nevada, and Oregon, where they may do so voluntarily. There are no forms to fill out, and no records need be kept.

Even if the purchaser is a prohibited person, let alone a non-prohibited person with criminal intent, a private party may sell him a firearm without committing a crime. The key is that while it is always illegal for a prohibited person to buy a firearm, it is only illegal to sell a firearm to a prohibited person if the seller knows or has "reasonable cause to believe" that he is doing so (U.S. Code).

How did this come to pass? The provisions of the federal Gun Control Act apply only to those who are "engaged in the business" of selling firearms. Any clear understanding of what "engaged in the business" might mean was abolished by the 1986 Firearm Owners' per style sheet Protection Act (U.S. Code). FOPA specifically excluded from the scope of engagement in the business a person who makes "occasional sales, exchanges, or purchases of firearms for the enhancement of a personal collection or for a hobby, or who sells all or part of his personal collection of firearms" (U.S. Code).

The practical result was to make it much more difficult to set an upper limit to the number of firearm sales that an individual could make without being required to have a license and comply with the safeguards described above (Braga and Kennedy 2000, Wintemute 2007, 2009b). ATF summarized the situation this way in a 1999 study of gun shows: "Unfortunately, the effect of the 1986 amendments has often been to frustrate the prosecution of unlicensed dealers masquerading as collectors or hobbyists but who are really trafficking firearms to felons or other prohibited persons" (Bureau of Alcohol, Tobacco and Firearms 1999b).

State Regulation of Firearm Sales

In 33 states, statutes regulating firearm sales do not go beyond those enacted by Congress. But 17 states regulate at least some private-party sales, usually by requiring that the seller have the transaction processed by a licensed retailer (Table 7.1) (Bureau of Justice Statistics 2006). Such transactions are then subject to the same procedural safeguards that apply to the retailer's own sales that identity is confirmed, a background check is performed, and a record is kept. Six states require background checks for all firearm sales, regardless of firearm type or place of sale, and another nine do so for all handgun sales.

In at least 17 states, the background check can be waived for holders of permits to carry concealed weapons and similar permits, whether at gun shows or elsewhere (Bowling et al. 2010). This has adverse consequences that will be discussed later in this essay.

Table 7.1   State regulation of private-party firearm sales

State	Handgun sales		Long gun sales	
	All sales	Gun shows only	All sales	Gun shows only
California	•		•	
Colorado		•		•
Connecticut	•			•
Hawaii	•		•	
Illinois	•		•	
Iowa	•			
Maryland	•			
Massachusetts	•		•	
Michigan	•			
Missouri	•			
Nebraska	•			
New Jersey	•		•	
New York	•			•
North Carolina	•			
Oregon		•		•
Pennsylvania	•			
Rhode Island	•		•	

Source: From *Survey of state procedures related to firearm sales, 2005.*
Washington, DC: Bureau of Justice Statistics, 2006. NCJ 214645.
  Note: In the remaining 33 states, private-party firearm sales are not
regulated.

In California, a comprehensive background check and recordkeeping policy has been in place since 1991. In essence, private-party sales must be routed
through a licensed retailer. At gun shows, designated retailers serve as transfer agents to facilitate sales between individual attendees.

All firearm types are covered, but there are exceptions for certain transactions. These include a transfer between spouses or vertically between other
immediate family members, such as from a parent to a child or a grandparent
to a grandchild. Temporary transfers, such as infrequent and short-term loans
between persons who are personally known to each other, are also exempted.

There are no exemptions for holders of concealed weapon or other permits. Private parties are still allowed to sell firearms in small numbers, involving a licensed retailer to satisfy the background check and recordkeeping requirements.

There is no requirement that the seller and buyer be present at the licensed retailer simultaneously. Many sales are done on consignment; the seller deposits firearms with the retailer for sale, and the seller and buyer never meet. Some retailers maintain separate a display space for consignment firearms.

The retailer is allowed to charge a fee of up to $10 per firearm for serving as a transfer agent (the fee is less per firearm for transfers involving multiple firearms). Whether the sale occurs at a gun show or elsewhere, the purchaser may take delivery of his firearm from the retailer only after the state's 10-day waiting period has expired. The increased foot traffic at participating retailers provides opportunities to develop new customers. As one retailer explained, "when they come in to do the paper, everybody needs bullets and cleaning supplies" (Matthews 2009).

The system does not appear to impair the operations of California's legal firearms market. More than 601,000 firearms were sold in the state in 2011 (California Department of Justice). Trends in the California market reflect those occurring nationwide. Firearm sales increased 15.6% per year, on average, over the last five years for which we have data (California Department of Justice 2012). A leading industry newsletter has described California's market as "lucrative" (Anonymous 2007).

Criminal Acquisition of Firearms from Private Parties

Private-party firearm sales are quick—they can be completed in less than a minute—and convenient. Even a law-abiding purchaser might appreciate the absence of paperwork that characterizes private-party sales. Their anonymity attracts those who put privacy at a premium.

But these same attributes make private-party sales the only viable option for prohibited persons and the principal option for purchasers with criminal intent, for whom a record of the sale would be hazardous. Again, it is only illegal to sell a firearm to a prohibited person if the seller knows or has "reasonable cause to believe" that he is doing so (U.S. Code). The matter is easily finessed. As one private-party seller said while contemplating a possibly illegal handgun sale at a gun show, "Of course, if I don't ask, nobody knows" (Wintemute 2009b).

Private-party sales are critical to illegal commerce in firearms. As discussed earlier, perhaps 40% of all firearm sales nationwide are private-party transactions. For those who commit crimes with firearms, that percentage at least doubles. Four large-scale surveys of persons incarcerated for firearm-related felonies in the 1990s asked inmates where they acquired the firearm they used in the crime for which they were incarcerated. Between 12% and 21% of these inmates acquired their weapons from licensed retailers (Harlow 2001, Scalia 2000, Wright and Rossi 1986). An analysis of more recent data also considered whether the inmates were prohibited from possessing firearms at the time of acquisition (Vittes, Vernick, and Webster). Overall, 13.4% of respondents obtained their firearms from licensed retailers. For prohibited persons, purchases from licensed retailers fell to just 3.9%.

For juveniles, direct purchase of any type of firearm from a licensed retailer is illegal, as are handgun purchases for people aged 18 to 20. Private-party sales are essentially their only source of firearms (Ash et al. 1996, Webster et al. 2002).

Private-party sales are also an important component of firearm trafficking operations. Of 1,530 trafficking investigations conducted by ATF during 1996 to 1998, 314 (20.5%) involved unlicensed sellers (Bureau of Alcohol, Tobacco and Firearms 2000b). A related study evaluated data for trafficking operations involving juveniles and youth (Braga and Kennedy 2001). Of 648 such operations, 92 (14.2%) involved private-party sellers.

There is no current estimate of the proportion of private-party sales that involve prohibited persons. But when background checks for licensed retailer sales were first required in some states by the Brady Act, as many as 9.4% of prospective purchasers were prohibited persons (Manson and Gilliard 1997). It is reasonable to estimate that the proportion is similar or higher for private-party sales that do not involve background checks.

At gun shows, some private-party handgun sellers make a point of checking the buyer's driver's license to be sure that they are not making an illegal sale to an out-of-state resident (Wintemute 2009b). But asking questions about the buyer's eligibility to purchase firearms, theoretically something that private-party sellers could do, guarantees unpleasantness (or worse) and risks the loss of the sale. In observational research at nearly 80 gun shows, such questioning was never observed (Wintemute 2009b). Other private party vendors serve as "hotspots," making repeated sales that serve criminal purposes

(Bureau of Alcohol, Tobacco and Firearms 2000b, Braga and Kennedy 2000, Wintemute 2009b).

Criminal Acquisition of Firearms at Gun Shows

Gun shows present a special case, in that large numbers of licensed retailers and private-party sellers are active in the same setting and competing for customers (Bureau of Alcohol, Tobacco and Firearms 1999b, Wintemute 2007, 2009b). Between 25% and 50% of firearm sellers who rent table space at gun shows are private parties (Bureau of Alcohol, Tobacco and Firearms 1999b, Wintemute 2007). Such tables frequently carry "Private Sale" signs implying that purchases require no paperwork, no background check, no waiting period, and no recordkeeping. Individual attendees who do not rent table space but bring firearms to sell are common. In a study by the author, as many as 31.6% of gun show attendees were armed, and many of these attendees were unambiguously offering their firearms for sale (Wintemute 2007).

While there are no data on the frequency of illegal private-party sales at gun shows, it is clear that some sellers are willing to make them. Private investigators recently conducted "integrity tests" of 30 private-party sellers at seven gun shows in Nevada, Ohio, and Tennessee (City of New York 2009). The subjects were selected after observation suggested they were effectively in the business of selling firearms. An investigator then negotiated the purchase of a firearm with each seller, but during the negotiation said that he "probably could not pass a background check." Of the 30 sellers, 19 completed the sales despite the clear indication that the buyer was a prohibited person.

As a highly visible marketplace for private-party sales, gun shows have received a great deal of attention. As detailed elsewhere, however, three points suggest a more nuanced understanding of the role gun shows play in legal and illegal commerce in firearms (Wintemute 2009b).

Gun shows account for a small proportion of firearm sales. According to the National Survey of Private Ownership of Firearms, discussed earlier, 3.9% of firearms are acquired at gun shows (Cook and Ludwig 1996). Unpublished data from the National Firearms Survey (Hepburn et al. 2007) yield a similar result; 9% of firearm owners acquired their most recent firearms at a gun show.

Most sales at gun shows probably involve licensed retailers. Most vendors at gun shows are licensed retailers, as are nearly all of the largest and most active vendors (Wintemute 2009b). Again, unpublished data from the National

Firearms Survey agree (Hepburn et al. 2007). Of respondents who purchased firearms at gun shows, more than 75% bought them from licensed retailers.

Licensed retailers are the primary source of firearms acquired at gun shows that are later used in crime. A study of 314 ATF trafficking investigations involving gun shows reported that while an unlicensed seller was the main subject in most of the investigations (54.1%), two thirds of the trafficked firearms were linked to investigations involving a licensed retailer (Braga and Kennedy 2000).

Effectiveness of Background Checks

The evidence suggests that background checks and denials of purchases by prohibited persons reduce risk of arrest among the individuals who are directly affected and interfere with the operations of criminal firearm markets, particularly with firearm trafficking. This essay considers observational evidence on the latter point from gun shows, where large numbers of firearm sales can be observed directly in a short period of time (Wintemute 2009b, 2007).

The best such evidence comes from a study comparing gun shows in California, with its comprehensive background check policy and separate regulations for gun shows, to shows in four states without such policies (Arizona, Nevada, Texas, and Florida) that are leading sources of firearms used in crime in California (Wintemute 2007). Altogether, 28 shows were included. Events in all states were well attended, and commerce was brisk. Shows in California were smaller than those in the comparison states, whether measured by number of firearm vendors or number of attendees, but the number of attendees per vendor was larger.

No direct private-party sales between attendees were observed in California. Instead, private-party sales were completed with the assistance of a licensed retailer serving as transfer agent (Wintemute 2007). In the comparison states, such transactions occurred frequently; an appropriately-stationed observer could see several occurring at any one time.

One unintended effect of California's policies may have been to displace illegal sales to nearby and more permissive states. At some shows in Reno, Nevada, which is a short distance across the border, more than 30% of the vehicles in the parking lot were from California (Wintemute 2007). Such undermining of more rigorous regulation in some states by lack of regulation in others has long been an argument for more rigorous regulation at the federal level. However, an unexpected finding suggests diffusion of benefit. Though surrogate, or "straw man," purchases are illegal nationwide under federal law, they were more than six times as common in the comparison states as in California (Wintemute 2007).

Commenting on this study, *Shooting Sports Retailer*, a firearm industry trade magazine, agreed that "there is some evidence that gun shows with restrictive regulations mandating background checks have less illegal activity than shows in states or jurisdictions without this requirement" (Matthews 2009).

Recommendations

Anonymous, undocumented private-party sales are an important contributor to firearm violence in the United States. Comprehensive background check requirements restore a simple, single, equitable structure to retail commerce in firearms. They have been shown to be feasible, and the evidence is that they provide concrete benefits. The United States should adopt a comprehensive background check requirement for firearm sales.

The primary direct effect of such a requirement will be to prevent, or make substantially more difficult, the criminal acquisition of firearms. Many prohibited persons attempting to purchase firearms from private parties will be detected by the background checks, and their purchases will be denied. Background checks and denials reduce risk of violent and firearm-related crime among prohibited persons (Wintemute et al. 2001, Wright, Wintemute, and Rivara 1999). Non-prohibited buyers with criminal intent will be deterred by the new requirements for purchaser identification and record keeping. Recall that 80% of felons incarcerated for firearm-related crimes who were *not* prohibited persons nonetheless acquired their firearms from private parties (Vittes, Vernick, and Webster 2012).

Some prohibited persons and others with criminal intent will continue to seek firearms from private-party sellers. There will still be individuals willing to sell firearms to prohibited persons. There are likely to be fewer, however, because a comprehensive background check policy changes the rules for sellers as well. Private parties will no longer be able to sell firearms legally, at least, without determining whether buyers can legally purchase them. Direct sales will now be crimes and could be made prohibiting offenses.

These effects at the individual level, taken together, will interfere with the operation of criminal firearm markets and disrupt firearm trafficking operations (Webster, Vernick, and Bulzacchelli 2009, Pierce et al. 2012). Mapping trafficking networks and investigating individual crimes will be aided by more complete records of firearm transfers. Increasingly, it will be possible for law enforcement agencies to identify the most recent purchaser of a crime-involved firearm, not the first (Wintemute et al. 2004, Pierce et al. 2012).

California's policies provide a suitable model. Reasonable exemptions from the background check are allowed, and private-party sales may be made in small numbers if a licensed retailer is involved.

In order to avoid a massive increase in delayed denials, the current three-day limit to the waiting period for firearm purchases should be lifted. Firearm acquisition should be allowed once the buyer has passed the background check.

Pitfalls to Avoid
Closing the "Gun Show Loophole"

Requiring background checks for private-party sales only at gun shows is known as closing the "gun show loophole." There is no such loophole in federal law, in the limited sense that the law does not exempt private-party sales at gun shows from regulation that is required elsewhere. The fundamental flaw in the gun show loophole proposal is its failure to address the great majority of private-party sales, which occur at other locations and increasingly over the Internet at sites where any non-prohibited person can list firearms for sale and buyers can search for private-party sellers.

Creating an Exemption for Permit Holders

The Fix Gun Checks Act, introduced in the 112th Congress and expected to be reintroduced in 2013, is described as requiring a background check for all firearm purchases. It does not. A prospective purchaser in at least 17 states may avoid a background check by presenting an unexpired permit to carry a concealed weapon, or similar permit, for which a background check was required at the time of issuance. Such permits remain valid for as long as five years. An important fraction of permit holders become prohibited persons during that time (Wright and Wintemute 2010). Nationwide, there would be many thousands each year. Their new prohibitions will most often result from new convictions for serious crimes.

No state routinely recovers permits that have not reached their nominal expiration dates from people who are no longer eligible to have them. Thus, under the Fix Gun Checks Act, those permits will allow newly prohibited individuals who are at high risk for committing further crimes to avoid background checks and acquire firearms. Moreover, a permit exemption is unnecessary; several states operate comprehensive background check systems without it.

Drawbacks, Costs, and Uncertainties

A comprehensive background check policy would make private-party sales less convenient. Airport security screening provides a useful analogy. All of us, regardless of our individual risk of committing violence in the air, are subjected to this inconvenience in one form or another. We tolerate it because it is one of the ways terrorists do get caught.

There would be a financial cost to firearm purchasers. In California, retailers may charge $10 per firearm, in addition to other fees required by the state. This is a small fraction of the purchase price of all but the least expensive firearms, however.

Some private-party sellers will object, finding the new requirements burdensome. The great majority of individuals who sell firearms have no interest in providing weapons for use by criminals. They will see the value of background checks and recordkeeping as means to prevent violent crime. It is unreasonable to expect private parties to question potential buyers about their eligibility, initiate background checks, and retain records. Private parties who sell firearms infrequently, who are hobbyists or collectors, will encounter the new requirements infrequently. Those who sell more often are in the business and should obtain licenses.

Retailers will object if the fee they are allowed to charge is too low to cover their costs. In California, $10 per firearm has proved satisfactory. Retailers will see an offsetting benefit in increased opportunities to develop new customers.

There will be costs to governments as they conduct background checks for nearly all firearm sales and issue more denials. The checks will only be as good as the data on which they rely. Efforts to improve the quality and completeness of these data must continue.

Implementing a comprehensive background check policy will be more a matter of substantial scaling up than of developing qualitatively new programs, which would be more expensive. In 11 states, including populous California, New York, and Pennsylvania, such policies are in effect now. Feasibility is proven.

REFERENCES

Anonymous. 2007. "California Market Still Lucrative." *The New Firearms Business*, 15 March, 5.
Ash, Peter, et al. 1996. "Gun Acquisition and Use by Juvenile Offenders." *Journal of the American Medical Association*, no. 275: 1754–1758.
Bowling, Michael, et al. 2010. Background Checks for Firearms Transfers, 2009—Statistical Tables. Washington, DC: Bureau of Justice Statistics.
Braga, Anthony A., et al. 2002. "The Illegal Supply of Firearms." In *Crime and Justice: A Review of Research*, ed. Michael Tonry. Chicago, IL: University of Chicago Press, 319–352.
Braga, Anthony A., and David M. Kennedy. 2000. "Gun Shows and the Illegal Diversion of Firearms." *Georgetown Public Policy Review*, no. 6: 7–24.
Braga, Anthony A., and David M. Kennedy. 2001. "The Illicit Acquisition of Firearms by Youth and Juveniles." *Journal of Criminal Justice*, no. 29: 379–388.
Bureau of Alcohol, Tobacco and Firearms. 1999b. Gun Shows: Brady Checks and Crime Gun Traces. Washington, DC: Bureau of Alcohol, Tobacco and Firearms.
Bureau of Alcohol, Tobacco and Firearms. 2000b. Following the Gun: Enforcing Federal Laws against Firearms Traffickers. Washington, DC: Bureau of Alcohol, Tobacco and Firearms.
Bureau of Justice Statistics. 2006. Survey of State Procedures Related to Firearm Sales, 2005. Washington, DC: Bureau of Justice Statistics.
California Department of Justice. 2012. Dealers Record of Sale Transactions.
City of New York. 2009. Gun Show Undercover: Report on Illegal Sales at Gun Shows. New York, NY: City of New York.
Cook, Philip J., and Jens Ludwig. 1996. *Guns in America: Results of a Comprehensive National Survey on Firearms Ownership and Use*. Washington, DC: The Police Foundation.
Cook, Philip J., Jens Ludwig, and Anthony A. Braga. "Criminal Records of Homicide Offenders." *Journal of the American Medical Association*, no. 294 (2005): 598–601.
Cook, Philip J., Stephanie Molliconi, and Thomas B. Cole. 1995. "Regulating Gun Markets." *Journal of Criminal Law and Criminology*, no. 86: 59–92.
Federal Bureau of Investigation. 2012b. National Instant Criminal Background Check System (NICS) Operation 2011. Washington, DC: Federal Bureau of Investigation.
Harlow, Caroline Wolf. 2001. Firearm Use by Offenders. Washington, DC: Bureau of Justice Statistics.
Hepburn, Lisa M., et al. 2007. "The U.S. Gun Stock: Results from the 2004 National Firearms Survey." *Injury Prevention*, no. 13: 15–19.
Manson, D., and D.K. Gilliard. 1997. Presale Handgun Checks, 1996: A National Estimate. Washington, DC: Bureau of Justice Statistics.
Matthews, Jim. 2009. "In Defense of the Neighborhood Gun Show." *Shooting Sports Retailer*, January, 58–62.
Pierce, Glenn L., et al. 2012. New Approaches to Understanding and Regulating Primary and Secondary Illegal Firearms. Washington, DC: National Institute of Justice.

Scalia, John. 2000. *Federal Firearm Offenders, 1992–98.* Washington, DC: Bureau of Justice Statistics.

Title 18, *U.S. Code,* Part 1, Chapter 44, Section 921(a)(21)(C).

Title 18, *U.S. Code,* Part 1, Chapter 44, Section 922(d).

Vittes, Katherine A., Jon S. Vernick, and Daniel W. Webster. 2012. "Legal Status and Source of Offenders' Firearms in States with the Least Stringent Criteria for Gun Ownership [Published Online Ahead of Print June 23, 2012]." *Injury Prevention.* DOI: 10.1136/injuryprev-2011-040290.

Webster, Daniel W., et al. 2002. "How Delinquent Youths Acquire Guns: Initial versus Most Recent Gun Acquisitions." *Journal of Urban Health,* no. 79: 60–69.

Webster, Daniel W., Jon S. Vernick, and Maria T. Bulzacchelli. 2009. "Effects of State-Level Firearm Seller Accountability Policies on Firearm Trafficking." *Journal of Urban Health,* no. 86: 525–537.

Wintemute, Garen J. 2007. "Gun Shows across a Multistate American Gun Market: Observational Evidence of the Effects of Regulatory Policies." *Injury Prevention,* no. 13: 150–156.

Wintemute, Garen J. 2009b. *Inside Gun Shows: What Goes on When Everybody Thinks Nobody's Watching.* Sacramento, CA: Violence Prevention Research Program.

Wintemute, Garen J., et al. 2004. "The Life Cycle of Crime Guns: A Description Based on Guns Recovered from Young People in California." *Annals of Emergency Medicine,* no. 43: 733–742.

Wintemute, Garen J., et al. 2001. "Subsequent Criminal Activity among Violent Misdemeanants Who Seek to Purchase Handguns: Risk Factors and Effectiveness of Denying Handgun Purchase." *Journal of the American Medical Association,* no. 285: 1019–1026.

Wright, James D., and Peter H. Rossi. 1986. *Armed and Considered Dangerous: A Survey of Felons and Their Firearms.* New York, NY: Aldine de Gruyter.

Wright, Mona A., and Garen J. Wintemute. 2010. "Felonious or Violent Criminal Activity That Prohibits Gun Ownership among Prior Purchasers of Handguns: Incidence and Risk Factors." *Journal of Trauma,* no. 69: 948–955.

Wright, Mona A., Garen J. Wintemute, and Frederick A. Rivara. 1999. "Effectiveness of Denial of Handgun Purchase to Persons Believed to Be at High Risk for Firearm Violence." *American Journal of Public Health,* no. 89: 88–90.

8

Preventing the Diversion of Guns to Criminals through Effective Firearm Sales Laws

Daniel W. Webster, Jon S. Vernick, Emma E. McGinty, and Ted Alcorn

Weaknesses in Federal Gun Laws Which Enable Criminals to Get Guns

Preventing individuals who are deemed too risky or dangerous from obtaining firearms is arguably the most important objective of gun control policies. Many perpetrators of gun violence are prohibited by federal law from purchasing firearms from a licensed dealer due to prior felony convictions or young age. Other contributions to this book provide compelling evidence that existing conditions for disqualifying someone from legally possessing firearms are justifiable and should be expanded (Vittes, Webster, and Vernick, in this volume). Wintemute (chap. 7 in this volume) and Zeoli and Frattaroli

Daniel W. Webster, ScD, MPH, is a professor in the Department of Health Policy and Management at the Johns Hopkins Bloomberg School of Public Health. Jon S. Vernick, JD, MPH, is an associate professor and associate chair in the Department of Health Policy and Management at the Johns Hopkins Bloomberg School of Public Health. Emma E. McGinty, MS, is a research assistant and fourth-year PhD candidate in Health Policy and Management at the Johns Hopkins Bloomberg School of Public Health. Ted Alcorn, MA, MHS, is a senior policy analyst in the Office of the Mayor of New York City.

(in this volume) provide evidence that laws which prohibit firearm possession by persons convicted of violent misdemeanors and those who are subject to restraining orders for domestic violence can reduce violence.

Some prohibited persons will voluntarily refrain from having a firearm in order to avoid criminal sanctions. But policies that enhance firearm seller and purchaser accountability are likely to determine how effectively gun control laws prevent prohibited individuals from acquiring guns. The federal Brady Law serves as a foundation, albeit incomplete, for preventing prohibited persons from acquiring firearms by making firearm purchases from federally licensed firearm dealers contingent upon the prospective purchaser passing a background check (Cook and Ludwig, in this volume). Licensed dealers must check purchasers' IDs, submit purchase applications to the FBI's National Instant Check System (NICS), and maintain records of all firearms acquisitions and sales so that ATF auditors can assess the dealers' compliance with gun sales laws.

Data on guns recovered by police and traced by the U.S. Bureau of Alcohol, Tobacco and Firearms (ATF) have indicated that about 85% of criminal possessors were not the retail purchaser (Bureau of Alcohol, Tobacco and Firearms 2002). This is consistent with our analysis of data from the most recent (2004) Survey of Inmates in State Correctional Facilities (SISCF) to determine the source for the handguns acquired by the 1,402 inmates incarcerated for an offense committed with a handgun. The largest proportions of offenders got their handguns from friends or family members (39.5%) or from street or black market suppliers (37.5%), sales for which there are no federal background check requirements. Licensed gun dealers were the direct source for 11.4% of the gun offenders. One in 10 offenders in our sample reported that they had stolen the handgun that they used in their most recent crime. Handgun acquisitions by offenders at gun shows and flea markets were rare (1.7 %).

It is easy to understand why offenders would prefer private sellers over licensed firearms dealers. Under federal law and laws in most states, firearm purchases from unlicensed private sellers require no background check or record keeping. The lack of record keeping requirements helps to shield an offender from law enforcement scrutiny if the gun were used in a crime and recovered by police. Indeed, of the offenders in the SISCF who were not prohibited from possessing a handgun prior to the crime leading to their incarceration, two-thirds had obtained their handguns in a transaction with a private seller.

That only 11% of handgun offenders reported acquiring their handguns from a licensed gun dealer does not mean that licensed dealers play a negligible role in the diversion of guns to criminals. Federal gun trafficking investigations indicate that corrupt licensed dealers represent one of the largest channels for the illegal gun market (Bureau of Alcohol, Tobacco and Firearms 2000), and a national phone survey of gun dealers found a willingness to make gun sales likely to be illegal relatively common (Sorenson and Vittes 2003). As articulated by Vernick and Webster (in this volume) and Braga and Gagliardi (in this volume), current federal laws provide many protections to licensed firearm sellers, and the Bureau of Alcohol, Tobacco, Firearms and Explosives lacks the resources and political power to serve as a robust deterrent to illegal gun sales.

Prior Evidence That Better Regulation of Gun Sellers Reduces Diversions of Guns to Criminals

Weaknesses in federal gun sales laws may cause skepticism about whether gun control can work in the United States. However, states vary greatly in the nature of their gun sales laws. For example, many states extend conditions for firearm prohibitions beyond those covered in federal law to include additional high-risk groups and place additional regulations on firearm sales to prevent illegal transfers. Twelve states require retail firearm sellers to be licensed by state or local governments and allow law enforcement to conduct audit inspections of gun dealers (Vernick, Webster, and Bulzachelli 2006). Fifteen states extend firearms sales regulations to sales by private, unlicensed sellers, and two additional states require background checks for firearms sold at gun shows. Nine states have some form of licensing system for handgun purchasers, five require applicants to apply directly with a law enforcement agency and be photographed and fingerprinted, and three allow agencies to use their discretion to deny an application if they deem it to be in the interest of public safety. Additional laws enacted by states to keep guns from prohibited persons include mandatory reporting of loss or theft of private firearms, limiting handgun sales to one per person per month, and banning the sale of low-quality "junk guns" that are overrepresented in crime (Wintemute 1994; Wright, Wintemute, and Webster 2010).

A study which used crime gun trace data from 53 U.S. cities for the years 2000–2002 examined the association between state gun sales regulations and the diversion of guns to criminals (Webster, Vernick, and Bulzacchelli 2009). Diversion of guns to criminals was measured by the number of guns recovered by police within one year of retail sale unless the criminal possessor was the legal retail purchaser. In addition to examining state laws, this study also surveyed state and local law enforcement officials to ascertain their policies for conducting compliance inspections or undercover stings of licensed dealers. Strong regulation and oversight of licensed gun dealers—defined as having a state law that required state or local licensing of retail firearm sellers, mandatory record keeping by those sellers, law enforcement access to records for inspection, regular inspections of gun dealers, and mandated reporting of theft of loss of firearms—was associated with 64% less diversion of guns to criminals by in-state gun dealers. Regulation of private handgun sales and discretionary permit-to-purchase (PTP) licensing were each independently associated with lower levels of diversion of guns sold by in-state dealers. The finding on private sales regulations is consistent with the results of a systematic observational study of gun sales at gun shows that found anonymous undocumented firearms sales to be ubiquitous and illegal "straw man" sales more than six times as common in states that do not regulate private sales compared with California that does regulate such sales (Wintemute 2007; Wintemute, chap. 7 in this volume).

Diversions of Guns to Criminals Following Missouri's Repeal of Permit to Purchase Licensing

The associations between state gun sales laws and diversions of guns to criminals cited above are cross-sectional and therefore do not capture changes in gun diversions following changes in state gun sales laws. The strong association between at least some forms of PTP licensing and lower rates of gun diversions to criminals could potentially be confounded by some variable omitted from the analyses that distinguishes states that enact the most comprehensive firearm sales regulations from those that do not. There have been few noteworthy changes in gun sales laws during a period when crime gun tracing practices were more common and the data were available to track changes over time. An exception is the repeal of Missouri's PTP law effective August 28, 2007. This law had required handgun purchasers to apply for a PTP through their local county sheriff's office and required a PTP for all handgun sales, whether by licensed or unlicensed sellers. Following the repeal, handgun purchasers could purchase handguns without a background check or record keeping if the seller was not a licensed dealer, and licensed gun dealers rather than sheriff's deputies processed applications to purchase handguns.

Using annual state-level data on crime guns recovered by police in Missouri and traced by the ATF for the period 2002–2011, we examined changes in commonly used indicators of illegal gun diversion—the number and proportion of guns with short sale-to-crime intervals—before and after the state repealed its PTP law. If Missouri's PTP law had been curtailing the diversion of guns to criminals, the repeal of the law should result in more short sale-to-crime guns recovered by police, and the shift in increasing crime guns should coincide with the length of time between the repeal of the law and a crime gun's recovery by police.

Such a pattern is clearly evident in the data presented in Table 8.1. The percentage of traced crime with a sale-to-crime interval of less than three months begins to increase from a pre-repeal stable mean of 2.8% to 5.0% in 2007 when the repeal was in effect for four months, and then jumps up to a mean of 8.5% for 2008 through 2011. The percentage of crime guns with sale-to-crime intervals of three to twelve months increased sharply beginning in 2008 from a pre-repeal mean of 6.2% to 14.0% for 2008–2011 when all such guns were purchased after the law's repeal. If the PTP repeal increased the diversion of guns to criminals, the percentage of crime guns recovered at a

Table 8.1   Percentage of Missouri Crime Guns with
Short Time Intervals between Retail Sale and Recovery
by Police for Years 2002–2011

Year	Up to 3 months (%)	3–12 months (%)	1–2 years (%)
2002	2.9	5.2	5.2
2003	3.2	5.3	6.1
2004	2.1	5.6	5.7
2005	3.3	5.1	6.6
2006	3.2	7.5	7.2
2007	4.5	7.9	7.1
2008	9.4	12.6	6.7
2009	8.1	15.0	12.7
2010	7.6	13.7	13.0
2011	8.5	14.3	12.7

one to two years sale-to-crime interval should increase beginning in 2009. Indeed, that is what happened. These guns increased sharply from a mean of 6.4% to 13.0%. The sharp increase in very short sale-to-crime intervals for guns in Missouri was not part of a national trend; in fact, the average sale-to-crime interval increased nationally from 10.2 years in 2006 to 11.2 years in 2011.

Because states with stronger gun sales laws tend to attract guns originating in states with weaker gun laws (Cook and Braga 2001; Webster, Vernick, and Hepburn 2001), we also compared trends in the proportion of Missouri's crime guns that were initially purchased in Missouri versus those that had been purchased outside of the state. Consistent with our hypotheses that Missouri's PTP had been preventing guns from being diverted to criminals, the share of crime guns originating from Missouri increased from a mean of 55.6% when the PTP law was in place to 70.8% by 2011, while the proportion that had originated from out of state gun dealers decreased from 44.4% before the repeal, began dropping in 2008, and was 29.2% in 2011. This is a remarkable change for an indicator that tends to change very little over time.

Effects of State Gun Sales Laws on the Export of Guns to Criminals across State Borders

In 2009, 30% of crime guns traced by the ATF were recovered in states other than the state where they were originally sold; however, there is great variation across states with respect to the proportion of crime guns which were originally sold by gun dealers in other states. Mayors Against Illegal Guns (2010) published a report showing great disparities across states in the number of crime guns exported per capita. Bivariate analyses indicated that each of ten selected gun control laws were associated with exporting fewer guns per capita that were used by criminals in other states. In a National Bureau of Economic Research (NBER) working paper, Knight used an index of eleven laws developed by MAIG to examine the flow of guns to and from states with strong versus weak gun laws and found that states with weak gun laws tended to export guns to states with strong gun laws (Knight 2011).

The present study adds to this literature by using crime gun trace data from the Bureau of Alcohol, Tobacco, Firearms and Explosives (ATF) to examine the cross-sectional association between state gun laws and the per capita rate of exporting crime guns across the 48 contiguous U.S. states. The following state gun sales laws were considered: strong regulations of retail gun dealers[1]; permit-to-purchase (PTP) licensing; private sales regulations (mandatory background checks of sellers or valid PTP); handgun registration; mandatory reporting to law enforcement of theft and loss of firearms by private owners; whether the state has criminal penalties for dealers who fail to conduct background checks or has penalties for illegal straw purchasers; one-gun-per-month restrictions; assault weapon bans; and junk gun bans. Three variations of PTP laws were examined: (1) discretionary PTP laws which give law enforcement the discretion to refuse to issue permits; (2) PTP with fingerprinting which requires applicants to appear at the law enforcement agency that issues the permits to be photographed and fingerprinted; and (3) nondiscretionary PTP laws which require a permit to purchase a firearm but do not require applicants to go to agencies to be fingerprinted.

We used negative binomial regression models with robust standard errors to estimate the association between state gun laws and the per capita rate of crime guns exported to criminals in other states after controlling for potential confounders. Key confounders controlled for in the analyses were the prevalence of gun ownership, out-of-state population migration, and the number of people living near the border of states with strong gun laws. State population served as an offset variable so that transformed regression coefficients could be interpreted as incident rate ratios (IRR) and percentage reductions in risk.

Data on crime gun exports were obtained from the 2009 state-level crime gun trace data posted on the ATF's website. ATF defines crime guns as recovered firearms that were "illegally possessed, used in a crime, or suspected to have been used in a crime." In 2009, 61% of the guns that police submitted to ATF were successfully traced to the first retail sale.

Data on state gun laws were obtained through legal research and from ATF and U.S. Department of Justice Publications. Oak Ridge National Laboratory's LandScan global population distribution data was used with arcGIS Version 10 to calculate state border population variables used as control variables in statistical models. These control variables included population within 50 miles of a bordering states with the strongest gun control laws[2] and states with medium level of gun control.[3] Household prevalence of firearm ownership was obtained from the Behavioral Risk Factor Surveillance System 2001 survey (Centers for Disease Control and Prevention 2001), and measures of state migration[4] were obtained from the American Community Survey (ACS) 2005–2009 five-year estimates. Finally, we measured two variables indicating that a state borders Canada or Mexico, respectively.

States that exported the most crime guns per 100,000 population were Mississippi (50.4), West Virginia (47.6), Kentucky (35.0), and Alabama (33.4). Of these four states, three (Mississippi, West Virginia, and Kentucky) had none of the state gun laws we examined. Alabama penalized gun dealers who failed to conduct background checks but had no other laws of interest in place. States that exported the fewest crime guns per capita—New York (2.7), New Jersey (2.8), Massachusetts (3.7), and California (5.4)—each had strong gun dealer oversight, regulated private sales, and handgun registries. New York, New Jersey, and Massachusetts also had discretionary PTP and required reporting of firearm theft/loss.

Data from the regression analysis are presented in Table 8.2. Due to high collinearity (Variance Inflation Factor > 10), assault weapons bans and handgun registration laws were dropped from the final models. Statistically significant lower per capita export of crime guns across state borders was found for

Table 8.2   Estimates of association between state gun laws and crime gun exports

	IRR	Robust SE	*p* value
State gun laws			
Discretionary purchase permits	0.24	0.10	.001
Purchase permits with fingerprinting	0.55	0.15	.02
Nondiscretionary permits	0.75	0.15	.15
Strong dealer regulation[a]	1.45	0.30	.07
Penalty for failure to conduct background checks	0.76	0.12	.07
Penalty for straw purchasers	1.46	0.30	.07
Junk guns banned	0.68	0.13	.04
Private sales regulated	0.71	0.11	.03
Firearm theft/loss reported	0.70	0.10	.02
One gun per month	0.81	0.26	.51
Covariates			
Household gun ownership	6.05	4.20	.009
Border population in states with strong gun laws[b]	1.00	1.82E-08	.50
Border population in states with medium gun laws[c]	1.00	2.57E-08	.14
Migration out of state	0.99	5.04E-07	.50
Borders Canada	0.68	0.065	<.001
Borders Mexico	0.84	0.19	.43

Note: IRR = incidence rate ratio. Model also includes state population offset term.

[a]States were considered to have strong dealer regulation if they require licensing of gun dealers, allow inspection of dealer records, and penalize dealers who falsify records.

[b]States were considered to have strong gun laws if they have a discretionary permit-to-purchase law.

[c]States were considered to have medium gun laws if they regulate private sales, require licensing of gun dealers, and allow inspections of dealer records.

discretionary PTP laws (IRR=0.24, lowered risk 76%), nondiscretionary PTP laws requiring fingerprinting at a law enforcement agency (IRR=0.55, −45%), junk gun bans (IRR=0.68, −32%), regulation of private sales (IRR=0.71, −29%), and required reporting of firearm theft or loss by private gun owners (IRR=0.70, −30%) were each associated with statistically significantly lower rates of crime gun exports. Effects for penalties for gun dealers' failure to conduct background checks (IRR=0.76) and penalties for straw purchases (IRR=1.24) approached statistical significance at the .05 level but in opposite directions. Although billed as a deterrent to interstate gun trafficking, one-gun-per-month restrictions were unrelated to trafficking and neither were strong dealer regulations, penalties for failure to conduct background checks, or penalties for straw purchasing. Household gun ownership (IRR=6.05) was associated with higher crime gun export rates and bordering Canada was associated with lower crime gun exports (IRR=0.84). States bordering other states where gun laws are relatively strict was unrelated to the rate of exporting crime guns after controlling for gun sales laws and other factors.

Conclusions and Policy Implications

Data presented here provide compelling evidence that the repeal of Missouri's permit-to-purchase (PTP) law increased the diversion of guns to criminals. The timing of the effects on our indicator of diversion, short intervals between sales, and recovery in crime was in exact correspondence with the timing of the law's repeal. The changes observed in gun diversions in Missouri are likely related to the substantial change in how guns were sold following the law's repeal. Prospective purchasers of handguns being sold by private individuals no longer had to pass a background check and sellers were no longer required to document the sale. Prospective purchasers, including illegal straw purchasers, interested in buying handguns from licensed dealers applied to purchase the gun at the place that profited from the sale rather than at a law enforcement agency. Repealing the PTP law made it less risky for criminals, straw purchasers, and persons willing to sell guns to criminals and to their intermediaries, and these individuals appear to have taken advantage of the opportunities afforded to them by the repeal.

In our study of state gun sales laws in the 48 contiguous states, discretionary PTP laws were the most dramatic deterrent to interstate gun trafficking. This finding is consistent with prior research showing a negative association between these laws and intrastate diversion of guns to criminals; however, the effects were either mediated by or explained by lower levels of gun ownership in states with these laws (Webster, Vernick, and Bulzachelli 2009). Discretionary permitting procedures such as in-depth and direct scrutiny by law enforcement, longer waiting times, higher fees, and stricter standards for legal ownership may depress gun ownership and reduce opportunities for criminals to find individuals who have guns that they would be willing to sell or who would be targets for gun theft. The strong negative association between nondiscretionary PTP laws and exporting guns to criminals in other states after statistically controlling for gun ownership levels, geography, and other gun laws suggests that PTP laws deter gun trafficking.

Perhaps most relevant to current debates about federal gun policy, we found that states which regulated all handgun sales by requiring background checks and record keeping, not just those made by licensed dealers, diverted significantly fewer guns to criminals in other states. This finding is consistent with the results of a prior study of intrastate diversions of guns to criminals (Webster, Vernick, and Bulzachelli 2009) and the findings of an observational study of sales practices gun shows (Wintemute 2007; chap. 7 in this volume). The importance of fixing this flaw in current gun law is highlighted by data first reported here which indicate that nearly 80% of handgun offenders incarcerated in state prisons reported purchasing or trading for their handgun from an unlicensed seller who, in most states, was not legally obligated to ensure that the purchaser passed a background check or to keep a record of the transaction.

Our examination of state firearms regulations and the interstate diversion of guns to criminals considered a larger array of laws than prior studies. Laws requiring private gun owners to promptly report theft or loss of firearms to police are intended to increase private gun seller accountability and provide law enforcement with a tool to combat illegal straw purchases when such purchasers accept no responsibility for the gun being in the hands of a prohibited person with dubious claims of unreported gun theft. Having this measure of accountability significantly reduced interstate gun trafficking, as did bans of junk guns. Junk guns are the least expensive guns, and their low price enables traffickers to invest relatively little money in guns that can sell for nearly five times more than retail prices on the streets in states with the most restrictive gun laws. Prior research on the effects of Maryland's ban of junk guns found the banned guns used much less in Baltimore, Maryland, than in cities without such bans, seven years after Maryland's law was enacted (Vernick, Webster, and Hepburn 1999), and gun homicides were 9% lower than projected had the law not been enacted (Webster, Vernick, and Hepburn 2002).

Interestingly, a policy designed specifically to deter interstate gun trafficking—one-gun-per-month limits for gun buyers—was not associated with the export of guns to criminals in other states. Strong gun dealer regulations were also unrelated to exporting of crime guns across state lines. A prior study of intrastate trafficking found that strong dealer regulations by themselves were not effective unless law enforcement reported that they had a policy of regular compliance inspections. Unfortunately, we had no measure of enforcement for the current study.

Our assessment of the effects of state gun control laws on the export of guns to criminals in other states had several limitations. First, the cross-sectional study design precludes an assessment of whether changes in gun control laws prompt subsequent changes in crime gun exports. Longitudinal crime gun trace data could not be obtained, as many of the state laws of interest were in place before crime gun tracing become common practice. The sharp increase in diversions of guns to criminals following the repeal of Missouri's law, however, lessens this concern. Second, our outcome data does not include all crime gun exports. Not all crime guns are submitted to the ATF for tracing. In 2009, gun traces could not be completed for nearly 40% of crime guns due to insufficient or incorrect data. Third, although reducing the diversion of guns to criminals is a key objective of some gun control laws, there is currently insufficient research to discern the degree to which reductions in diverted guns affects gun violence, and it appears as though some have had no impact.

In spite of these limitations, our study is the first to estimate independent associations between a number of state gun control laws and crime gun export rates while controlling for confounders, and it is the first longitudinal assessment of the impact of permit-to-purchase licensing that regulates all handgun sales. Our findings on cross-state diversions of crime guns underscores the importance of having more comprehensive federal regulation of firearm sales because lax laws in many states facilitate the arming of criminals beyond state borders. At a minimum, federal law should require background checks and record keeping for all firearms sales. Regulating many private sellers is a challenge, yet the data suggest that it is necessary to deter the diversion of guns to criminals, and requiring gun owners to report theft or loss of firearms provides additional accountability to prevent illegal sales.

ACKNOWLEDGMENTS

Funding for this research was provided by grants from the Joyce Foundation and Bloomberg Philanthropies.

NOTES

1. Licensing of gun dealers, inspection of dealer records allowed, and criminal penalties for dealers who falsified records.
2. PTP laws or in the District of Columbia with what could be considered a ban on firearm ownership until 2008.
3. Regulate private sales, require licensing of gun dealers, and allow inspections of dealer records.
4. The number of people who moved out of each state between 2005 and 2009.

REFERENCES

Bureau of Alcohol, Tobacco and Firearms (ATF). 2000. *Following the Gun.* Washington, DC: U.S. Department of the Treasury.
Bureau of Alcohol, Tobacco and Firearms (ATF). 2002. *Crime Gun Trace Reports (2000): The Youth Crime Gun Interdiction Initiative.* Washington, DC: U.S. Department of the Treasury.
Bureau of Justice Statistics. 2004. *Survey of Inmates in State Correctional Facilities (SISCF).* Washington, DC: U.S. Department of Justice.
Centers for Disease Control and Prevention (CDC). 2001. *Behavioral Risk Factor Surveillance System Survey Data.* Atlanta, GA: U.S. Department of Health and Human Services.
Cook, Philip J., and Anthony A. Braga. 2001. "Comprehensive Firearms Tracing: Strategic and Investigative Uses of New Data on Firearms Markets." *Arizona Law Review* 43 (2): 277–309.
Cook, Philip J., Jens Ludwig, and Anthony A. Braga. 2005. "Criminal Records of Homicide Offenders." *Journal of the American Medical Association* 294: 598–601.
Environmental Systems Research Institute (ESRI). 2011. ArcGIS Desktop: Release 10. Redlands, CA.
Knight, Brian G. 2011. "State Gun Policy and Cross-State Externalities: Evidence from Crime Gun Tracing." National Bureau of Economic Research Working Paper no. 17469. Cambridge, MA.
Mayors Against Illegal Guns. 2010. *Trace the Guns: The Link Between Gun Laws and Interstate Gun Trafficking.* http://www.mayorsagainstillegalguns.org/downloads /pdf/trace_the_guns_report.pdf.
Sorenson, Susan B., and Katherine A. Vittes. 2003. "Buying a Handgun for Someone Else: Firearm Dealer Willingness to Sell." *Injury Prevention* 9:147–150. doi:10.1136 /ip.9.2.147.

Vernick, Jon S., Daniel W. Webster, and Maria T. Bulzacchelli. 2006. "Regulating Firearms Dealers in the United States: An Analysis of State Law and Opportunities for Improvement." *Journal of Law, Medicine & Ethics* 34: 765–775.

Vernick, Jon S., Daniel W. Webster, and Lisa M. Hepburn. 1999. "Effects of Maryland's Law Banning Saturday Night Special Handguns on Crime Guns." *Injury Prevention* 5: 259–263.

Vittes, Katherine A., Jon S. Vernick, and Daniel W. Webster. 2012. "Legal Status and Source of Offenders' Firearms in States with the Least Stringent Criteria for Gun Ownership." *Injury Prevention*. Published Online First: 23 June. doi:10.1136/injuryprev-2011-040290.

Webster, Daniel W., Jon S. Vernick, and Maria T. Bulzacchelli. 2009. "Effects of State-Level Firearm Seller Accountability Policies on Firearms Trafficking." *Journal of Urban Health* 86: 525–537.

Webster, Daniel W., Jon S. Vernick, and Lisa M. Hepburn. 2001. "The Relationship between Licensing, Registration and Other State Gun Sales Laws and the Source State of Crime Guns." *Injury Prevention* 7: 184–189.

Webster, Daniel W., Jon S. Vernick, and Lisa M. Hepburn. 2002. "Effects of Maryland's Law Banning Saturday Night Special Handguns on Homicides." *American Journal of Epidemiology* 155: 406–412.

Wintemute, Garen J. 1994. *Ring of Fire: The Handgun Makers of Southern California.* Sacramento, CA: Violence Prevention Research Program.

Wintemute, Garen J. 2007. "Guns Shows across a Multistate American Gun Market: Observational Evidence of the Effects of Regulatory Policies." *Injury Prevention* 13: 150–155. Erratum in: *Injury Prevention* 13: 286.

Wright, Mona A., Garen J. Wintemute, and Daniel W. Webster. 2010. "Factors Affecting a Recently Purchased Handgun's Risk for Use in Crime under Circumstances That Suggest Gun Trafficking." *Journal of Urban Health* 87: 352–364.

9

Spurring Responsible Firearms Sales Practices through Litigation

The Impact of New York City's Lawsuits against
Gun Dealers on Interstate Gun Trafficking

Daniel W. Webster and Jon S. Vernick

Surveys of criminals indicate that "street or illegal sources," family, and friends are the most common proximate sources for criminals to obtain guns (Webster et al., in this volume; Harlow 2004). However, there are little data on how guns are initially diverted into the illegal market and into the hands of direct suppliers for criminals. Data from gun trafficking investigations indicate that licensed gun dealers play an important role in the diversion of guns from the legal to the illegal market. Gun dealers facilitate blatantly illegal sales by straw purchasers (individuals who buy guns on behalf of prohibited purchasers), or sell guns to traffickers or directly to criminals (Bureau of Alcohol, Tobacco and Firearms 2000). Phone surveys of licensed gun dealers, in which callers asked whether the dealer would sell them a handgun intended for their boyfriend, found between 20% and 50% were willing to make what would have been an illegal sale (Sorenson & Vittes 2003; Wintemute 2010).

Daniel W. Webster, ScD, MPH, is a professor in the Department of Health Policy and Management at the Johns Hopkins Bloomberg School of Public Health. Jon S. Vernick, JD, MPH, is an associate professor and associate chair in the Department of Health Policy and Management at the Johns Hopkins Bloomberg School of Public Health.

Research has shown that gun dealers' sales practices can have a powerful effect on the illicit market. Although some licensed gun dealers rarely sell guns that are subsequently recovered from criminals, others have been identified as the origin of hundreds of crime guns in a given year (Americans for Gun Safety 2004; Wintemute, Cook, & Wright 2005). In Milwaukee, for example, a single gun dealer was linked to the majority of the city's crime guns which were recovered within a year of the first retail sale (Webster, Vernick, & Bulzachelli 2006). In response to negative publicity about the gun shop's frequent connection to guns used in crime, that gun dealer voluntarily changed his shop's sales practices—including eliminating the sale of so-called "junk guns." This change was followed by an immediate 76% reduction in the flow of new guns from that gun shop to criminals in Milwaukee, and a 44% reduction in new crime guns citywide (Webster, Vernick, & Bulzacchelli 2006).

A recent study found that comprehensive state or local regulation of licensed gun dealers (e.g., state or local licensing, record-keeping requirements, mandating or allowing inspections) coupled with routine law enforcement compliance efforts was associated with less intrastate trafficking of guns (Webster, Vernick, & Bulzacchelli 2009). Litigation is another policy tool that has been used to deter gun sales practices which could enable criminals to obtain guns (Vernick, Rutkow, & Salmon 2007). Beginning in the late 1990s, several local governments began to sue gun manufacturers, wholesalers, and retail gun shops for engaging in sales practices that, according to the plaintiffs, facilitated the diversion of guns from the legal to the illegal gun market. In support of their claims that retail gun dealers were engaging in negligent sales practices which enabled criminals to obtain guns, the plaintiffs presented data from the United States Bureau of Alcohol, Tobacco, Firearms and Explosives (ATF) which indicated that a relatively small number of gun dealers had long histories of selling a large number of guns that police later recovered from criminals. Some cities, including Chicago and Detroit, initiated a series of undercover stings of gun shops in their area which were linked to the most crime guns. These stings involved undercover police officers posing as gang members and blatantly attempting to illegally purchase firearms using straw purchasers. The videotapes of these stings were presented as evidence in the lawsuits and, in the case of Chicago, were also used in criminal cases against individuals who broke state gun sales laws. A study which tracked illegal gun trafficking indicators over time found that the Chicago and

Detroit lawsuits were associated with significant reductions in the flow of new handguns to criminals. Guns recovered by police within a year of retail sale by an in-state gun dealer dropped 62% in Chicago and 36% in Detroit. There were no significant changes in gun trafficking indicators in three comparable Midwestern cities that had not sued local gun dealers (Webster et al. 2006).

As discussed in the essay by Jon Vernick et al. (in this volume), in 2005 a new federal law was enacted which made it much more difficult for individuals or municipalities to bring lawsuits against firearm makers and sellers. Under the Protection of Lawful Commerce in Arms Act (PLCAA), lawsuits against firearm manufactures or dealers "resulting from the criminal or unlawful misuse" of a firearm "by the person or a third party" may not be brought in state or federal court (15 U.S.C. §7903(A)(5) (2010)). Thus, if a city were to sue a gun dealer alleging harm caused by the criminal (i.e., "third party") use of firearms in that city, the lawsuit would be dismissed unless one of the limited exceptions to the PLCAA applied. Even lawsuits pending at the time the PLCAA was enacted were to be "immediately dismissed." As a result, nearly all lawsuits brought by cities against gun dealers and manufacturers were dismissed (Vernick, Rutkow, & Salmon 2007).

One exception to the PLCAA's protection of the firearm industry involves lawsuits where the plaintiff can show that harm was caused by a firearm dealer or manufacturer who "knowingly violated a State or Federal statute applicable to the sale or marketing of the product . . ." (15 U.S.C. §7903(a)(5) (2010)). Under this exception, if the damages alleged in the lawsuit are associated with the knowing violation of a firearms sales law *by the defendant* whether or not another criminal act, such as a homicide or assault by the gun buyer, was also involved—then the lawsuit may proceed.

This exception was used by New York City in its 2006 litigation against 27 gun dealers who were videotaped facilitating illegal straw gun purchases in undercover stings. This essay describes New York City's use of litigation to compel these gun dealers to adopt new business practices designed to prevent the diversion of guns to criminals and other prohibited persons. It also presents data from 10 of the dealers who had maintained electronic sales records showing a dramatic reduction in the number of guns sold by these dealers that were subsequently recovered by the New York Police Department (NYPD).

New York City's Lawsuits against Selected Gun Dealers

Following shooting deaths of two NYPD officers and the fatal shooting of a young child caught in crossfire, in 2006 New York City Mayor Michael Bloomberg made fighting illegal guns a top priority of his administration. The success of the undercover stings and lawsuits in Chicago and Detroit in reducing the flow of new guns to criminals encouraged New York City officials to undertake a similar effort. The city hired private investigators to stage and secretly videotape undercover stings of 55 gun dealers located across seven states that were among the most common source states for guns recovered by police from criminals and crime scenes in New York City. The seven states were Alabama, Georgia, North Carolina, Ohio, Pennsylvania, South Carolina, and Virginia. Some of the targeted gun dealers had also sold guns to individuals prosecuted for crimes related to gun trafficking.

All of the stings were conducted in a similar manner. A male and a female investigator entered the gun stores together. The male investigator engaged sales staff with questions about different firearms and selected one or more to purchase. The female investigator, who had not been involved in the selection of the gun, would then attempt to complete the federal form for a background check of prospective firearm purchasers. The male investigator would attempt to pay for the firearm and receive it from the sales person after the instant background check was completed. Transactions of this type violate federal firearms laws; this was acknowledged by many of the gun dealers who were stung and refused to make the sale.

Of the 55 gun dealers, 27 were caught facilitating illegal sales in the undercover stings and were sued by New York City. Nearly all of the dealers came to an agreement with the city to change their business practices to prevent illegal gun sales. As part of the settlements, a special master was appointed to ensure that each gun dealer complied with all applicable firearm sales laws. Gun dealers were required to allow the special masters to use in-store observation (including use of videotape surveillance); records monitoring, including: all crime gun trace requests made by ATF since the date of the settlement; inventory inspections; random and repeated sales integrity testing; and instructional programs designed to provide best practices sales training to all employees involved in firearms sales. Gun dealers were also required to file a performance bond with the Court that was considered by the city to be satisfactory. The performance bond required the gun dealer, usually within

15 days of its signing, to forfeit a designated amount of money to New York City anytime the special master found that the dealer sold a gun to a straw purchaser or violated other applicable gun sales laws and regulations. Evidence of such a violation could have resulted from an indictment against a straw purchaser indicating circumstances under which a reasonable person would have recognized that a straw purchase was occurring, observation of a straw purchase from reviews of videotape monitors, or a sale made to an investigator conducting a simulated straw purchase. The performance bond lasted until the special master certified that three consecutive years of full compliance by the gun dealership had occurred.

Assessing Program Effects on the Diversion of Guns to Criminals

Electronic sales data for specific guns sold (i.e., make, model, caliber, serial number, date of sale) for the period from January 1, 2003 through June 30, 2007 were made available to the special master by 10 of the gun dealers sued by New York City. The special master shared the data with the New York City Law Department which then provided it to researchers. To ascertain whether any of the guns sold by these 10 dealers were subsequently recovered by NYPD, we obtained NYPD's database for firearms it recovered from criminals, crime scenes, and other settings from January 1, 2003 through June 30, 2008. The NYPD database contained data on manufacturer/make, model, caliber, and serial number for each gun as well as the date on which it was recovered. The gun sales and police recovery databases were subsequently merged. To identify guns that were sold by the 10 gun dealers of interest and later recovered by NYPD, we looked for matches based on make, caliber, and serial number.

The primary goal of the analysis was to compare the likelihood of NYPD recovery for guns sold before and after the lawsuits were announced. Guns sold during the pre-lawsuit period had much greater opportunity for NYPD recovery than guns sold after the lawsuits due to more follow-up time for the pre-lawsuit-sold guns compared with post-lawsuit sales. Guns sold prior to the lawsuit had from 25 to 66 months (mean = 43 months) of follow-up time, whereas guns sold after the lawsuits had 13 to 25 months (mean = 18 months) of follow-up time. Researchers were only provided sales data for 13.5 months following the announcement of the lawsuits and had between 12 and 25.5 months of follow-up time for police recovery data for post-lawsuit sales.

Therefore, we constrained the follow-up time for the pre-lawsuit-sold guns to make it roughly equivalent to that of the post-lawsuit cohort of guns. Specifically, we selected all guns sold during the 13.5 months immediately prior to the lawsuits for comparison with the post-lawsuit-sold guns. We then determined which of these guns had been subsequently recovered by NYPD, and if the recovery occurred within a follow-up time period that was within the bounds of the appropriate follow-up period for guns sold during the post-lawsuit period. For example, a gun sold on May 16, 2006—the first day following the announcement of the first lawsuits—had a follow-up time of 776 days during which recovery was determined. Similarly, a 776-day window of exposure was examined for guns sold on the first day of the pre-lawsuit cohort of gun sales (April 15, 2005). In contrast, post-lawsuit sales which took place on the last day for which gun sales data were available (June 30, 2007) had a maximum follow-up period of 365 days. We, therefore, constrained the follow-up period for guns sold on the last day prior to the lawsuits' announcement (May 14, 2006) to 365 days.

To test whether the odds of NYPD recovery for guns sold after the lawsuits were announced was different from the odds of NYPD recovery for guns sold before the lawsuits, we calculated the crude odds ratio, its 95% confidence interval, and Pearson's chi-square statistic. In addition, we performed a logistic regression to estimate the relationship between the time period in which a gun was sold (before lawsuits = 0; after lawsuits = 1) after controlling for the exposure or days of follow-up and a set of indicator variables for the specific dealer that sold the gun.

For the 10 gun dealers included in the study, we identified sales records for 12,267 guns—6,081 before the lawsuits and 6,186 after the lawsuits. The mean follow-up time for post-lawsuit-sold gun sales was slightly longer than that of pre-lawsuit-sold guns (565.7 versus 542.3, $p < .001$). The number of recorded sales varied greatly across the 10 dealers from a low of 91 to a high of 2,337.

Only 5 of the 6,186 (0.008%) guns sold after the lawsuit were subsequently recovered by NYPD compared with 31 of the 6,081 (0.005%) guns sold during the period immediately before the lawsuit ($\chi^2 = 19.28$, df = 1, $p < .001$). The odds of a NYPD recovery was 84.2% lower during the post-lawsuit sales period than the pre-lawsuit sales period (OR = 0.16, 95% CI: 0.02, 0.41). The adjusted odds ratio for NYPD recovery for post-lawsuits guns versus pre-lawsuits guns estimated from the logistic regression which controlled for follow-up time and dealer-specific effects (OR = 0.18, 95% CI: 0.07, 0.46) was similar to the crude odds ratio indicating the odds a gun sold following the lawsuits was recovered by NYPD relative to the odds of a gun sold before the lawsuits was recovered by NYPD.

Discussion and Policy Implications

This study has several limitations which restrict our ability to ascertain the full effects of the lawsuits and any subsequent changes in business practices resulting from the settlement agreements. First, we only had access to police gun recovery data for New York City. Most gun dealers sued by the city were located in many states that were hundreds of miles from New York including Georgia, Alabama, South Carolina, North Carolina, Virginia and Ohio. Although illegal gun markets vary across states, it seems likely that the new policies and practices instituted by the gun dealers to reduce the illegal diversion of guns to criminals would reduce the flow of guns to criminals within their home states as well as that of other states. Access to crime gun trace data from ATF would have allowed us to examine broader effects of the lawsuits; however, congressionally imposed restrictions on access to these data make such research extremely difficult if not impossible (Webster et al. 2012).

Agreements with the special master for the settlements against the gun dealers prevented us from knowing the identity of any of the dealers being studied. Knowing which dealers were included and the dates of the settlements would have allowed us to more precisely measure pre- and post-lawsuit periods. We believe that our estimates of the association between the lawsuits and probability of gun sales leading to subsequent recovery of the gun by NYPD are somewhat conservative because we assumed that any protective effects would be realized immediately following the announcement of the lawsuits against the first 15 gun dealers sued. Among the five post-lawsuit-sold guns later recovered by NYPD, one had been sold the day after the first lawsuits were announced and another was sold 10 days after the first lawsuits. Certainly, the agreements to institute an array of business practices designed to reduce the diversion of guns to criminals had not been reached or implemented within 10 days of the first lawsuits.

With the available data, it is impossible to determine the degree to which the sharp reduction in the risk of NYPD recovery following gun sales is due to the active oversight of the gun dealers by the special masters for their settlements or to new sales policies and practices. Marketing researchers have theorized about and studied the countermarketing of products—rejection of unwanted demand by getting rid of undesirable customers or the prevention of risky transactions—that pose a special risk to consumers or the public at large if there is great risk of the product causing consumer or public harm if misused. They have found evidence of countermarketing effects among retail firearm sellers (Gundlock, Bradford, & Wilkie 2010). Walmart, the largest seller of firearms in the United States, has adopted a 10-point, voluntary code for responsible sales practices to prevent guns they sell from getting into the hands of criminals (Mayors Against Illegal Guns 2013).

The findings from our study are consistent with a growing body of research evidence which indicates that gun dealers' sales practices affect the probability of guns getting to criminals (Webster, Vernick, & Bulzachelli 2006), and that policies designed to hold gun sellers accountable can curtail the diversion of guns to criminals (Webster et al. 2009; Webster et al., this volume). Conversely, there is evidence that the federal policy which curtailed the use of crime gun trace data in lawsuits or in decisions about firearm dealers' licensure, so that gun dealers are less accountable, can increase the diversion of guns to criminals by problem dealers (Webster et al. 2012). While the current study focused narrowly on the effects of lawsuits—and presumably the gun sales reforms agreed to by the gun dealers—on the dealers who were sued, a prior study demonstrated citywide reductions in the flow of new guns to criminals in Chicago and Detroit following undercover stings and lawsuits against area gun dealers (Webster et al. 2006). These findings suggest that, to prevent the flow of large numbers of guns to criminals, policymakers should eliminate special protections for gun dealers from lawsuits and law enforcement oversight.

REFERENCES

Americans for Gun Safety Foundation. 2004. *Selling Crime: High Crime Gun Stores Fuel Criminals.* Washington, DC, January.

Bureau of Alcohol, Tobacco and Firearms. 2000. *Following the Gun: Enforcing Federal Firearms Laws Against Firearms Traffickers.* Washington, DC: U.S. Department of the Treasury, June.

Bureau of Alcohol, Tobacco, Firearms and Explosives. 2008. *ATF New York City.* New York: U.S. Department of Justice, New York Division of the BATF, ATF Gun Center, February.

Gundlach, G.T., K.D. Bradford, W.L. Wilkie. 2010. "Countermarketing and Demarketing Against Product Diversion: Forensic Research in the Firearms Industry." *Journal of Public Policy & Marketing* 29: 103–122.

Harlow, Caroline W. 2004. *Survey of Inmates in State Correctional Facilities (SISCF)*. Washington, DC: Bureau of Justice Statistics, United States Department of Justice.

Koper, C.S. 2006. "Federal Legislation and Gun Markets: How Much Have Recent Reforms of the Federal Firearms Licensing System Reduced Criminal Gun Suppliers?" *Criminology and Public Policy* 1: 151–178.

Mayors Against Illegal Guns. 2013. Responsible Firearms Sellers Partnership: A 10-Point Voluntary Code. http://www.mayorsagainstillegalguns.org/downloads /pdf/partnership.pdf

Sorenson, Susan B., and Katherine A. Vittes. 2003. "Buying a handgun for someone else: firearm dealer willingness to sell." *Injury Prevention* 9(2): 147–150.

Vernick, J.S., L. Rutkow, D.A. Salmon. 2007. "Availability of Litigation as a Public Health Tool for Firearm Injury Prevention: Comparison of Guns, Vaccines, and Motor Vehicles." *American Journal of Public Health* 97: 1991–1997.

Webster, D.W., J.S. Vernick, and M.T. Bulzacchelli. 2006. "Effects of a Gun Dealer's Change in Sales Practices on the Supply of Guns to Criminals." *Journal of Urban Health* 83: 778–787.

Webster, D.W., J.S. Vernick, and M.T. Bulzacchelli. 2009. "Effects of State-Level Firearm Seller Accountability Policies on Firearms Trafficking." *Journal of Urban Health* 86: 525–537.

Webster, DW, Vernick JS, Bulzacchelli MT, Vittes KA. 2012. "Recent federal gun laws, gun dealer accountability and the diversion of guns to criminals in Milwaukee." *Journal of Urban Health* 89: 87–97.

Webster, D.W., A.M. Zeoli, M.T. Bulzacchelli, and J.S. Vernick. 2006. "Effects of Police Stings of Gun Dealers on the Supply of New Guns to Criminals." *Injury Prevention* 12: 225–230.

Wintemute, Garen. 2010. "Firearm retailers' willingness to participate in an illegal gun purchase." *Journal of Urban Health* 87(5): 865–78.

Wintemute, G.J., P.J. Cook, M.A. Wright. 2005. "Risk Factors Among Handgun Retailers for Frequent and Disproportionate Sales of Guns Used in Violent and Firearms Crimes." *Injury Prevention* 11:357: 363.

10

Curtailing Dangerous Sales Practices by Licensed Firearm Dealers

Legal Opportunities and Obstacles

Jon S. Vernick and Daniel W. Webster

It is an enlightening truism of gun policy that, in the United States, the vast majority of guns used in crime were originally sold by federally licensed firearm dealers. The primary exceptions are the modest number of guns stolen from manufactures or dealers or illegally imported from abroad. This does not mean that most gun dealers flout the law or knowingly sell guns to criminals. But it does suggest that one potentially fruitful approach to make it harder for firearms to flow from the legal to the illegal market is through enhanced regulation and oversight of firearm dealers.

There are approximately 55,000 federally licensed gun dealers in the United States (ATF 2013). Yet data from a 2000 analysis indicate that just over 1% of these dealers sold more than half (57%) of the guns later traced to crime (BATF 2000a). This disproportionate supply of crime guns is not explained solely by the dealers' sales volume, local crime rates, or buyer demographics

Jon S. Vernick, JD, MPH, is an associate professor and associate chair in the Department of Health Policy and Management at the Johns Hopkins Bloomberg School of Public Health. Daniel W. Webster, ScD, MPH, is a professor in the Department of Health Policy and Management at the Johns Hopkins Bloomberg School of Public Health.

(Wintemute, Cook, and Wright 2005). In addition, analyses of gun trafficking investigations have found that licensed gun dealers accounted for the largest single source of guns diverted to the illegal market (BATF 2000b; Braga et al. 2012). From a policy perspective, this concentration of crime gun suppliers among a relatively small group of licensed dealers bolsters the case for increased oversight. It suggests that focusing enforcement resources on this set of dealers has the potential for substantial payoff in reducing the diversion of guns to criminals.

Interventions more widely focused on a larger set of dealers are also needed. For example, there is evidence that a substantial proportion of gun dealers are willing to make a sale under conditions of questionable legality. In one national study, more than half (52.5%) of dealers surveyed were willing to make a "straw sale," where one person unlawfully buys a gun intended for another (Sorenson and Vittes 2003). In another study of California firearm dealers, 20% were willing to participate in a straw sale (Wintemute 2010).

This essay examines some of the law and policy opportunities for improved regulation and oversight of firearm dealers. Existing law also creates certain obstacles for law enforcement efforts. Recommendations to address these legal obstacles are provided.

Dealer Licensing and Inspection

Under federal law, persons "engaged in the business" of selling firearms must obtain a dealer's license from the Bureau of Alcohol, Tobacco, Firearms and Explosives (ATF). The initial license costs $200 and is good for three years. Licensed dealers may purchase firearms directly from manufactures or distributors and may transfer a firearm to another licensed dealer, even across state lines, without a background check.

Seventeen U.S. states and the District of Columbia also require a state-level firearm dealer's license. Criteria for obtaining the license vary widely. Some states impose conditions such as minimum age, criminal history standards, and fingerprinting. Others simply mandate the completion of a form and payment of a licensing fee (Vernick, Webster, et al. 2006).

Regular inspection of licensed gun dealers can serve to identify those who fail to account for their inventory, violate record keeping rules, or otherwise disobey the law. Frequent or serious violations can result in revocation of a dealer's license. Even if no violation is found, regular inspection sends the message that law enforcement takes its dealer oversight mission seriously and that dealers are at greater risk if they break the law.

At the federal level, dealer oversight and inspection are the responsibility of ATF. Under the federal Firearm Owners' Protection Act (FOPA) of 1986, however, ATF is limited to one routine inspection of licensed gun dealers per year (18 U.S.C. 923(g)(1)(B)(ii)(I)). Resources for dealer oversight are also modest. As a result, most dealers are inspected much less frequently (Office of the Inspector General 2004). In 2007, ATF reported that it inspected each dealer on average only once every 17 years, though this figure may have improved more recently (Mayors Against Illegal Guns 2008). FOPA also raised the legal standard for revocation of a dealer's license to require a "willful" violation of the law—a much higher standard than the law usually imposes (18 U.S.C. § 923 (e)).

At the state level, just two states (Massachusetts and Rhode Island) mandate regular inspections of dealers. Overall, 23 states permit but do not require such inspections (Vernick, Webster, et al. 2006).

Research clearly demonstrates that enhanced dealer oversight reduces illegal gun trafficking. Webster et al. studied guns recovered by the police in 54 U.S. cities from 2000 to 2002 to identify factors associated with intrastate gun trafficking (defined as the share of guns with an interval between retail sale and recovery by the police, from someone other than the buyer, of less than one year). The authors defined strong gun dealer regulation and oversight as requiring under state law (1) a dealer's license; (2) record keeping of firearm sales; (3) dealers' premises to be open for inspections; and (4) prompt reporting of firearm thefts from dealers. After controlling for other factors, cities in states with strong dealer regulation had a much lower measure of intrastate gun trafficking (Webster, Vernick, and Bulzacchelli 2009).

Regarding *interstate* gun trafficking, research by Mayors Against Illegal Guns has demonstrated that states neither requiring nor permitting inspections of gun dealers are much more likely to export crime guns to other states than are jurisdictions with these laws. In fact, the average exporting rate for states without dealer inspection laws is 50% greater than for states with these laws (Mayors Against Illegal Guns 2008). Other research has also demonstrated that comprehensive enforcement of gun sales laws reduced gun trafficking in Boston (Braga and Pierce 2005).

Undercover Stings and Lawsuits against Gun Dealers

In some jurisdictions, police have used crime gun trace data to identify local firearm dealers selling disproportionate numbers of guns used in crime. Law enforcement has then conducted targeted enforcement efforts.

In 1998 and 1999, law enforcement in Chicago, Detroit, and Gary, Indiana, conducted undercover stings of retail gun stores suspecting of facilitating large numbers of illegal firearm sales. Police posed as gang members looking to "settle scores" or as straw buyers. After a number of the dealers were video-taped making illegal sales, the cities each separately sued those gun dealers. The lawsuits in Chicago and Detroit received substantial press coverage. An evaluation of the stings and lawsuits in Chicago, Detroit, and Gary compared gun trafficking indicators in these cities with three comparable midwestern cities (Cincinnati, Cleveland, and St. Louis) that did not conduct stings. The researchers found a 62% reduction in trafficked guns sold by in-state retailers in Chicago ($p < 0.001$); a 36% decline in Detroit ($p = 0.051$); and a nonsignificant increase in Gary, where the intervention and publicity were less robust (Webster, Bulzacchelli, et al. 2006).

The ability for litigation to serve as an important public health tool to address scofflaw gun dealers and the supply of crime guns was diminished in 2005 with the enactment of the federal Protection of Lawful Commerce in Arms Act (PLCAA). Under the PLCAA, gun makers and dealers received substantial protection against lawsuits "resulting from the criminal or unlawful misuse of a qualified product by the person or a third party." Following the PLCAA, numerous lawsuits brought by municipalities and individuals arguing, in part, that firearm manufacturers failed to adequately supervise their dealers, were dismissed (Vernick, Rutkow, and Salmon).

One important exception to the PLCAA allows lawsuits against gun dealers to proceed if the dealer "knowingly" violated laws governing firearm sales. A series of undercover stings and lawsuits brought by New York City took advantage of this exception. In 2006, New York City identified 55 gun dealers in seven states who were supplying guns used in crime in the city. During an undercover sting operation, 27 of these dealers were caught facilitating illegal sales and were sued by the city. Nearly all agreed to settle their case by agreeing to a number of changes to their business practices to reduce illegal gun sales. These changes were overseen by a special master. Webster and Vernick studied the effects of the settlement on crime guns recovered from

10 dealers. The odds that a crime gun sold by one of these 10 dealers was later recovered in New York City were 84% lower after the change in business practices (Webster and Vernick, in this volume).

Access to Trace Data and the Tiahrt Amendment

Firearm trace data supplied by ATF have been critical to identifying problem dealers in need of enhanced oversight. The case of a prominent gun dealer in the Milwaukee area, Badger Guns and Ammo, provides a powerful example of the potential utility of trace data. In May 1999, ATF publicly released information that Badger led the nation in the number of guns sold that were later traced to crime. Just a few days later, Badger announced that it would no longer sell small, poorly made handguns, known as "junk guns" or "Saturday Night Specials," which are favored by some criminals and disproportionately traced to crime (Vernick, Webster, and Hepburn 1999; Webster, Vernick, and Hepburn 2002). Following this change in sales practices, there was a 71% decline in the number of new Saturday Night Special crime guns recovered in Milwaukee and an overall 44% decline in the recovery of all guns with indicia of trafficking (i.e., recovery within one year from a user other than the initial buyer) (Webster et al. 2006).

However, beginning in 2003, an amendment to ATF's annual appropriation by Congress has limited the release of trace data. Named after its sponsor, Representative Todd Tiahrt (R-KS), the Tiahrt Amendment began modestly, stating: "No funds appropriated under this Act . . . shall be available to take any action based upon . . . [the Freedom of Information Act] with respect to records . . . maintained pursuant to [the Gun Control Act] . . . or provided by . . . law enforcement agencies in connection with . . . the tracing of a firearm" (Pub. L. No. 108-7 § 644 (2003)). From 2003 to 2008, the Tiahrt Amendment was slowly expanded to prohibit any release of individual trace data by ATF to the public (including researchers); use of trace data in civil litigation; requiring dealers to conduct a physical inventory of their firearms as part of a compliance inspection; and maintaining records of background checks from firearm purchase applications for more than 24 hours (Tang 2009; Mayors Against Illegal Guns 2013).

In addition to impeding research on illegal gun trafficking, there is evidence that the Tiahrt Amendment may have emboldened some gun dealers who no longer needed to fear disclosure of trace data to the public. Researchers were able to obtain trace information directly from the Milwaukee police department (though not for comparison cities) for the period from 2003 to 2006 to study the effects of the Tiahrt Amendment on Badger Guns and Ammo. The adoption of the Tiahrt Amendment was associated with a 203% increase in the number of guns diverted to criminals within one year of retail sale by Badger (Webster et al. 2012).

Recommendations

The law has an important opportunity to either hinder or facilitate greater oversight of licensed gun dealers. Importantly, such oversight need not interfere with law-abiding citizens' rights under the Constitution's Second Amendment (Vernick et al. 2011).

The following six recommendations are based on the research findings described in this essay.

1. *Portions of the Firearm Owners' Protection Act (FOPA) should be repealed.* These portions limit routine dealer inspections by ATF to one per year and raise the legal standard for revocation of a dealer's license. Honest firearm dealers do not need these protections and they impede identification and prosecution of the minority of dealers who violate the law.

2. *Funds should be allocated to permit ATF to conduct regular routine inspections of gun dealers.* These inspections can identify inventory or record keeping irregularities and generally send the message that gun dealers face an increased risk of being caught if they flout the law.

3. *ATF should be granted authority to impose a range of sanctions—including license suspension, fines, or other penalties—for dealers who violate gun sales or other laws.* ATF needs the authority to impose a range of administrative sanctions, short of criminal prosecution, to address problems with scofflaw dealers before they escalate.

4. *All states should mandate a state-level firearm dealer's license in addition to the federal license.* This would provide states with leverage to revoke a license if a dealer is caught making illegal sales, without needing to rely upon the often lengthy federal revocation process. All 50 U.S. states require a license for persons engaged in practices as mundane as cosmetology. Businesses with the public safety implications of dealing in firearms merit at least as much state-level oversight.

5. *The Protection of Lawful Commerce in Arms Act (PLCAA) should be repealed.* The PLCAA interferes with litigation's ability to serve as a restraint on the dangerous practices of firearm dealers and manufacturers. There is no evidence that the firearm industry needs or merits this unprecedented liability protection.

6. *The Tiahrt Amendment should be repealed.* Researchers should have access to trace data to understand how illegal gun markets respond to changes in business practices, law enforcement efforts, or new legislation. Requiring dealers to conduct a physical inventory of their firearms as part of compliance inspections can help to identify those who sell guns off-the-books or who otherwise cannot account for their stock.

ACKNOWLEDGMENTS

The authors wish to thank the Johns Hopkins University for supporting the development of this essay. Much of the research described, conducted by Johns Hopkins faculty, was supported by the Joyce Foundation of Chicago or by gifts from an anonymous donor.

REFERENCES

Braga, Anthony A., Pierce, Glen L. 2005. "Disrupting Illegal Firearms Markets in Boston: The Effects of Operation Ceasefire on the Supply of New Handguns to Criminals." *Criminology and Public Policy* 4:717–748.

Braga, Anthony A., Wintemute, Garen J., Pierce, Glenn L., Cook, Philip J., Ridgeway, Greg. 2012. "Interpreting the Empirical Evidence on Illegal Gun Market Dynamics." *Journal of Urban Health* 89:779–793.

Bureau of Alcohol, Tobacco, Firearms and Explosives (BATF). 2000a. *Commerce in Firearms in the United States.* Washington, DC: US Department of the Treasury.

Bureau of Alcohol, Tobacco, Firearms and Explosives (BATF). 2000b. *Following the Gun: Enforcing Federal Gun Laws against Firearms Traffickers.* Washington, DC: US Department of the Treasury.

Bureau of Alcohol, Tobacco, Firearms and Explosives. Listing of Federal Firearm Licensees. http://www.atf.gov/about/foia/ffl-list.html.

Mayors Against Illegal Guns. 2008. *The Movement of Illegal Guns in America.* New York: Mayors Against Illegal Guns, December.

Mayors Against Illegal Guns. 2013. *The Tiahrt Amendments.* http://www.mayors againstillegalguns.org/html/federal/tiahrt.shtml.

Office of the Inspector General, US Department of Justice. 2004. *Inspection of Firearm Dealers by the Bureau of Alcohol, Tobacco, Firearms, and Explosives.* Report Number I-2004–005 (July).

Sorenson, Susan B., and Vittes, Katherine A. 2003. "Buying a Handgun for Someone Else: Firearm Dealer Willingness to Sell." *Injury Prevention* 9:147–150.

Tang, Angela J. 2009. "Taking Aim at Tiahrt." *William and Mary Law Review* 50: 1787–1829.

Vernick, Jon S., Rutkow, Lainie, Salmon, Daniel A. 2007. "Availability of Litigation as a Public Health Tool for Firearm Injury Prevention: Comparison of Guns, Vaccines, and Motor Vehicles." *American Journal of Public Health* 97:1991–1997.

Vernick, Jon S., Rutkow, Lainie, Webster, Daniel W., Teret, Stephen P. 2011. "Changing the Constitutional Landscape for Firearms: The Supreme Court's Recent Second Amendment Decisions." *American Journal of Public Health* 101:2021–2026.

Vernick, Jon S., Webster, Daniel W., Bulzacchelli, Maria T., Mair, Julie S. 2006. "Regulation of Firearm Dealers in the United States: An Analysis of State Law and Opportunities for Improvement." *Journal of Law, Medicine & Ethics* 765–775.

Vernick, Jon S., Webster, Daniel W., Hepburn, Lisa M. 1999. "Effects of Maryland's Law Banning Saturday Night Special Handguns on Crime Guns." *Injury Prevention* 5:259–263.

Webster, Daniel W., Bulzacchelli, Maria T., Zeoli, April M., Vernick, Jon S. 2006. "Effects of Undercover Police Stings of Gun Dealers on the Supply of New Guns to Criminals." *Injury Prevention* 12: 225–230.

Webster, Daniel W., Vernick, Jon S., Bulzacchelli, Maria T. 2006. "Effects of a Gun Dealer's Change in Sales Practices on the Supply of Guns to Criminals." *Journal of Urban Health* 83:778–787.

Webster, Daniel W., Vernick, Jon S., Bulzacchelli, Maria T. 2009. "Effects of Firearm Seller Accountability Policies on Firearm Trafficking." *Journal of Urban Health* 86:525–537.

Webster, Daniel W., Vernick, Jon S., Bulzacchelli, Maria T., Vittes, Katherine A. 2012. "Temporal Association between Federal Gun Laws and the Diversion of Guns to Criminals in Milwaukee." *Journal of Urban Health* 89:87–97.

Webster, Daniel W., Vernick, Jon S., Hepburn, Lisa M. 2002. "Effects of Maryland's Law Banning Saturday Night Special Handguns on Homicides." *American Journal of Epidemiology* 155: 406–412.

Wintemute, Garen. 2010. "Firearm Retailers' Willingness to Participate in an Illegal Gun Purchase." *Journal of Urban Health* 87:865–878.

Wintemute, Garen J., Cook, Phillip J., Wright, Mona A. 2005. "Risk Factors among Handgun Retailers for Frequent and Disproportionate Sales of Guns Used in Violent and Firearm Related Crimes." *Injury Prevention* 11:357–363.

Part II / Making Gun Laws Enforceable

Enforcing Federal Laws against Firearms Traffickers

Raising Operational Effectiveness by Lowering Enforcement Obstacles

Anthony A. Braga and Peter L. Gagliardi

Research suggests that only about one of every six firearms used in a crime was obtained legally (Reiss and Roth 1993) and that most serious gun violence is committed by a relatively small number of very active criminals (Braga 2003; Cook, Ludwig, and Braga 2005). Clearly, the United States has a large problem with the illegal acquisition of guns by high-risk individuals who should not have access to them. Criminal demand for guns is influenced by a number of factors such as fear of victimization and status concerns, technological concerns (e.g., concealment, caliber), and economic concerns (e.g., affordability) (Sheley and Wright 1995; Wright and Rossi 1994). While semi-automatic assault rifles have been misused in some high-profile tragedies, such as the horrific school shooting in Newtown, Connecticut, handguns are most frequently recovered in crime by law enforcement agencies (Cook, Braga, and Moore 2011).

Anthony A. Braga, PhD, is the Don M. Gottfredson Professor of Evidence-Based Criminology in the School of Criminal Justice at Rutgers University and a Senior Research Fellow in the Program in Criminal Justice Policy and Management at Harvard University. Peter L. Gagliardi is the Senior Vice President, Forensic Technology Inc.

One broad class of gun control policy instruments are those designed to influence who has access to different kinds of firearms (Braga, Cook, et al. 2002; Cook, Braga, and Moore 2011). In essence, these "supply-side" interventions seek to reduce gun crimes by keeping guns out of the wrong hands without denying access to legitimate owners or infringing on legitimate uses of guns. In maintaining legal firearms commerce for law-abiding citizens, there is the serious problem of preventing illegal transfers. That prevention currently is being handled very poorly. Loopholes in existing gun laws weaken accountability of licensed gun dealers and private sellers; this facilitates illegal transfers by scofflaw licensed gun dealers, generates difficulty in screening out ineligible buyers, and, most important, results in a vigorous and largely unregulated secondary market—gun sales by private individuals—in which used guns change hands (Cook, Molloconi, and Cole 1995).

Unfortunately, no rigorous field experiments have tested whether supply-side strategies would reduce criminal gun acquisition and use. While guns used in crimes are stolen from legal owners, the available scientific evidence suggests that a noteworthy portion of crime guns are illegally diverted from legal commerce. Research also suggests that supply-side interventions have promise in limiting criminal access to firearms. A key element of supply-side interventions involves the investigation, apprehension, and prosecution of illegal gun traffickers and others who illegally divert guns to criminals. Unfortunately, the investigation of illegal gun traffickers is hampered by a variety of enforcement obstacles.

In this essay, we briefly review the available research on the workings of illegal gun markets and the potential efficacy of supply-side interventions designed to disrupt the flow of illegal guns to criminals. We then make policy and legislative recommendations to improve the enforcement of federal firearms laws against gun traffickers.

Evidence

Much of the evidence in support of supply-side interventions comes from analyses of U.S. Bureau of Alcohol, Tobacco, Firearms and Explosives (ATF) firearm trace data and firearms trafficking investigations that indicate some percentage of the guns used in crime were recently diverted from legal firearms commerce (ATF 1997, 2000, 2002; Braga, Wintemute et al. 2012; Cook and Braga 2001; Pierce et al. 2004). Firearm tracing makes it possible, at least in principle, to determine the chain of commerce for a firearm from the point of import or manufacture to the first retail sale (and beyond, in states that maintain records of gun purchases). Unfortunately, not all firearms can be traced and firearm trace data have some widely recognized limits. The National Academies' Committee to Improve Research Information and Data on Firearms, however, suggests that the validity of conclusions drawn from firearm trace data research depends on the care taken in the application and analyses of these data (National Research Council 2005).

Among the main findings of these research studies are (1) new guns are recovered disproportionately in crime (Cook and Braga 2001; Pierce et al. 2004; Zimring 1976). (2) Some licensed firearm retailers are disproportionately frequent sources of crime guns; these retailers are linked to more guns traced by ATF than would be expected from their overall volume of gun sales (there could be many reasons for these patterns; see Wintemute 2005). (3) Under test conditions, significant proportions of licensed retailers and private party gun sellers will knowingly participate in illegal gun sales (Sorenson and Vittes 2003; Wintemute 2010). (4) On average, about one-third of guns used in crime in any community are acquired in that community, another third come from elsewhere in the same state, and a third are brought from other states (ATF 1997, 2002; Cook and Braga 2001). (5) There are longstanding interstate trafficking routes for crime guns, typically from states with weaker gun regulations to states with stronger ones. The best known of these is the "Iron Pipeline" from the Southeast to the Middle Atlantic and New England (Cook and Braga 2001; Pierce et al. 2004).

Analyses of ATF firearm trafficking investigation data reveal that illegal gun traffickers exploit an incredibly leaky legal firearms commerce system. For instance, a 2000 report examining 1,530 gun trafficking investigations made by ATF between July 1, 1996, and December 31, 1998, found that more than 84,000 firearms were diverted from legal to illegal commerce (ATF 2000). The report identified the primary gun trafficking pathways as scofflaw and negligent firearms dealers, "straw man" legal purchasers who provide guns to criminals, and illegal diversions through secondary market sources such as gun shows, flea markets, and want ads. The analysis also revealed the organized theft of firearms from licensed dealers, common carriers, and residences as illegal diversion pathways. Moreover, ATF (2000) found that 61 percent of the cases involved the diversion of twenty or fewer firearms, and it concluded that most but not all gun trafficking investigations involve a relatively small number of firearms. The two largest gun trafficking cases involved the illegal diversion of some 11,000 and 10,000 firearms, respectively.

While survey research highlights the importance of theft and secondary market acquisitions in supplying adult criminals and juveniles with guns, these studies also complement analyses of firearm trace and investigation data in suggesting a fairly substantial role, either direct or indirect, for retail outlet sales in supplying criminals with guns. About 27 percent of state prisoners in a U.S. Bureau of Justice Statistics survey said they acquired their most recent handgun from a retail outlet (Beck and Gilliard 1993). Similarly, Wright and Rossi (1994) reported that 21 percent of male prisoners had acquired their most recent handgun from a licensed dealer. Sheley and Wright (1995) found that 32 percent of juvenile inmates had asked someone, typically a friend or family member, to straw purchase a gun for them in a gun shop, pawnshop, or other retail outlet. All three survey studies also found that "street" and "black market" sources are important, sources that may well include traffickers who are buying from retail outlets and selling on the street.

Despite multiple illegal sources of firearms for criminals, ethnographic research suggests that illegal gun markets may not work well in particular urban environments. Cook, Ludwig, and Braga (2005) found evidence of considerable frictions in the underground market for guns in Chicago. These frictions existed mainly because the underground gun market was both illegal and "thin"—the number of buyers, sellers, and total transactions was small, and relevant information on reliable sources of guns was scarce. The research further found that Chicago street gangs helped to overcome these market frictions, but the gangs' economic interests caused gang leaders to limit their supply primarily to gang members, and even then transactions were usually loans or rentals with strings attached. Thin underground gun markets may be particularly vulnerable to focused gun market disruption strategies.

A growing body of evaluation evidence suggests that enforcement and regulatory interventions focused on retail sales practices can generate subsequent reductions in new guns recovered in crime. In Detroit and Chicago, the number of guns recovered within a year of first retail sale from someone other than the original purchaser was sharply reduced after undercover police stings and lawsuits targeted scofflaw retail dealers (Webster, Zeoli, et al. 2006). In Boston, a gun market disruption strategy that focused on the illegal diversion of new handguns from retail outlets in Massachusetts, southern states along Interstate 95, and elsewhere resulted in a significant reduction in the percentage of new handguns recovered in crime by the Boston Police Department (Braga and Pierce 2005).

In Milwaukee, the number of guns recovered within a year of first retail sale from someone other than the original purchaser dramatically decreased after voluntary changes in the sales practices of a gun dealer that received negative publicity for leading the United States in selling the most guns recovered by police in crime (Webster, Vernick, and Bulzacchelli 2006). In Chicago, an analysis of recovered crime handguns found that the 1994 implementation of the Brady Handgun Violence Prevention Act was associated with a marked decrease in crime handguns imported from states that were required to institute the provisions of the Act (Cook and Braga 2001). The Brady Act mandated licensed dealers to conduct a criminal background check on all handgun buyers and required a one-week waiting period before transferring the gun to a criminal.

Policy Implications

Research suggests that supply-side interventions could be used to good effect in reducing the illegal supply of firearms to criminals. It is the responsibility of ATF, often working with state and local law enforcement, to investigate criminal firearms trafficking, arrest the perpetrators, and refer them to U.S. Attorneys for prosecution. Unfortunately, some major obstacles hinder federal law enforcement efforts to hold gun traffickers accountable for their crimes (Braga 2001). ATF is essentially working with one hand tied behind its back because of the way the federal firearms laws are written, cuts to its operating budgets, and persistent political interference. Here, we make six policy and legislative recommendations to improve the capacity of the U.S. Department of Justice to enforce federal laws against gun traffickers. This list should not be considered exhaustive as other opportunities certainly exist.

1. *Require the Execution of Private Sales through Federal Firearms Licensees.* The lack of background checks and transaction paperwork in the secondary market makes it easy for prohibited persons to acquire firearms and difficult for law enforcement agencies to prevent, detect, and prosecute illicit buyers and sellers who operate in the secondary market. Secondary market transactions are legal but not subjected to any federal requirement that the transaction be formally recorded or paperwork maintained. Most states do not have laws that require a record of secondary market transactions. The

main federal legal requirement is that the private seller may not knowingly transfer firearms to proscribed persons such as felons, fugitives, drug users, and illegal aliens. The provisions of the 1994 Brady Act do not apply to secondary firearms market transactions; therefore, criminal background checks of the prospective buyer are not conducted during these private transactions. Requiring private sales to be executed through federally licensed gun dealers would effectively close a major legal loophole exploited by gun traffickers and criminals. As part of these reforms, mandatory reporting of multiple purchases of handguns should be extended to include multiple purchases of certain long guns (e.g., semi-automatic rifles capable of accepting high-capacity magazines), similar to current practices in states along the southwest border of the United States with Mexico.

The enforcement of laws against gun trafficking is also hindered by the cumbersome procedure ATF uses to trace firearms. Most of the relevant firearms transaction records are not centralized but kept piecemeal, much in paper form, by the dealers, distributors, and manufacturers. This arrangement reflects the intention of Congress to ensure that there would be no national registry of firearms owners while maintaining some mechanism to allow crime investigators to trace a firearm. Modest changes to the system could make a big difference (Travis and Smarrito 1992). For example, a requirement for licensed dealers to report serial numbers for all gun transfers to ATF would greatly facilitate the tracing process without creating a central registry of gun owners. Electronic exchange of this information by means of a web portal would significantly expedite the process.

2. *Enact Effective Firearms Diversion/Trafficking Statutes.* There are no federal laws that specifically prohibit firearms trafficking and that adequately reflect the public safety risks of straw purchasing of weapons. For instance, there are no defined elements of gun trafficking in existing federal statutes such as the identification of a threshold number of illegally diverted guns and the establishment of a nexus to criminal activity. While there are nearly 40 federal statutes that touch on the various relevant areas of the illegal diversion of firearms (see ATF 2009), ATF agents commonly rely upon two statutes when investigating gun trafficking crimes: engaging in the business of dealing firearms without a license (Title 18, Section 922(a)(1)(A)) and falsifying the ATF Form 4473 (Title 18, Section 922(a)(6)).

The 1986 McClure-Volkmer Firearm Owners' Protection Act (FOPA) makes it very difficult to prosecute gun traffickers for dealing firearms without a license. Individuals who make occasional gun sales, buy guns as a hobby, or sell firearms from their private collections are exempt from acquiring a federal firearms license. Gun traffickers exploit this gaping hole in licensing law to illegally divert guns to criminals and juveniles. Since the telltale paperwork is not available for these unregulated transactions, firearms traffickers operating in the secondary market can easily avoid prosecution by claiming that they were selling only a handful of firearms from their private collection. Although federal law penalizes individuals who make false statements on firearms transfer paperwork, it is difficult for ATF agents to prove that straw purchasers are falsifying paperwork, purchasing firearms for proscribed persons rather than buying firearms for their personal collections and subsequently selling them lawfully on the unregulated secondary market. The problem is compounded because document falsification violations are seldom viewed by prosecutors as appealing cases to bring before a jury.

A telling analysis of the disposition of 1,530 ATF firearms trafficking investigations suggests that prosecuting unlicensed dealers for engaging in the business of selling firearms and for straw purchasing presents a significant challenge in court (ATF 2000). Although ATF agents reported that dealing without a license and falsifying paperwork violations were occurring in cases accepted for prosecution, the prosecutor was able to charge at least one defendant with these violations in less than 38% of cases involving dealing without a license and less than 45% of the straw purchasing cases. In these cases, defendants were charged with being a convicted felon in possession of firearms, drug offenses, or other crimes revealed during the investigation.

3. *Revisit Sentencing Guidelines for Firearm Diversion/Trafficking Crimes.* Penalties for the illegal diversion of firearms should reflect the serious public safety consequences of these crimes. Since guns are durable goods, even one illegal gun can have repetitive and dire consequences. For instance, ballistic imaging analysis of a single handgun recovered by the Boston Police Department revealed that, in one year, it had been used in 14 violent crimes across four cities in two states (Gagliardi 2010). Prosecuting scofflaw dealers, who are associated with the illegal diversion of multiple guns, is often frustrating for U.S. Attorneys and ATF investigators. For instance, corrupt licensed dealers illegally divert firearms through record keeping violations such as making false entries in their records and failing to keep the required transfer information. Although a corrupt licensed dealer may illegally divert hundreds of guns to the street, these record keeping violations are primarily misdemeanors.

Gun traffickers are often prosecuted for associated criminal conduct because trafficking charges are difficult to prove and sometimes carry lesser penalties when compared to other crimes such as being a felon in possession of a firearm or drug trafficking (ATF 2000). One quarter of firearms traffickers in the ATF analyses were charged with being a convicted felon in possession of a firearm and another 6% were charged with other prohibited persons charges. More than 27% were charged with conspiracy charges and over 12% were charged with a narcotics violation. Gun trafficking investigations are sometimes prosecuted as drug trafficking cases because prosecutors prefer the mandatory minimum sentencing provisions. For instance, using a firearm during the commission of a drug trafficking or violent crime (Title 18, Section 924(c)) carries a mandatory five-year imprisonment sentence.

Most gun criminals, unfortunately, do not have prior felony convictions (Greenfeld and Zawitz 1995). Corrupt licensed dealers and individuals who execute straw purchases are legally entitled to engage in firearm transfers and, by definition, not felons or drug abusers. Therefore, although prosecutors and ATF agents are creatively using the existing federal laws to make cases against gun traffickers, this type of prosecution strategy clearly has its limits.

4. *Develop and Implement Regional Crime Gun–Processing Protocols.* Gun crime investigations are seriously undermined when local jurisdictions do not comprehensively process all recovered crime guns and related evidence (see IACP 2011). Without these comprehensive data, federal, state, and local agencies are not able to develop an accurate assessment of the sources of illegal guns and their use in violent crime. Law enforcement agencies at the local, state, and federal level should conduct a thorough review of their internal directives on the processing of the crime guns and related evidence. Policy procedures should include processing for ballistic evidence as well as DNA, latent fingerprints, and trace evidence from firearms; processing projectiles and casings through the ATF National Integrated Ballistics Information Network (NIBIN); conducting firearms traces; and reporting to the National Crime Information Center (NCIC) (see Gagliardi 2010). The various law enforcement agencies operating within a given region should collaborate on the design of mutually agreeable crime gun–processing protocols.

5. *Create a Strong and Effective ATF.* ATF is underfunded, often without stable leadership, and routinely whipsawed by special interests and Congress. Despite the number of gun dealers having reached nearly 130,000 federal licensees, ATF's budget has been largely stagnant, increasing from $850 million in FY

2002 to only $1.1 billion in FY 2012. ATF had to eliminate more than $2 million in field contractor support and shut down 66% of its ballistic-imaging workstation sites across the United States for its NIBIN program in FY 2012. ATF has only some 2,500 special agents and roughly 800 inspectors. In terms of law enforcement personnel, the agency is roughly the same size as a city police department (the Boston Police Department has an authorized strength of some 2,250 officers). ATF has only enough inspectors to check every licensed firearms dealer once every ten years. Finally, ATF has been led by an acting director since the last confirmed director, Carl Truscott, resigned in August 2004.

In their roles as guardians of the Second Amendment, the National Rifle Association (NRA) and gun-rights politicians consistently meddle in ATF investigative initiatives. For instance, in February 2006, Congress convened two hearings on ATF's enforcement activities at eight gun shows in Richmond, Virginia, that resulted in an Inspector General's review of ATF's gun show investigation operations. Four witnesses testified that ATF agents used aggressive and harassing techniques. These individuals included the gun show promoter, a federal firearms licensee, a salesman working for a licensed gun dealer, and a private investigator hired by the NRA. The hearings did not reveal any illegal activities or other violations by ATF.

ATF needs to be properly funded to perform its mission now and in the future as newly mandated responsibilities are added. The agency clearly needs stable leadership now. Like the director of the Federal Bureau of Investigation, the ATF director's position should be a fixed ten-year term. This would ensure that the position is professional and nonpartisan and that it spans the political turnover of four-year presidential election cycles. ATF should also be able to more closely regulate the business practices of licensed dealers and set standards for secure storage and common carrier transportation of firearms and ammunition.

6. *Publish an Annual National Crime Gun-Tracing Report.* Rational debate on gun policy requires detailed information on crime guns. ATF currently produces only modest summaries of the characteristics of crime gun traces for the 50 states, the District of Columbia, U.S. territories, Canada, Mexico, and the Caribbean (www.atf.gov/statistics/index.html). Unlike the national and city-level trace reports generated by the now-defunct Youth Crime Gun Interdiction Initiative (e.g., ATF 1997, 2002), ATF's current state-level crime gun summaries do not involve external academics and do not provide more rigorous and detailed analyses of crime gun sources, trends, and patterns.

ATF should return to publishing these more detailed annual crime gun trace reports overseen by external academics.

To complement the routine reporting of detailed crime gun statistics, the U.S. government should also lift restrictions on the release of ATF trace data as mandated by the Tiahrt Amendment, remove ideological and politically motivated barriers to conducting basic gun research through grants from the Centers for Disease Control and Prevention (CDC) and the National Institutes of Health (NIH), and increase funding for gun violence reduction research through the National Institute of Justice (NIJ). Indeed, much of the research evidence reviewed here was initiated prior to the passage of the Tiahrt Amendment.

Conclusion

The available evidence suggests that reducing the flow of guns to criminals may indeed disrupt their capacity to kill. Better record keeping and improved regulation of gun transactions can reduce access to guns by criminals and assist law enforcement agencies in launching investigations and prosecuting gun criminals. However, a measurable impact on firearms trafficking and related violence requires an adequate commitment of resources in terms of people, processes, and technology. For further gains, the firearms supply chain must be made more secure. The operational capacity of ATF must be strengthened. Success against firearms trafficking will be achieved only by separating firearms trafficking strategy from gun politics.

Reflecting upon the research and development experiences from the Clinton administration and early days of the George W. Bush administration, we suggest there should be a reinvigoration of the fusion of all-source information on crime gun sources along with comprehensive analysis and reporting, in which all sides of the gun control debate can be confident. Increased law enforcement–academic analysis and reporting of ATF firearms trace can begin the effort. Public safety and the public debate in the United States and other countries will surely benefit from the best possible information on the illegal sources of guns to criminals. Without credible data and rigorous analyses, the broader gun control policy debate will be based on ideology and conjecture. The case for a supply-side approach to gun violence is well supported by the empirical evidence on illegal gun market dynamics. To date, however, there is little empirical evidence that such an approach reduces rates of gun crime. We believe that it is time to develop experimental evidence on whether interventions designed to limit illegal transfers of firearms can reduce gun violence.

REFERENCES

Beck, Allen, and Darrell Gilliard. 1993. *Survey of State Prison Inmates, 1991*. Washington, DC: U.S. Bureau of Justice Statistics.

Braga, Anthony A. 2001. More Gun Laws or More Gun Law Enforcement? *Journal of Policy Analysis and Management* 20: 545–549.

Braga, Anthony A. 2003. Serious Youth Gun Offenders and the Epidemic of Youth Violence in Boston. *Journal of Quantitative Criminology*, 19: 33–54.

Braga, Anthony A., Philip J. Cook, David M. Kennedy, and Mark H. Moore. 2002. The Illegal Supply of Firearms. In *Crime and Justice: A Review of Research*, vol. 29, edited by Michael Tonry. Chicago: University of Chicago Press.

Braga, Anthony A., and Glenn L. Pierce. 2005. Disrupting Illegal Firearms Markets in Boston: The Effects of Operation Ceasefire on the Supply of New Handguns to Criminals. *Criminology & Public Policy* 4: 717–748.

Braga, Anthony A., Garen J. Wintemute, Glenn L. Pierce, Philip J. Cook, and Greg Ridgeway. 2012. Interpreting the Empirical Evidence on Illegal Gun Market Dynamics. *Journal of Urban Health* 89: 779–793.

Cook, Philip J., and Anthony A. Braga. 2001. Comprehensive Firearms Tracing: Strategic and Investigative Uses of New Data on Firearms Markets. *Arizona Law Review* 43: 277–309.

Cook, Philip J., Anthony A. Braga, and Mark H. Moore. 2011. Gun Control. In *Crime and Public Policy*, rev. ed., edited by James Q. Wilson and Joan Petersilia. New York: Oxford University Press.

Cook, Philip J., Jens Ludwig, and Anthony A. Braga. 2005. Criminal Records of Homicide Offenders. *Journal of the American Medical Association* 294: 598–601.

Cook, Philip J., Jens Ludwig, Sudhir Venkatesh, and Anthony A. Braga. 2007. Underground Gun Markets. *Economic Journal* 117: 558–588.

Cook, Philip J., Stephanie Molloconi, and Thomas Cole. 1995. Regulating Gun Markets. *Journal of Criminal Law and Criminology* 86: 59–92.

Gagliardi, Peter L. 2010. *The 13 Critical Tasks: An Inside-Out Approach to Solving More Gun Crime*. Montreal, Quebec: Forensic Technology Inc.

Greenfeld, Lawrence, and Marianne Zawitz. 1995. *Weapons Offenses and Offenders*. Washington, DC: U.S. Bureau of Justice Statistics.

International Association of Chiefs of Police (IACP). 2011. *Reducing Gun Violence in Our Communities*. Alexandria, VA: IACP.

National Research Council. 2005. *Firearms and Violence: A Critical Review*. Committee to Improve Research and Information on Firearms. Washington, DC: National Academies Press.

Pierce, Glenn L., Anthony A. Braga, Raymond R. Hyatt, and Christopher S. Koper. 2004. The Characteristics and Dynamics of Illegal Firearms Markets: Implications for a Supply-Side Enforcement Strategy. *Justice Quarterly* 21: 391–422.

Reiss, Albert J., and Jeffrey Roth, eds. 1993. *Understanding and Preventing Violence.* Washington, DC: National Academies Press.

Sheley, Joseph, and James D. Wright. 1995. *In the Line of Fire: Youth, Guns, and Violence in Urban America.* New York: Aldine de Gruyter.

Sorenson, Susan and Katherine Vittes. 2003. Buying a Handgun for Someone Else: Firearm Retailer Willingness to Sell. *Injury Prevention* 9: 147–150.

Travis, Jeremy, and William Smarrito. 1992. A Modest Proposal to End Gun Running in America. *Fordham Urban Law Journal* 19: 795–811.

U.S. Bureau of Alcohol, Tobacco and Firearms (ATF). 1997. *Crime Gun Trace Analysis Reports (1997): The Illegal Firearms Market in 17 Communities.* Washington, DC: Bureau of Alcohol, Tobacco and Firearms.

U.S. Bureau of Alcohol, Tobacco and Firearms (ATF). 2000. *Following the Gun: Enforcing Federal Laws against Firearms Traffickers.* Washington, DC: ATF.

U.S. Bureau of Alcohol, Tobacco and Firearms (ATF). 2002. *Crime Gun Trace Analysis (2000): National Report.* Washington, DC: ATF.

U.S. Bureau of Alcohol, Tobacco, Firearms and Explosives (ATF). 2009. *Firearms Trafficking Investigation Guide.* Washington, DC: U.S. Department of Justice.

Webster, Daniel W., Jon Vernick, and Maria Bulzacchelli. 2006. Effects of a Gun Dealer's Change in Sales Practices on the Supply of Guns to Criminals. *Journal of Urban Health* 83: 778–787.

Webster, Daniel W., April Zeoli, Maria Bulzacchelli, and Jon Vernick. 2006. Effects of Police Stings of Gun Dealers on the Supply of New Guns to Criminals. *Injury Prevention* 12: 225–230.

Wintemute, Garen J. 2005. Risk Factors among Handgun Retailers for Frequent and Disproportionate Sales of Guns Used in Violent and Firearm Related Crimes. *Injury Prevention* 11: 357–363.

Wintemute, Garen J. 2010. Firearm Retailers' Willingness to Participate in an Illegal Gun Purchase. *Journal of Urban Health* 87: 865–878.

Wright, James D., and Peter H. Rossi. 1994. *Armed and Considered Dangerous.* 2nd ed. New York: Aldine de Gruyter.

Zimring, Franklin E. 1976. Street Crime and New Guns: Some Implications for Firearms Control. *Journal of Criminal Justice* 4: 95–107.

Part III / Gun Policy Lessons from the United States

High-Risk Guns

America's Experience with the Federal Assault Weapons Ban, 1994–2004

Key Findings and Implications

Christopher S. Koper

In 1994, the federal government imposed a ten year ban on military-style semi-automatic firearms and ammunition-feeding devices holding more than ten rounds of ammunition. This legislation, commonly known as the federal assault weapons ban, was intended in the broadest sense to reduce gunshot victimizations by limiting the national stock of semi-automatic firearms with large ammunition capacities and other features conducive to criminal uses. Reflecting America's general political divisions over the issue of gun control, the debate over the law was highly contentious. Ten years later, Congress allowed the ban to expire.

More recently, there have been growing calls for a reexamination of the assault weapons issue. This debate has been fueled by a series of mass shooting incidents involving previously banned firearms or magazines. Since 2007, for example, there have been at least 11 incidents in which offenders using

Christopher S. Koper, PhD, is an associate professor in the Department of Criminology, Law and Society at George Mason University and a senior fellow and co-director of the Research Program on Evidence-Based Policing at George Mason's Center for Evidence-Based Crime Policy.

assault weapons or other semi-automatics with magazines larger than 10 rounds have wounded or killed eight or more people (Violence Policy Center 2012). Some of the most notorious of these incidents have been a 2007 shooting on the college campus of Virginia Tech that left 33 dead and 17 wounded; a 2011 shooting in an Arizona parking lot that killed 6 and wounded 13, including Congresswoman Gabrielle Giffords; a 2012 shooting in an Aurora, Colorado, movie theatre that left 12 dead and 58 wounded; and, most recently, a shooting in a Newtown, Connecticut, elementary school that left 26 victims dead, 20 of whom were children (an additional victim was killed elsewhere).

To help inform the new dialogue on this issue, this essay examines America's experience with the 1994 assault weapons law. During the course of the ban, the National Institute of Justice (NIJ) funded a series of studies on the law's impacts for the U.S. Department of Justice and the U.S. Congress (Koper 2004; Koper and Roth 2001, 2002; Roth and Koper 1997, 1999). I present highlights from those studies, with an emphasis on findings from the final evaluation reported in 2004 (Koper 2004). These studies sought to assess the law's impacts on (1) the availability of assault weapons (AWs) and large-capacity magazines (LCMs) as measured by price and production (or importation) indices in legal markets; (2) trends in criminal uses of AWs and LCMs; and (3) trends in the types of gun crimes that seemed most likely to be affected by changes in the use of AWs and LCMs. (The latter two issues are emphasized in this summary.) Finally, the research team examined studies of gun attacks more generally in order to estimate the ban's potential to produce longer-term reductions in shootings.

In summary, the ban had mixed effects in reducing crimes with the banned weaponry because of various exemptions and loopholes in the legislation. The ban did not appear to affect gun crime during the time it was in effect, but some evidence suggests it may have modestly reduced gunshot victimizations had it remained in place for a longer period. The ban's most important provision was arguably its prohibition on ammunition magazines holding more than 10 rounds. Policymakers considering a new version of the ban might particularly focus on this aspect of the previous legislation and reconsider the exemptions and loopholes that undermined the effectiveness of the original ban.

Provisions of the Assault Weapons Ban

Enacted on September 13, 1994, Title XI, Subtitle A of the Violent Crime Control and Law Enforcement Act of 1994 imposed a ten-year ban on the "manufacture, transfer, and possession" of certain semi-automatic firearms designated as assault weapons. The AW ban did not prohibit all semi-automatics; rather, it was directed at semi-automatics having features that appear to be useful in military and criminal applications but unnecessary in shooting sports or self-defense. Examples of such features include pistol grips on rifles, flash hiders, folding rifle stocks, threaded barrels for attaching silencers, and the ability to accept ammunition magazines holding large numbers of bullets. The law specifically prohibited 18 models and variations by name (e.g., the Intratec TEC-9 pistol and the Colt AR-15 rifle), as well as revolving cylinder shotguns (see Koper 2004, 5). This list included a number of foreign rifles that the federal government had banned from importation into the country beginning in 1989 (e.g., Avtomat Kalashnikov models). In addition, the ban contained a generic "features test" provision that generally prohibited other semi-automatic firearms having two or more military-style features, as described in Table 12.1. In total, the federal Bureau of Alcohol, Tobacco, Firearms and Explosives (ATF) identified 118 model and caliber variations that met the AW criteria established by the ban.

The law also banned "copies or duplicates" of the named gun makes and models, but federal authorities emphasized exact copies. Relatively cosmetic changes, such as removing a flash hider or bayonet mount, were thus sufficient to transform a banned weapon into a legal substitute. In this sense, the law is perhaps best understood not as a gun ban but as a law that restricted weapon accessories. A number of gun manufacturers began producing modified, legal versions of some of the banned guns, though not all of these substitute weapons proved as popular as the banned versions.[1] In other respects (e.g., type of firing mechanism, ammunition fired, and the ability to accept a detachable magazine), the banned AWs did not differ from other legal semi-automatic weapons.

The other major component of the assault weapons legislation was a ban on most ammunition-feeding devices holding more than 10 rounds of ammunition (referred to as large-capacity magazines).[2] The LCM ban was arguably the most important part of the assault weapons law for two reasons. First, an LCM is the most functionally important feature of an AW-type firearm. As noted by the U.S. House of Representatives, most prohibited AWs came equipped with magazines holding 30 rounds and could accept magazines holding as

Table 12.1   Features test of the federal assault weapons ban

Weapon category	Military-style features (2 or more qualified a firearm as an assault weapon)
Semi-automatic pistols accepting detachable magazines	1) ammunition magazine that attaches outside the pistol grip 2) threaded barrel capable of accepting a barrel extender, flash hider, forward handgrip, or silencer 3) heat shroud attached to or encircling the barrel 4) weight of more than 50 ounces unloaded 5) semiautomatic version of a fully automatic weapon
Semi-automatic rifles accepting detachable magazines	1) folding or telescoping stock 2) pistol grip that protrudes beneath the firing action 3) bayonet mount 4) flash hider or a threaded barrel designed to accommodate one 5) grenade launcher
Semi-automatic shotguns	1) folding or telescoping stock 2) pistol grip that protrudes beneath the firing action 3) fixed magazine capacity over 5 rounds 4) ability to accept a detachable ammunition magazine

many as 50 or 100 rounds (United States Department of the Treasury 1998, 14). Removing LCMs from these weapons thus greatly limits their firepower.

Second, the reach of the LCM ban was much broader than that of the AW ban because many semi-automatics that were not banned by the AW provision could accept LCMs. Approximately 40 percent of the semi-automatic handgun models and a majority of the semi-automatic rifle models that were being manufactured and advertised prior to the ban were sold with LCMs or had a variation that was sold with an LCM (calculated from Murtz and the Editors of Gun Digest 1994). Still others could accept LCMs made for other firearms and/or by other manufacturers. A national survey of gun owners in 1994 found that 18% of all civilian-owned firearms and 21% of civilian-owned handguns were equipped with magazines having 10 or more rounds (Cook and Ludwig 1996, 17). The AW provision did not affect most LCM-compatible guns, but the LCM provision limited the capacities of their magazines to 10 rounds.

The AW ban also contained important exemptions. AWs and LCMs manufactured before the effective date of the ban were "grandfathered" and thus legal to own and transfer. Though not precise, estimates suggest there were upward of 1.5 million privately owned AWs in the United States when the ban took effect (American Medical Association Council on Scientific Affairs 1992; Cox Newspapers 1989, 1; Koper 2004, 10). Gun owners in America possessed an estimated 25 million guns that were equipped with LCMs or 10-round magazines in 1994 (Cook and Ludwig 1996, 17), and gun industry sources estimated that, including aftermarket items for repairing and extending magazines, there were at least 25 million LCMs available in the United States as of 1995 (Gun Tests 1995, 30). Moreover, an additional 4.8 million pre-ban LCMs were imported into the country from 1994 through 2000 under the grandfathering exemption, with the largest number arriving in 1999. During this same period, importers were also authorized to import another 42 million pre-ban LCMs that may have arrived after 2000.

Criminal Use of Assault Weapons and Large-Capacity Magazines Prior to the Ban

During the 1980s and early 1990s, AWs and other semi-automatic firearms equipped with LCMs were involved in a number of highly publicized mass shootings that raised public concern about the accessibility of high-powered, military-style weaponry and other guns capable of rapidly discharging high numbers of bullets (Cox Newspapers 1989; Kleck 1997, 124–126, 144; Lenett 1995; Violence Policy Center 2012). Perhaps most notably, AWs or other semi-automatics with LCMs were used in 6, or 40%, of 15 particularly severe mass shooting incidents between 1984 and 1993 that resulted in at least 6 deaths or at least 12 killed or wounded (Kleck, 1997, 124–126, 144). Early studies of AWs, though sometimes based on limited and potentially unrepresentative data, also suggested that AWs recovered by police were often associated with drug trafficking and organized crime (Cox Newspapers 1989, 4; also see Roth and Koper 1997, chap. 5), fueling a perception that AWs were guns of choice among drug dealers and other particularly violent groups. These events intensified concern over AWs and other semi-automatics with LCMs and helped spur the 1989 federal import ban on selected semi-automatic rifles (implemented by executive order) and the passage of the 1994 federal AW ban (the states of California, New Jersey, Connecticut, Hawaii, and Maryland also passed AW legislation between 1989 and 1994).

Looking at the nation's gun crime problem more broadly, numerous studies of AW-type weapons conducted prior to the federal ban found that AWs typically accounted for up to 8% of guns used in crime, depending on the specific AW definition and data source used (e.g., see Beck et al. 1993; Hargarten et al. 1996; Hutson, Anglin, and Pratts 1994; Hutson et al. 1995; McGonigal et al. 1993; New York State Division of Criminal Justice Services 1994; Roth and Koper 1997, chap. 2; Zawitz 1995). A compilation of 38 sources indicated that AWs accounted for about 2% of crime guns on average (Kleck 1997, 112, 141–143). Similarly, the most common AWs prohibited by the 1994 federal ban accounted for between 1% and 6% of guns used in crime according to most of several national and local data sources examined for the NIJ-funded studies summarized here (Koper 2004, 15).

As with crime guns in general, the majority of AWs used in crime were assault pistols rather than assault rifles. Among AWs reported by police to ATF during 1992 and 1993, for example, assault pistols outnumbered assault rifles by a ratio of three to one.

The relative rarity of AW use in crime can be attributed to a number of factors. Many of these models are long guns, which are used in crime much less often than handguns. Also, as noted, a number of the rifles named in the 1994 law were banned from importation into the United States in 1989. Further, AWs in general are more expensive and more difficult to conceal than the types of handguns that are used most frequently in crime.

Criminal use of guns equipped with LCMs had not been studied as extensively as criminal use of AWs at the time of the ban. However, the overall use of guns with LCMs, which is based on the combined use of AWs and non-banned guns with LCMs, is much greater than the use of AWs alone. Based on data examined for this and a few prior studies, guns with LCMs were used in roughly 13% to 26% of most gun crimes prior to the ban, though they appeared to be used in 31% to 41% of gun murders of police (see summary in Koper 2004, 18; also see Adler et al. 1995; Fallis 2011; New York Division of Criminal Justice Services 1994).

The Ban's Effects on Crimes with Assault Weapons and Large-Capacity Magazines

Although there was a surge in production of AW-type weapons as Congress debated the ban in 1994, the law's restriction of the new AW supply and the interest of collectors and speculators in these weapons helped to drive prices higher for many AWs (notably assault pistols) through the end of the 1990s

Table 12.2   Assault weapons as a percentage of guns recovered by police

City	Pre-ban	Post-ban	% change
Baltimore, MD	1.88% (1992–1993)	1.25% (1995–2000)	−34%
Boston, MA	2.16% (1991–1993)	0.6% (2000–2002)	−72%
Miami, FL	2.53% (1990–1993)	1.71% (1995–2000)	−32%
St. Louis, MO	1.33% (1992–1993)	0.91% (1995–2003)	−32%
Anchorage, AK	3.57% (1987–1993)	2.13% (1995–2000)	−40%
Milwaukee, WI	5.91% (1991–1993)	4.91% (1995–1998)	−17%

Note: Figures for Baltimore, Boston, Miami, and St. Louis are based on all recovered guns. Figures for Anchorage and Milwaukee are based on, respectively, guns tested for evidence and guns recovered in murder cases. Changes in Baltimore, Boston, Miami, and St. Louis were statistically significant at $p < .05$. See Koper (2004) for further details about the data and analyses.

and appeared to make them less accessible and/or affordable to criminal users.[3] Analyses of several national and local databases on guns recovered by police indicated that crimes with AWs declined following the ban.

To illustrate, the share of gun crimes involving the most commonly used AWs declined by 17% to 72% across six major cities examined for this study (Baltimore, Miami, Milwaukee, Boston, St. Louis, and Anchorage), based on data covering all or portions of the 1995–2003 post-ban period (Table 12.2). (The number of AW recoveries also declined by 28% to 82% across these locations and time periods; the discussion here focuses on changes in AWs as a share of crime guns in order to control for general trends in gun crime and gun seizures.) Similar patterns were found in a national analysis of recovered guns reported by law enforcement agencies around the country to ATF for investigative gun tracing.[4] The percentage of gun traces that were for AWs fell 70% between 1992–1993 and 2001–2002 (from 5.4% to 1.6%), though the interpretation of these data was complicated by changes that occurred during this time in gun tracing practices (see Koper 2004 for further discussion).

The decline in crimes with AWs was due primarily to a reduction in the use of assault pistols. Assessment of trends in the use of assault rifles was complicated by the rarity of crimes with such rifles and by the substitution in some cases of post-ban rifles that were very similar to the banned models. In general, however, the decline in AW use was only partially offset by substitution of post-ban AW-type models. Even counting the post-ban models as AWs, the share of crime guns that were AWs fell 24% to 60% across most of the local jurisdictions studied. Patterns in the local data sources also suggested that crimes with AWs were becoming increasingly rare as the years passed.

The decline in crimes with AWs appeared to have been offset throughout at least the late 1990s by steady or rising use of other semi-automatics equipped with LCMs. Assessing trends in LCM use was difficult because there is no national data source on crimes with LCMs and few contacted jurisdictions maintained such information. It was possible, nonetheless, to examine trends in the use of guns with LCMs in four jurisdictions: Baltimore, Milwaukee, Anchorage, and Louisville (KY). Across the different samples analyzed from these cities (some databases included all recovered guns and some included only guns associated with particular crimes), the share of guns with an LCM generally varied from 14% to 26% prior to the ban. In all four jurisdictions, the share of crime guns equipped with LCMs rose or remained steady through the late 1990s (Table 12.3). These trends were driven primarily by handguns with LCMs, which were used in crime roughly three times as often as rifles with LCMs (though crimes with rifles having LCMs also showed no general decline). Generalizing from such a small number of jurisdictions must be done very cautiously, but the consistency of the findings across these geographically diverse locations strengthens the inference that they reflected a national pattern.

Failure to reduce LCM use for at least several years after the ban was likely because of the immense stock of exempted pre-ban magazines, which, as noted, was enhanced by post-ban imports. The trend in crimes with LCMs may have been changing by the early 2000s, but the available data were too limited and inconsistent to draw clear inferences (post-2000 data were available for only two of the four study sites).

Table 12.3   Guns with large-capacity magazines as a percentage of guns recovered by police (selected years)

City	Pre-ban	Late 1990s	Early 2000s
Baltimore, MD	14.0% (1993)	15.5% (1998)	15.7% (2003)
Anchorage, AK	26.2% (1992–1993)	30.0% (1999–2000)	19.2% (2001–2002)
Milwaukee, WI	22.4% (1993)	36.4% (1998)	N/A
Louisville, KY	N/A	20.9 (1996)	19.0% (2000)

Note: Figures for Baltimore and Milwaukee are based on, respectively, guns associated with violent crimes and with murders. Figures for Anchorage and Louisville are based on guns submitted for evidentiary testing. The Anchorage figures are based on handguns only. See Koper (2004) for further details about the data and analyses.

A later media investigation of LCM use in Richmond, Virginia, suggests that the ban may have had a more substantial impact on the supply of LCMs to criminal users by the time it expired in 2004. In that city, the share of recovered guns with LCMs generally varied between 18% and 20% from 1994 through 2000 but fell to 10% by 2004 (Fallis 2011). It is not clear whether the Richmond results represented a wider national or even regional trend. (The data from this study also show that after the ban was lifted, the share of Richmond crime guns with an LCM rose to 22% by 2008.)

The Ban's Impacts on Gun Violence

Because offenders could substitute non-banned guns and small magazines for banned AWs and LCMs, there was not a clear rationale for expecting the ban to reduce assaults and robberies with guns. But by forcing this weapon substitution, it was conceivable that the ban would reduce the number and severity of shooting deaths and injuries by reducing the number of shots fired in gun attacks (thus reducing the number of victims per gunfire incident and the share of gunshot victims sustaining multiple wounds). Based on this logic, the research team examined several indicators of trends in the lethality and injuriousness of gun violence for different portions of the 1995–2002 post-ban period. These included national-level analyses of gun murders, the percentage of violent gun crimes resulting in death, the share of gunfire cases resulting in wounded victims, the percentage of gunshot victimizations resulting in death, and the average number of victims per gun homicide incident. For selected localities, the team also examined trends in wounds per gunshot victim or the percentage of gunshot victims sustaining multiple wounds.

On balance, these analyses showed no discernible reduction in the lethality or injuriousness of gun violence during the post-ban years (see Koper 2004, Koper and Roth 2001, and Roth and Koper 1997). Nationally, for example, the percentage of violent gun crimes resulting in death (based on gun homicides, gun assaults, and gun robberies reported to the Uniform Crime Reports) was the same for the period 2001–2002 (2.9%) as it was for the immediate pre-ban period 1992–1993 (Koper 2004, 82, 92). Accordingly, it was difficult to credit the ban with contributing to the general decline in gun crime and gun homicide that occurred during the 1990s.

However, the ban's exemption of millions of pre-ban AWs and LCMs meant that the effects of the law would occur only gradually. Those effects were still unfolding when the ban was lifted and may not have been fully realized until several years beyond that, particularly if importation of foreign, pre-ban LCMs had continued in large numbers. In light of this, it was impossible to make definitive assessments of the ban's impact on gun violence.

It was also difficult to judge the ban's effects on the more specific problem of mass shootings. The research team attempted to assess changes in mass shootings during the first few years of the ban, but this effort was hampered by the difficulty of counting these incidents (results can be sensitive to the definitions and data sources used) and identifying the specific types of guns and magazines used in them (Roth and Koper 1997, app. A). There is no national data source that provides detailed information on the types of guns and magazines used in shooting incidents or that provides full counts of victims killed and wounded in these attacks. Studying mass shootings in particular poses a number of challenges with regard to defining these events, establishing the validity and reliability of methods for measuring their frequency and characteristics (particularly if done through media searches, as is often necessary), and modeling their trends, as they are particularly rare events (e.g., see Duwe 2000; Roth and Koper 1997, app. A).

Nonetheless, the issue of mass shootings continues to be a catalyst to the debate surrounding AW legislation. A recent media compilation of 62 mass shooting incidents that involved the death of four or more people over the period 1982–2012, for instance, suggests that 25% of the guns used in these attacks were AW-type weapons (these were not precisely defined) and another 48% were other types of semi-automatic handguns (Follman, Aronsen, and Pan 2012). Continuing improvements in media search tools and greater attention to the types of guns and magazines used in multiple-victim attacks may improve prospects for examining this issue more rigorously in future studies.

Assessing the Potential Long-Term Effects of Banning Assault Weapons and Large-Capacity Magazines

Although available evidence is too limited to make firm projections, it suggests that the ban may have reduced shootings slightly had it remained in place long enough to substantially reduce crimes with both LCMs and AWs. A small number of studies suggest that gun attacks with semi-automatics—including AWs and other guns equipped with LCMs—tend to result in more shots fired, more persons wounded, and more wounds inflicted per victim than do attacks with other firearms (see reviews in Koper 2004; Koper and Roth 2001; also see McGonigal et al. 1993; Richmond et al. 2003; Reedy and Koper 2003; Roth and Koper 1997). For example, in mass shooting incidents that resulted in at least 6 deaths or at least 12 total gunshot victims from 1984 through 1993, offenders who clearly possessed AWs or other semi-automatics with LCMs (sometimes in addition to other guns) wounded or killed an average of 29 victims in comparison to an average of 13 victims wounded or killed by other offenders (see Koper and Roth's [2001] analysis of data compiled by Kleck [1997, 144]).

Similarly, a study of handgun attacks in Jersey City, New Jersey, during the 1990s found that the average number of victims wounded in gunfire incidents involving semi-automatic pistols was in general 15% higher than in those involving revolvers (Reedy and Koper 2003). The study also found that attackers using semi-automatics to fire more than 10 shots were responsible for nearly 5% of the gunshot victims in the sample. Used as a tentative guide, this implies that the LCM ban could have eventually produced a small reduction in shootings overall, perhaps up to 5%, even if some gun attackers had the foresight to carry more than one small magazine (or more than one firearm) and the time and poise to reload during an attack.

Effects of this magnitude might be difficult to measure reliably, but they could nonetheless yield significant societal benefits. Consider that in 2010 there were 11,078 gun homicides in the United States and another 53,738 non-fatal assault-related shootings according to the federal Centers for Disease Control and Prevention (see the CDC's web-based injury statistics query and reporting system at http://www.cdc.gov/injury/wisqars/index.html). At these levels, reducing shootings by just 1% (arguably a reasonable ballpark estimate for the long-term impact of substantially reducing AW and LCM use) would amount to preventing about 650 shootings annually. The lifetime medical costs of assault-related gunshot injuries (fatal and nonfatal) were estimated to be about $18,600 per injury in 1994 (Cook et al. 1999). Adjusting for inflation, this amounts to $28,894 in today's dollars. Moreover, some estimates suggest that the full societal costs of gun violence—including medical, criminal justice, and other government and private costs (both tangible and intangible)— could be as high as $1 million per shooting (Cook and Ludwig 2000). Hence, reducing shootings by even a very small margin could produce substantial long-term savings for society, especially as the shootings prevented accrue over many years.

Lessons and Implications from the 1994 Ban

Studies of America's previous assault weapons ban provide a number of lessons that can inform future policymaking. A new law similar to the old ban will have little impact on most gun crimes, but it may prevent some shootings, particularly those involving high numbers of shots and victims. It may thus help to reduce the number and severity of mass shooting incidents as well as produce a small reduction in shootings overall.

The most important feature of the previous ban was the prohibition on large-capacity ammunition magazines. A large magazine is arguably the most critical feature of an assault weapon, and restrictions on magazines have the potential to affect many more gun crimes than do those on military-style weapons. Restrictions focused on magazine capacity may also have a greater chance of gaining sufficient public and political support for passage than would new restrictions on assault weapons, though current polling suggests that both measures are supported by three-quarters of non-gun owners and nearly half of gun owners (Barry et al., in this volume). To enhance the potential impact of magazine restrictions, policymakers might also consider limiting magazine capacity to fewer than 10 rounds for all or selected weapons (for example, lower limits might be set for magazines made for semi-automatic rifles).[5] It is unknown whether further restrictions on the outward features of semi-automatic weapons, such as banning weapons having any military-style features, will produce measurable benefits beyond those of restricting magazine capacity.

Policymakers must also consider the implications of any grandfathering provisions in new legislation. Assessing the political and practical difficulties of registering all assault weapons and large magazines or establishing turn-in or buyback programs for them is beyond the scope of this essay. Policymakers should note, however, that it may take many years to attain substantial reductions in crimes with banned weapons and/or magazines if a new law exempts the existing stock (which has likely grown considerably since the time of the original ban). Policies regarding exemptions must also explicitly address the status of imported guns and magazines.

Past experience further suggests that public debate on reinstating the ban or crafting a new one will raise prices and production of the guns and magazines likely to be affected. This could temporarily saturate the market for the guns and magazines in question (particularly if close substitutes emerge) and delay desired reductions in crimes with some categories of the banned weaponry (this appeared to happen with assault rifles that were banned by the 1994 law and may have contributed as well to the observed trends in use of large magazines).

A new ban on assault weapons and/or large-capacity magazines will certainly not be a panacea for America's gun violence problem nor will it stop all mass shootings. However, it is one modest measure that, like federal restrictions on fully automatic weapons and armor-piercing ammunition, can help to prevent the further spread of particularly dangerous weaponry.

NOTES

1. In general, the AW ban did not apply to semi-automatics possessing no more than one military-style feature listed under the ban's features test provision. Note, however, that firearms imported into the country still had to meet the "sporting purposes test" established under the federal Gun Control Act of 1968. In 1989, ATF determined that foreign semi-automatic rifles having any one of a number of named military features (including those listed in the features test of the 1994 AW ban) fail the sporting purposes test and cannot be imported into the country. In 1998, the ability to accept an LCM made for a military rifle was added to the list of disqualifying features. Consequently, it was possible for foreign rifles to pass the features test of the federal AW ban but not meet the sporting purposes test for imports (U.S. Department of the Treasury 1998).

2. Technically, the ban prohibited any magazine, belt, drum, feed strip, or similar device that has the capacity to accept more than 10 rounds of ammunition or which can be readily converted or restored to accept more than 10 rounds of ammunition. The ban exempted attached tubular devices capable of operating only with .22 caliber rimfire (i.e., low velocity) ammunition.

3. See Koper (2004), Koper and Roth (2002), and Roth and Koper (1997) for more extensive discussions of the ban's impacts on prices and production of AWs, nonbanned firearms, and LCMs.

4. A gun trace is an investigation into the sales history of a firearm (e.g., see ATF 2000).

5. To support the formulation and evaluation of policy in this area, there are also a number of research needs worth noting. For one, it is important to develop better data on crimes with guns having LCMs. Policymakers should thus encourage police agencies to record information about magazines recovered with crime guns. Likewise, ATF should consider integrating ammunition magazine data into its national gun tracing system and encourage reporting of magazine data by police agencies that trace firearms. Second, there is a need for more studies that contrast the outcomes of attacks with different types of guns and magazines. Such studies would help to refine predictions of the change in gun deaths and injuries that would follow reductions in attacks with firearms having large-capacity magazines.

REFERENCES

Adler, Wendy, C., Frederick M. Bielke, David J. Doi, and John F. Kennedy. (1995). *Cops under Fire: Law Enforcement Officers Killed with Assault Weapons or Guns with High Capacity Magazines.* Washington, DC: Handgun Control, Inc.
American Medical Association Council on Scientific Affairs. 1992. "Assault Weapons as a Public Health Hazard in the United States." *JAMA* 267:3067–3070.
Beck, Allen, Darrell Gilliard, Lawrence Greenfeld, Caroline Harlow, Thomas Hester, Louis Jankowski, Tracy Snell, James Stephan, and Danielle Morton. 1993. *Survey of State Prison Inmates, 1991.* Washington, DC: Bureau of Justice Statistics, U.S. Department of Justice.
Bureau of Alcohol, Tobacco, and Firearms (ATF). (2000). *Commerce in Firearms in the United States.* Washington, DC: United States Department of the Treasury.
Cook, Philip J., Bruce A. Lawrence, Jens Ludwig, and Ted R. Miller. 1999. "The Medical Costs of Gunshot Injuries in the United States." *JAMA* 282:447–454.
Cook, Philip J., and Jens Ludwig. 1996. *Guns in America: Results of a Comprehensive National Survey on Firearms Ownership and Use.* Washington, DC: Police Foundation.
Cook, Philip J., and Jens Ludwig. 2000. *Gun Violence: The Real Costs.* New York: Oxford University Press.
Cox Newspapers. 1989. *Firepower: Assault Weapons in America.* Washington, DC: Cox Enterprises.
Duwe, Grant. 2000. "Body-Count Journalism: The Presentation of Mass Murder in the News Media." *Homicide Studies* 4:364–399.
Fallis, David. 2011. "VA Data Show Drop in Criminal Firepower During Assault Gun Ban." *Washington Post*, January 23.
Follman, Mark, Gavin Aronsen, and Deanna Pan. 2012. "A Guide to Mass Shootings in America." *Mother Jones*, Dec. 15. http://www.motherjones.com/politics/2012/07/mass-shootings-map.
Gun Tests. 1995. "Magazine Rule Change Unlikely." March.
Hargarten, Stephen W., Trudy A. Karlson, Mallory O'Brien, Jerry Hancock, and Edward Quebbeman. 1996. "Characteristics of Firearms Involved in Fatalities." *JAMA* 275:42–45.
Hutson, H. Range, Deirdre Anglin, Demetrios N. Kyriacou, Joel Hart, and Kelvin Spears. 1995. "The Epidemic of Gang-Related Homicides in Los Angeles County from 1979 through 1994." *JAMA* 274:1031–1036.
Hutson, H. Range, Deirdre Anglin, and Michael J. Pratts, Jr. 1994. "Adolescents and Children Injured or Killed in Drive-By Shootings in Los Angeles." *New England Journal of Medicine* 330:324–327.
Kleck, Gary. (1997). *Targeting Guns: Firearms and Their Control.* New York: Aldine de Gruyter.
Koper, Christopher S. 2004. *An Updated Assessment of the Federal Assault Weapons Ban: Impacts on Gun Markets and Gun Violence, 1994–2003.* Report to the National Institute of Justice, U.S. Department of Justice. Jerry Lee Center of Criminology, University of Pennsylvania, Philadelphia, PA.
Koper, Christopher S., and Jeffrey A. Roth. 2001. "The Impact of the 1994 Federal Assault Weapon Ban on Gun Violence Outcomes: An Assessment of Multiple

Outcome Measures and Some Lessons for Policy Evaluation." *Journal of Quantitative Criminology* 17:33–74.

Koper, Christopher S., and Jeffrey A. Roth. 2002. "The Impact of the 1994 Federal Assault Weapons Ban on Gun Markets: An Assessment of Short-Term Primary and Secondary Market Effects." *Journal of Quantitative Criminology* 18:239–266.

Lenett, Michael G. 1995. "Taking a Bite Out of Violent Crime." *University of Daytona Law Review* 20:573–617.

McGonigal, Michael D., John Cole, C. William Schwab, Donald R. Kauder, Michael F. Rotondo, and Peter B. Angood. 1993. "Urban Firearm Deaths: A Five-Year Perspective." *Journal of Trauma*: 35:532–537.

Murtz, H.A., and the Editors of Gun Digest. 1994. *Guns Illustrated 1994*. Northbrook, IL: DBI Books.

New York State Division of Criminal Justice Services. 1994. *Assault Weapons and Homicide in New York City*. Albany, NY.

Reedy, Darin C., and Christopher S. Koper. 2003. "Impact of Handgun Types on Gun Assault Outcomes: A Comparison of Gun Assaults Involving Semiautomatic Pistols and Revolvers." *Injury Prevention* 9:151–155.

Richmond, Therese S., Charles C. Branas, Rose A. Cheney, and C. William Schwab. 2003. *The Case for Enhanced Data Collection of Handgun Type*. Firearm and Injury Center at Penn, University of Pennsylvania, Philadelphia, PA.

Roth, Jeffrey A., and Christopher S. Koper. 1997. *Impact Evaluation of the Public Safety and Recreational Firearms Use Protection Act of 1994*. Washington, DC: The Urban Institute.

Roth, Jeffrey A., and Christopher S. Koper. 1999. *Impacts of the 1994 Assault Weapons Ban: 1994–96*. Washington, DC: National Institute of Justice, U.S. Department of Justice.

United States Department of the Treasury. (1998). *Department of the Treasury Study on the Sporting Suitability of Modified Semiautomatic Assault Rifles*. Washington, DC.

Violence Policy Center (2012). *Mass Shootings in the United States Involving High-Capacity Ammunition Magazines*. Washington, DC.

Zawitz, Marianne W. 1995. *Guns Used in Crime*. Washington, DC: Bureau of Justice Statistics, U.S. Department of Justice.

Personalized Guns

Using Technology to Save Lives

Stephen P. Teret and Adam D. Mernit

Gunfire took the lives of 31,672 Americans in 2010.[1] Death by gunfire occurs in homes, workplaces, shopping malls, churches, schools, and on the streets, and to Americans of all ages. Often, when possible solutions to this compelling public health problem are considered, conversations focus on troubled individuals who are at risk for becoming shooters, mental health interventions for these individuals, and securing the safety of vulnerable places such as schools. Little attention is paid to modifying the gun itself, which is the vehicle that causes the human damage, such as changing the design of guns so that they are inoperable by unauthorized users—that is, making all guns personalized. But product-oriented interventions have been highly effective with other public health problems, such as motor vehicle–related deaths.[2] In fact, the impressive reductions in highway fatalities are more attributable to

Stephen P. Teret, JD, MPH, is a professor in the Department of Health Policy and Management and director of the Center for Law and the Public's Health at the Johns Hopkins Bloomberg School of Public Health. Adam D. Mernit is an undergraduate senior in public health studies at Johns Hopkins University.

changes in the design of cars than to enhancing the driving skill of hundreds of millions of motorists.

This essay explores the topic of personalized guns, sometimes called smart guns or childproof guns. The definition we use for a personalized firearm is a gun that, by design integral to the gun itself as opposed to an external locking device, can be fired only by the authorized user or users. Our argument is that if all newly manufactured guns were personalized guns, there would be a meaningful reduction in gun deaths. This is not to imply that other efforts to regulate the sale, carrying, and use of guns should be ignored. Rather, changing the design of guns so that they are personalized would complement other policy interventions to reduce gun violence.

The Need for Personalized Guns

Of the 31,672 persons killed by firearms in 2010 in the United States, 61 percent were suicides, 35 percent were homicides, and most of the remaining deaths were unintentional or accidental deaths.[3] How many of these gun deaths would be averted if guns were personalized is difficult to assess, but it is reasonable to assume that there would be substantial saving of lives.

Perhaps the most understandable saving of lives would occur in the unintentional or accidental category of gun deaths, which in 2010 accounted for 606 fatalities, 9 percent of which were of young people aged zero to 19 years.[4] Although these unintended deaths are far fewer in number than gun suicides and homicides, when they occur to children, they are seen as particularly tragic. Children find guns in their homes, often handguns kept loaded for protection, and are able to fire them, shooting themselves, their siblings, and playmates. Wintemute et al.[5] examined the circumstances of 88 deaths involving children shooting children and concluded that changes in gun design, particularly of handguns, would be useful in preventing such deaths.

The National Rifle Association (NRA) has long argued that the way to prevent accidental gun deaths of children is to educate them about gun safety. In pursuit of this goal, the NRA has developed its Eddie Eagle GunSafe Program, for children in pre-K through third grades. It states that since the inception of the program, 18 million children have been trained.[6] The effectiveness of training young children in gun safety has been studied, and doubt has been cast as to whether such training is useful.[7]

Vernick et al.[8] studied a series (N=117) of unintentional, undetermined intent, and negligent homicide gun deaths that occurred in Maryland and Milwaukee County, Wisconsin, from 1991 to 1998. The purpose of the study was to assess what portion of these deaths would likely have been prevented if the guns used were personalized and, separately, if the guns had other safety devices (loaded chamber indicators and magazine disconnect devices). Most (81%) of these deaths occurred with a handgun, roughly half being revolvers and half being pistols. Using specific criteria to address preventability, the researchers determined that 37 percent of the deaths would have been preventable if the guns involved were personalized.

Unintentional deaths are not the only type of gun death that could be affected by a change to personalized guns. Children and teenagers also use guns found in the home to commit suicide. In 2010, 748 youths between the ages of 10 and 19 committed suicide with a firearm.[9] Such deaths, often stemming from depression, would be less likely if the gun in the home were inoperable by the young person. Some have argued that the depressed teenager would just find another means of committing suicide, but other forms of suicide attempts (e.g., poisoning) have lower case fatality rates. The lethality of self-inflicted gunshots leaves little opportunity for medical intervention.

Stolen guns are used in crime and therefore figure prominently in homicides and assaultive injuries involving firearms. Cook and colleagues,[10] using data from the National Crime Victimization Survey (NCVS), noted that there are nearly 350,000 incidents of firearm theft from private citizens annually. Further, there are approximately 1.5 firearms taken during each of these burglaries, resulting in about half a million gun thefts each year. NCVS and FBI data show that the majority of the guns stolen are handguns.[11] These guns would be inoperable to criminals if they had been made as personalized guns.

A Brief History of Personalized Guns

Danger from the unauthorized use of guns has long been recognized. Roy G. Jinks's *History of Smith & Wesson*[12] tells the story of D. B. Wesson, one of the founding partners of the renowned gun-making firm, learning in the early 1880s of an incident in which a child was hurt while playing with a Smith & Wesson revolver that discharged. Wesson asked his son, Joe, to design a revolver that a young child could not operate, and in 1886, Smith & Wesson began to sell a gun it believed to be childproof. The revolver employed what is now known as a grip safety—a metallic lever on the back of the gun that must be pressed inward in order for the gun to fire. In its marketing materials for this gun, Smith & Wesson stated that "no ordinary child under eight can possibly discharge it." The concern that Smith & Wesson had for the safety of children more than 125 years ago has not carried through to present times. Smith & Wesson stopped using its childproofing technology many decades ago, and neither it nor other leading gun makers have developed and put into widespread operation newer technologies to protect the public from unauthorized gun use.

Ninety years later, however, a minor gun maker was still concerned with the danger of unauthorized use; he applied for and received a U.S. patent for a combination lock built into a carbine, a long gun. The U.S. patent was issued to Gerald Fox on May 29, 1973, Patent Number 3,735,519. The Fox Carbine featured a three-digit combination lock. The advertisement for this gun noted that "accidental and unauthorized firing is prevented by a patented, built-in combination lock safety."[13]

During the 1980s and 1990s, there was increasing interest in personalizing guns. In 1984, a Massachusetts inventor was granted a patent for a device called a "personalized safety method and apparatus for a hand held weapon." It was described as "responsive to the palm or fingerprint of one or more individuals. The safety device is activated by heat sensed when the device is hand held. The pattern of the palm or fingerprint is stored in the firearm and must match the user's in order for the blocking safety mechanism to allow the weapon to fire.[14] The renewed attention to gun personalization coincided both with advancements in electronic technologies and highly publicized mass shootings.

In 1992, faculty at the Johns Hopkins Bloomberg School of Public Health, with a $2,000 grant, commissioned a team of undergraduate students at the university's School of Engineering to create a prototype of a personalized handgun. Using an existing revolver purchased for this purpose, the students employed touch memory technology, which worked through contact between a semiconductor memory chip and a reader embedded within the grip of the gun. The chip stored a serial number, which was placed on a ring worn by the authorized gun user. When the ring came in contact with the reader on the gun, an electronic current moved a blocking mechanism that kept the gun from being able to fire.

Other technologies, such as radio frequency identification and magnetic encoding, were used in experiments to develop a personalized gun.

On May 12, 2000, President Bill Clinton announced that the United States Justice Department, through its National Institute of Justice, would provide two grants of $300,000 each to Smith & Wesson and FN Manufacturing, Inc., for research and development of personalized gun technology. The press release from the White House stated: "Smart gun technologies have the potential to limit a gun's use to its proper adult owner—and could prevent accidental shooting deaths of children, deter gun theft, and stop criminals from seizing and using the guns of police officers against them."[15]

Work by Colt's on personalized, or smart gun, technology resulted in a prototype handgun that used radio frequency identification. Colt's viewed its smart gun as a major growth prospect for the corporation. But Colt's did not want the progress it was making on personalized guns to be widely known. Colt's formed a new company, iColt, to pursue the technology, and it hoped for additional funding from the federal government. In June 1999, a memo was prepared by Colt's, noting that remarkable progress was being made on personalization technology. The memo further stated that "Colt's is working in Washington to help put $20 million to $40 million in the federal budget for research on 'smart gun' technology. Depending on how the press reports the current state of the 'smart gun,' it could be perceived by Congress that further research dollars are not needed." This memo was uncovered during discovery in a lawsuit against Colt's.[16] Shortly after the memo was written, and during substantial litigation against Colt's and other gun makers, Colt's discontinued its work on personalized guns, and so did most of the major manufacturers in the gun industry.

Modern Personalized Gun Technology

Personalized firearms presently exist. Armatix GmbH, a German company, has produced the iP1 Pistol, which is a personalized .22 caliber handgun that works like a conventional pistol except that it is digital and battery operated, which allows for software flexibility depending on the needs of the consumer.[17] The handgun is sold with an Active RFID Wrist Watch (designated by Armatix as iW1), which uses radio frequencies to activate the handgun, making it operable. The watch uses a personal identification number (PIN) that must be entered in order to unlock the electromechanical firing pin lock, making the gun operable by the owner.[18] Microchips in both the iW1 watch and the iP1 pistol communicate with each other. If the watch is not within a specified distance from the pistol, the gun is inoperable, rendering it useless. If the gun is first unlocked by its authorized user but then is taken beyond the distance where it can communicate with the watch, the gun will lock itself and be inoperable until the authorized user gets the watch and the gun back together.

A system of colored lights on the gun is used to convey the firearm's status to the user. A green light indicates that the firearm is in sync with the iW1 watch and is operable by the user. A red light indicates a "safe mode" in which the gun is locked and has not been made active by the authorized user. Additionally, a blue light indicates a "safe mode" in which the gun's magazine has been removed.[19] This feature ensures that the user knows that the magazine containing the ammunition is removed, that the gun is inoperable, and that, even if there is a round in the chamber, it cannot be fired. The gun can be fired only if the light indicator is green.

The Armatix personalized handgun is now being sold on a limited edition basis throughout much of Western Europe, and Armatix has been granted permission from the United States Bureau of Alcohol, Tobacco, Firearms and Explosives to sell the firearm in the United States. The limited, collector's edition is selling in Europe for 7,000 Euro (about US$10,000). Planned sales in the United States will be for a significantly lower cost, and once the pistol is selling in greater numbers, economies of scale will further reduce the cost, bringing it within the price range of many gun buyers.

TriggerSmart, a Limited Liability Irish company, is using radio frequency identification (RFID) technology in the development of its personalized pistol. TriggerSmart realized that a past issue with wireless personalization technology has been that both the firearm and the transmitter used to communicate with the firearm required batteries. This raised questions of reliability and functionality.[20] The TriggerSmart high-frequency RFID system incorporates technology that is commonly used in identification cards and in library books to establish communication between the firearm and a bracelet in order to authenticate a user.[21] The firearm's battery, antenna, and electronic interface are built into the handgrip of the gun. Once the radio frequency tags in the bracelet fall within a distance where it can communicate with the antenna in the handgrip, the gun enters an "instant on" phase and can be fired.[22]

The moment that the radio frequency tags comes out of contact, breaking communication, the firing pin locks and the gun cannot be fired. There is no battery in the bracelet component of the system, which addresses concerns over reliability and functionality. The company claims that this system is useful because the closer the tags in the bracelet are to the antenna in the firearm, the less battery power is used, offering a dependable power source that will last for extended periods of time.

The New Jersey Institute of Technology, in the United States, has been working for years on a biometric version of a personalized gun. Their product employs "grip recognition." The handgun, after some period of use by its owner, recognizes the palm configuration of the owner and will work only when held by that authorized user.

Achieving Personalized Guns

The federal government of the United States does not comprehensively regulate firearms with regard to their safe design. The U.S. Consumer Product Safety Commission, which is the federal agency that protects the public from unsafe consumer products, has expressly been forbidden by Congress to address the safety of guns.[23] Thus, gun makers are, under federal law, able to choose the design of their products without regard to safety and to ignore the lifesaving potential of personalized guns.

With other products, a manufacturer's failure to design its product in a safe, feasible manner that could prevent foreseeable injuries would likely result in liability. The threat of litigation has provided a strong incentive to the makers of most products to utilize safety technology.[24] It was argued that the same exposure to liability would force gun makers to adopt personalization.[25] But, on October 26, 2005, President George W. Bush signed into law the Protection of Lawful Commerce in Arms Act (15 U.S.C. §§ 7901–7903), which provides to gun makers far-reaching immunity from product liability litigation.

As awareness of the need for personalized handguns increased, there was also more interest in state legislative efforts that would require personalized handguns. To aid in this process, a model law entitled "A Model Handgun Safety Standard Act" was developed by the Johns Hopkins Center for Gun Policy and Research. This model legislation could be used by states or municipalities to require that all handguns manufactured or sold within their jurisdiction after a certain date be personalized. Legislation patterned after the model law was passed in New Jersey in 2002 (New Jersey Statutes, Title: 2C; Chapter 58; Sections 2C:58-2.2 et seq.) The New Jersey law provides that once a personalized gun is introduced for sale in the state and is recognized by the New Jersey attorney general as complying with the statutory definition of a personalized or childproof gun, then three years later all new handguns sold in New Jersey must be personalized.

In addition to state legislation, there are several actions that Congress could take to introduce personalized guns into the marketplace. These actions, stated in increasing order of effectiveness, in our opinion, are:

1. Provide funds, through the National Institute of Justice or another agency, for research and development of personalized gun technology. But, because of prior difficulties involving gun manufacturers' use of such funds, the work of the gun makers must be closely monitored.

2. Use the federal government's purchasing power to create a market for personalized guns.

3. Provide states with financial incentives to enact personalized or child-proof gun laws, much as Congress has done with other areas of public safety, such as raising the drinking age.

4. Amend the Consumer Product Safety Act to give the Consumer Product Safety Commission (CPSC) jurisdiction over firearms as consumer products. Also, mandate the CPSC to promulgate a standard regarding childproof guns.

5. Enact technology-forcing legislation mandating that all newly manufactured or imported firearms be personalized, starting three years from the effective date of the legislation.

6. Amend the Protection of Lawful Commerce in Arms Act, permitting litigation against firearms manufacturers for injuries sustained by an unauthorized use of a recently manufactured firearm that was not personalized but also providing a safe haven of immunity if the firearm had been personalized.

Conclusion

Personalized guns are an idea whose time has come. The technology is now available to make guns a safer consumer product. To require all guns to be personalized does not interfere with Second Amendment rights—one can still keep and bear arms, but the arms would be designed in such a manner as to reduce the likelihood of being involved in mayhem.

Based on the longstanding behaviors of the gun industry, it would be naïve to expect them to voluntarily adopt even lifesaving technology. This means that legislation, regulation, and perhaps litigation are needed to provide the public with safer guns.

NOTES

1. CDC Web-based Injury Statistics Query and Reporting System (WISQARS): http://www.cdc.gov/injury/wisqars/index.html.

2. Lund AK, Ferguson SA. Driver Fatalities in 1985–1993 Cars with Airbags. J Trauma. 1995; 38:469–475.

3. CDC Web-based Injury Statistics Query and Reporting System (WISQARS): http://www.cdc.gov/injury/wisqars/index.html.

4. CDC Web-based Injury Statistics Query and Reporting System (WISQARS): http://www.cdc.gov/injury/wisqars/index.html.

5. Wintemute GJ, Teret SP, Kraus JF, Wright MA, Bradfield G. When Children Shoot Children: 88 Unintended Deaths in California. JAMA. 1987;257(22):3107–3109.

6. http://www.nra.org/Article.aspx?id=1353.

7. Hardy, M. Teaching Firearm Safety to Children: Failure of a Program. J. Developmental & Behavioral Pediatrics. 2002;23(2):71–76.

8. Vernick JS, O'Brien M, Hepburn LM, et al. Unintentional and Undetermined Firearm Related Deaths: A Preventable Death Analysis for Three Safety Devices. Injury Prevention. 2003; 9:307–311.

9. CDC Web-based Injury Statistics Query and Reporting System (WISQARS): http://www.cdc.gov/injury/wisqars/index.html.

10. Cook PJ, Mulliconi S, Cole TB. Regulating Gun Markets. J Crim L Criminology. 1995;86:59–91.

11. Zawitz MW. Guns Used in Crime: Firearms, Crime and Criminal Justice: Selected Findings. Washington, DC: U.S. Dept. of Justice; Bureau of Justice Statistics, NCJ-160093. 1996.

12. Jinks RG. *History of Smith & Wesson*. North Hollywood, CA: Beinfeld Publishing. 1977.

13. http://forums.vwvortex.com/showthread.php?5127428-the-DEMRO-Fox-Carbine-a-really-really-really-dumb-gun-design.

14. Shaw FA. Personalized Safety Method and Apparatus for a Hand Held Weapon. U.S. Patent 4,467,545: Aug. 28, 1984.

15. http://clinton4.nara.gov/WH/New/html/20000531_4.html.

16. Ivey, C. Judge Orders Release of Colt's Smart Gun Research. San Jose *Mercury News,* Apr. 18, 2003; www.mercurynews.com.

17. Armatix iP1 product description at http://www.armatix.de/iP1-Pistol.779.0.html?&L=1.

18. Armatix iW1 product description at http://www.armatix.de/iP1-Pistol779.0.html?&L=1.

19. Armatix iP1 product description at http://www.armatix.de/iP1-Pistol.779.0.html?&L=1.

20. Pers. comm., Robert McNamara, Jan. 6, 2013.

21. Pers. comm., Robert McNamara, Jan. 6, 2013.

22. Pers. comm., Robert McNamara, Jan. 6, 2013.

23. Pub. L. 94-284, §3(e), May 11, 1976, 90 Stat. 504 (1976).

24. Teret SP. Litigating for the Public's Health. Am J Public Health 1986;76:1027–1029.

25. Teret SP, Culross P. Product-oriented Approaches to Reduce Youth Gun Violence. The Future of Children, 2002;12(2):119–131.

Part IV / International Case Studies of Responses to Gun Violence

Gun Control in Great Britain after the Dunblane Shootings

Michael J. North

Dunblane

On March 13, 1996, a man with a grudge against the local community walked into Dunblane Primary School in central Scotland. He was armed with two semi-automatic pistols and two revolvers and carrying hundreds of rounds of ammunition loaded into high-capacity magazines, all legally held. Within minutes Thomas Hamilton had shot and fatally wounded one teacher and sixteen 5- and 6-year-old children. Another ten children and three teachers were injured. All of his victims were shot with a 9-mm semi-automatic pistol. Hamilton then killed himself with one of his revolvers.

Gun homicide is rare in Great Britain. The deaths at Dunblane accounted for nearly a quarter of the country's gun victims in 1996. The public outrage at this scale of violence by a legally armed gunman translated into a campaign for tighter gun control, and within two years all handguns had been prohibited.

Michael J. North, PhD, was a biochemistry academic at the University of Stirling in Scotland when in March 1996 his only daughter was killed in a mass shooting at Dunblane Primary School. Following that event he became an advocate for gun control.

This essay outlines events which led to the landmark legislative changes and summarizes their impact. Only the key elements are included and more details can be found in North (2000). Inevitably, this is an insider's account and a more thorough analysis of the issues is provided by Squires (2000).

Firearms Legislation

Firearms legislation is determined by the UK parliament, though the laws applying in Northern Ireland differ in some respects from those for Great Britain (England, Wales and Scotland), the focus of this essay.

British law permits the private ownership of guns for which an appropriate reason can be demonstrated (e.g., target shooting, hunting, vermin control), but the reasons exclude self-protection (except rarely in Northern Ireland). Under the Firearms Act (1968) handgun and rifle owners were required to hold a firearm certificate (license) issued by the local police force. Justification for the ownership of each individual weapon was needed (a different system applies to shotguns). A person had to show suitability to be entrusted with a firearm with the application counter-signed by a responsible person who knew the applicant. Hamilton held firearms certificates for nearly 20 years and owned a number of handguns, all for target shooting at an approved gun club, the "good reason" for ownership of most of the legally held handguns in Great Britain.

Applications for firearm certificates were rarely unsuccessful, with only 1% being refused. Nor were many certificates revoked. Hamilton's ownership of guns had been called into question, but the senior officer responsible for firearms licensing dismissed the concerns. He later admitted to have been worried that if his certificate had been revoked, Hamilton would have successfully appealed. Hamilton therefore retained his certificate and was able to buy and keep dangerous weapons.

Some other types of firearms were prohibited. In 1988 many self-loading and pump-action rifles and shotguns had been banned in the aftermath of a mass shooting in August 1987 in Hungerford, Berkshire, where another legal gun owner killed sixteen people, half of whom were shot with a semi-automatic rifle. However, the Conservative Party government failed to tighten controls over handguns even though the other victims were killed with a pistol. It did set up a Firearms Consultative Committee to advise the Home Secretary

(The United Kingdom's equivalent of the United States Attorney General), but the membership was biased in favor of those with interests in shooting. Victims' voices were absent and the Committee became a means by which the gun lobby could influence Home Office policy and its implementation. Traditionally the Conservative Party had close links with the shooting community and there were accusations that the post-Hungerford response had been watered down because of vested interests.

Immediate Response to Dunblane

The Conservatives were still in power in 1996, and the Government faced awkward questions about why it had not dealt with handguns after Hungerford. Michael Forsyth, the local Member of Parliament (MP) in Dunblane, was Secretary of State for Scotland, a connection which undoubtedly gave weight to the case for tighter gun control within government. One of his first moves was to set up a Public Inquiry chaired by a senior judge, Lord Cullen, which "sought to answer questions about the circumstances that led up to and surrounded the shootings and make recommendations with a view to safeguarding the public against the misuse of firearms and other dangers" (Cullen 1996).

In the United Kingdom, Public Inquiries are held after major disasters to shed light on the causes and to offer recommendations on the lessons that can be learned. The forthcoming Inquiry provided breathing space for the Government which could delay announcing its position. On legal advice, other interested parties also had to wait until after the Inquiry's hearings were over before commenting. In retrospect, this proved to be a good thing for the victims' families, giving time for their thoughts to be collected. However, aided by continuous media coverage a widespread debate on gun control had already begun. Campaigns for a ban on handguns were initiated.

At Parliament, backbench MPs on the Home Affairs Committee held an inquiry into the possession of handguns, but evidence was heard predominantly from those with shooting interests with no input from victims. The MPs' report exposed a political split, the Conservative majority proposing that no significant new controls were necessary, and the Labour minority advocating a ban. The Government had hoped to keep politics out of the debate but the report reinforced a widely held perception that the Conservatives gave too much weight to the views of the shooters.

The ongoing national debate ensured that by the time the Cullen Report was published most groups and political parties had already established their positions, making it unlikely that anything Lord Cullen recommended would make a difference.

Campaign for a Handgun Ban

During the early 1990s there was a perception, supported by official crime data, that handgun crime was on the increase leading to anxieties about an "American-style" gun culture taking hold, something that had little appeal to the British. There was speculation about the provenance of guns used in crime and varying estimates of the numbers of illegal weapons. Firearms enthusiasts argued that the crime problem was entirely the result of unlicensed guns. To them, and indeed many policy makers, legal guns posed no problems. Hungerford, and then Dunblane, were reminders this was not the case.

Gun ownership is low in Great Britain, with most of the population unfamiliar with what weapons can be owned legally. There was widespread shock, including among politicians, at the amount of firepower that Hamilton had available to him. Shooting with handguns in gun clubs had been on the rise and increasingly involved weapons more powerful than those used for traditional Olympics-style target shooting. In his report Cullen commented on the growth of activities like combat shooting and said that its trappings "caused others to feel uneasy about what appears to be the use of guns as symbols of personal power" (Cullen 1996).

Campaigns in support of a handgun ban began almost immediately, reflecting a majority public view confirmed in opinion polls, that handguns were too dangerous for private possession because they were easily concealable, rapidly fired, not justifiable for shooting game and criminals' weapon of choice. Most of those who became active campaigners had little, if any, prior knowledge of guns. Gun enthusiasts argued that this precluded them from influencing policy and that only those with a working knowledge of guns were qualified to discuss firearms legislation. Advocates for gun control were said to be too emotional and seeking an ill-informed knee-jerk response. For many, including the Dunblane victims' families the Inquiry hearings were, however, providing a crash course in gun-related issues.

The prime motivation of the campaigners was to minimize the risk of another shooting like Dunblane. Most thought that a minority sport (target shooting with handguns) was insufficient justification for compromising public safety through the private ownership of dangerous weapons. Hamilton's own history with guns suggested it was impossible to design a licensing system which would ensure handguns were never owned by those who would potentially misuse them. Psychological testing, something favored by the shooting organizations to eliminate potential "madmen," was said by the British Medical Association to have no predictive measure. Campaigners concluded that in the interest of public safety it was better to keep handguns out of all private hands.

Most national newspapers immediately called on the Government to introduce tighter gun controls, and media support during the various campaigns ensured a continuous source of pressure on politicians. Individual campaigns arose spontaneously and independently around the country. Two petitions in particular gained national prominence, one launched by a Scottish tabloid newspaper, the *Sunday Mail*, and the Dunblane Snowdrop Petition, organized by parents of young families living in Central Scotland. Each called for a handgun ban and was eventually supported by hundreds of thousands of signatures before being handed into Parliament. The Snowdrop Campaign gained considerable media coverage. Gun Control Network (GCN), whose aim was to provide a permanent voice for gun control beyond the current campaign, was also set up and its founding members included parents of victims of both the Hungerford and Dunblane shootings together with lawyers and academics. The campaigns ran on limited budgets, occasionally accepting *pro bono* help from PR companies, but relying mostly on the efforts of volunteers. They never came to depend on large organizations or high-profile celebrities.

Although unable to be directly involved during the initial stages, many of the Dunblane families became active participants once the Inquiry hearings were over. Each family made its own decision to join in, but without exception all came to support the aim of a handgun ban. The families' involvement in the Snowdrop Campaign and GCN ensured the various activities were coordinated. The families boosted the public profile of the campaign, which came to be portrayed, misleadingly, as entirely their own. It was critical that the issue was kept alive and, more than anyone else, the families could do this by talking to the media about themselves and their children as well as the handgun ban. They were able to gain access to politicians, and parliamentary lobbying would become a key activity.

Inevitably the shooting organizations were opposed to any change to the gun laws. They believed many were being punished for the actions of one man. They said Dunblane could be dismissed as another "one-off" event and were adamant that tighter controls would not stop it happening again. Pro-gun representatives gave evidence to the Public Inquiry and participated in media debates but probably believed their previous close political contacts would ensure that little would be changed. They told the Government not to react to special pleading of the Dunblane families, that a handgun ban would have no impact on gun crime, and that a "madman" cannot be stopped. The groups opposed to the ban failed to win over the general public or much of the media. Their rallies were only modestly attended, and when their tactics became more aggressive the media were quick to expose their personal attacks on gun control campaigners. The gun lobby could still rely on some support among parliamentarians, but the influence they had was limited. Some in the shooting community had, prior to Dunblane, been concerned by trends in handgun shooting that might be giving shooting the "wrong image," but all the groups stood firm against any legislative changes. Their intransigence made it inevitable that those seeking a tightening of controls would harden their position since any compromise over gun safety measures appeared impossible.

As the Cullen Report was awaited the political parties had been assessing the arguments and monitoring public opinion. The Government waited until the Report's publication, but the main opposition parties all announced that they were favoring a total ban.

Legislative Changes

The Cullen Report was published in October 1996, six months after the shootings. Although he did not recommend an outright ban on handguns, Cullen did recommend restrictions on how handguns were kept, suggesting measures such as disablement of guns when not in use and locked barrel blocks. However, he went on to add that "if such a system is not adopted the Government should consider restricting the availability of self-loading pistols and revolvers of any caliber by banning of the possession of such handguns by individual owners" (Cullen 1996).

At the time the Government was weak; its party divided on a number of issues, and had a very small parliamentary majority. Facing an imminent general election, Conservative MPs were sensitive to the public mood, which had been reflected in the campaigns, but they also had traditional links to the shooting community. The Government opted for a compromise. Choosing to go further than Cullen's recommendations, ministers proposed a partial ban—prohibiting all large-caliber handguns, though smaller guns (.22s) used by target shooters for events like the Olympic Games were still permitted with tighter restrictions. The compromise satisfied neither the campaigners nor the gun lobby, and within Parliament the Government faced opposition from both sides of the argument. Some MPs, mostly in the Government's own party, opposed any kind of ban whilst the main opposition parties wanted a total ban.

Through press conferences, interviews and lobbying, the Dunblane families immediately attempted to persuade more MPs to support a bill for a complete ban, highlighting the fact that .22 handguns could be just as lethal as other calibers. However, the Government retained sufficient support for the partial ban, and despite dissatisfaction from both sides of the debate a bill was passed to ban just the higher caliber handguns.

Three months after the bill had been enacted the Labour party won a general election with a huge majority. A number of the new Labour ministers had had the opportunity during the previous year to meet with the Dunblane families and listen to their views. As a result Labour had made a commitment in its election manifesto to prohibit the remaining small caliber handguns. A new law was duly passed and by February 1998 all handguns had become prohibited weapons. Handgun owners received compensation for the weapons they were required to surrender.

While there has since been a sustained attempt on the part of some shooting organizations to reverse the handgun ban this has been largely unsuccessful. The only concession was to allow an elite group of Olympic pistol shooters to practice on British soil during a limited period before the 2012 London Games.

In Great Britain the gun issue was not clouded by arguments over self-defense and the right to bear arms. Cullen's report had unambiguously rejected guns for self-defense. The United Kingdom's dominant view that guns were part of the problem, not part of the solution, remained intact and the eventual handgun ban was very much in keeping with this viewpoint (Squires 2000).

Impact and Legacy

The precise impact of the handgun ban on the complex pattern of gun crime would be impossible to quantify. The gun lobby, rightly pointing out that criminals were unlikely to surrender illegal handguns, claimed a handgun ban could have no effect on criminal activity. It was inevitable that it would take some time to reduce the pool of illegal handguns after the ban, but there is plenty of anecdotal evidence, for example from the National Ballistics Intelligence Service (Nabis), that there are now fewer guns on the street. In England and Wales gun crime did continue to rise during the period immediately following the ban, but after reaching a peak in 2003 and 2004 the total number of firearm offenses has fallen in every subsequent year (Lau 2012). In Scotland gun crime has decreased in almost every year since 1998 and is now less than a third of the 1996 level (Anon. 2012). Gun homicides are even rarer. In 2012 there were only six gun homicides in London reported in the media and a total of 32 across Great Britain. This is not the picture of a country in the grip of gun violence, and the risk for most of the British population remains extremely low. If there had been a drift towards an "American-style" gun culture in the 1990s the handgun ban stopped it.

Some concerns do remain, not least the difficulty some policy makers still have in recognizing any problems with other legal guns. There has been no other mass shooting involving handguns, but Britain did suffer another tragedy in 2010 when a man killed 12 people in Cumbria before killing himself. Derrick Bird's weapons, a shotgun and a rifle, were legally owned, raising questions about remaining inadequacies in Great Britain's gun laws.

Dunblane led to the birth of a gun control movement in Great Britain. Gun control advocates and campaign groups representing victims are now accepted as important participants in discussions on firearms, something which has ensured a far more balanced approach. GCN has been invited to give evidence to a number of Parliamentary Select Committees, has had regular meetings with ministers and shadow ministers and pressed for the introduction of further legislation which, since the handgun ban, has tightened controls over imitation firearms and airguns.

The handgun ban in Britain created interest around the world. It has been cited as an example of what can and should be done to stem gun violence elsewhere. The international gun lobby has sought to discredit the ban with distorted claims about its impact, especially on the level and type of violent crime in Britain. But for most of the British population it remains a positive step which has helped maintain a society that wishes to be as free as possible from the threat of gun violence.

ACKNOWLEDGMENTS

My daughter was one of the victims of the Dunblane shootings. I wish to acknowledge the support provided since 1996 by the other Dunblane families and express my thanks to my GCN colleagues, especially Peter Squires whose book has been an invaluable help in the preparation of this essay.

REFERENCES

Anon. 2012. *Recorded Crimes and Offenses Involving Firearms. Scotland, 2011–2012.* Edinburgh: Scottish Government.

Cullen, Lord W. Douglas. 1996. *The Public Inquiry into the Circumstances Leading up to and Surrounding the Events at Dunblane Primary School on Wednesday 13th March 1996.* Edinburgh: The Stationery Office.

Lau, Ivy. 2012. *Recorded Offences Involving the Use of Firearms.* In "Homicides, Firearm Offences and Intimate Violence 2010/11: Supplementary Volume 2 to Crime in England and Wales," ed. Kevin Smith. London: Home Office.

North, Mick. 2000. *Dunblane: Never Forget.* Edinburgh: Mainstream.

Squires, Peter. 2000. *Gun Culture or Gun Control.* London: Routledge.

15

Rational Firearm Regulation

Evidence-based Gun Laws in Australia

Rebecca Peters

Australians understand how Americans feel after the mass shooting at Sandy Hook Elementary School in Newtown, Connecticut, on December 14, 2012, because we had a similar experience in April 1996. In our case a disturbed young man with assault weapons killed 35 people at the Port Arthur historic site in Tasmania, one of Australia's most popular tourist destinations. Nineteen other people were seriously injured in the attack. Most of the victims were tourists from other states; some were local residents and workers. The guns used were legally available in Tasmania but banned in most other states.

It was the largest massacre by a single shooter ever recorded in the world and ignited an explosion of public sorrow and outrage as the nation demanded that the gun laws be overhauled. Responding to public pressure, the Prime Minister summoned the Australasian Police Ministers' Council (APMC) and proposed a plan for strict uniform gun laws. The Police Ministers also read the mood of the nation, and 12 days after the massacre they agreed to

Rebecca Peters is a violence prevention specialist who has worked for more than 20 years on arms control, women's rights, public health, and human security.

adopt the National Firearms Agreement into law in all eight states and territories.

Guns in Australia

Australia is a former frontier country, with a well-established gun culture. Guns are owned mainly for sport, recreational hunting, and for use on farms. Each state and territory has its own gun laws, and in early 1996 these varied widely between the jurisdictions. Guns that were banned in some states were legally available in others; some states required all guns to be registered while others did not. The license screening process also varied, so a person barred from owning guns in one state could legally own them in another. One important element was consistent across the nation: the relatively strict regulation of handguns. All jurisdictions limited these weapons to pistol club members and security guards, and all required the ownership and transfer of handguns to be registered with police. As a result of this restrictive approach, handguns made up only around 5% of the Australian stockpile (Harding 1988).

In 1996 Australia's firearm mortality rate was 2.7/100,000 (Mouzos 1999), or about one quarter the US rate. Australia had suffered mass shootings before Port Arthur. As in the United States, each tragedy provoked calls for stronger gun laws, and a grassroots campaign had been building for a decade. Until Port Arthur, however, gun law reform tended to advance in a piecemeal fashion, one tweak in one state at a time.

The Battle Over Firearm Regulation

The campaign for stronger laws was waged by hundreds of community and professional organizations which made up the National Coalition for Gun Control (NCGC): public health and medical societies, women's groups, senior citizens' associations, rural counselors, youth agencies, parents' groups, legal services, human rights organizations, churches, researchers, trade unions, and police. Participants ranged across the political spectrum, from the Country Women's Association to the Council for Civil Liberties, from the War Widows' Guild to the Gay & Lesbian Anti Violence Project.

This diversity reflected the multiplicity of dangers that guns pose in society: some NCGC members were especially concerned about domestic violence, others about crime on the streets, youth suicide, or workplace violence. Their common conviction was that guns are inherently dangerous products whose availability should be strictly regulated. However useful or enjoyable guns may be for their owners, the interests of public health and public safety must prevail.

The size and breadth of the coalition also reinforced the fact that gun law reform was a mainstream concern rather than the preserve of a single-issue lobby group. Opinion polls had long indicated that the overwhelming majority of Australians wanted tough uniform gun laws; yet the issue was usually framed by the media as a tug-of-war between gun control activists and the gun lobby.

Australia has a strong pro-gun lobby which for years had blocked proposed reforms by threatening parliamentarians whose seats were held by a slim electoral margin. Although most gun owners were not opposed to tighter gun laws, the gun lobby could count on a small number of zealots who were prepared to vote solely on this issue. Thus, despite legislators from both major political parties privately acknowledging the need for reform, neither party was prepared to make the first move publicly. Campaigners had long attempted to persuade the two parties to move simultaneously toward tighter laws, but the highly adversarial nature of Australian politics prevented this shift from occurring before 1996.

The breakthrough after Port Arthur came because John Howard, the newly elected Prime Minister, showed extraordinary leadership and took a stand for stronger gun laws. His courage was especially remarkable because his is the more conservative of our two major political parties, and traditionally considered the natural ally of the gun lobby. In fact this political configuration facilitated a bipartisan agreement: a conservative government inviting progressives to support gun control was more likely to succeed than vice versa. The bipartisan policy gave cover to state and federal parliamentarians from both parties, allowing them to support the reforms without fear of their opponents using the issue against them in an election. As one parliamentarian observed to me, "We go into public life to try to make things better, but then politics gets in the way. It's good to get the chance to do what's right without worrying about politics." John Howard still refers to reform of the gun laws as one of his proudest achievements (Howard 2012).

The bipartisan agreement was a major defeat for the gun lobby, but it continued to fight against the reforms. Rural communities were leafleted warning of total gun prohibition; government officials were harassed with floods of form letters; new political parties were formed to represent shooters.

Outlandish declarations, conspiracy theories, and threats voiced by pro-gun extremists made us realize Australia had its own "lunatic fringe"—and that it was heavily armed. Death threats were made against activists and parliamentarians. An image seared on the collective memory was our Prime Minister addressing a gathering of rural gun owners, obviously wearing a bullet-proof vest under his suit. This was said to be the first time such a precaution had been taken in Australia.

The Importance of Information and Research

In 1996 the World Health Assembly declared violence a leading worldwide public health problem, and urged countries to develop science-based solutions to prevent it (World Health Assembly 1996).

The National Coalition for Gun Control was seeking a comprehensive regulatory system based on prevention, designed to address the real nature of gun violence in Australia. That reality, according to public health, legal and criminology research, was

- Most gun deaths were suicides; though most suicides did not involve guns (Moller 1994).
- Guns were used in about 23% of all homicides, but more often in family killings and in multiple-victim attacks (Strang 1993; Wallace 1986; Bonney 1989).
- Most homicides involved victims and perpetrators who knew each other. Among these cases, most involved close personal relationships— the victim was a family member, current or former sexual partner or rival of the perpetrator, or a person attempting to assist someone in one of those categories (Strang 1993; Wallace 1986; Bonney 1989; Gallagher et al. 1994).
- Family homicides were usually preceded by a pattern of domestic violence (Wallace 1986; Law Reform Commission of Victoria 1991; Neal 1992); but most domestic violence was not reported to police (Department of Premier & Cabinet (Victoria) 1985; Queensland Domestic Violence Task Force 1988; Task Force on Domestic Violence (WA) 1986).
- Most homicide offenders had not previously been adjudicated mentally ill or convicted of criminal violence (Strang 1993; Wallace 1986).

The last two points highlighted the limitations of gun laws based on reacting after the fact. A system that waits until violence is officially recorded before taking any action will fail to assist most victims.

In addition, research from two similar jurisdictions, New Zealand and Canada, showed many firearm homicides involved weapons owned by licensed shooters (Alpers 1995; Dansys Consultants Inc. 1992).

The NCGC consulted closely with researchers and practitioners in academia, public agencies and service delivery organizations. The campaign's policy demands were based mainly on the reports of national and state expert review committees that had considered the regulation of firearms, either as a primary focus or as part of wider violence prevention (National Committee on Violence 1990; National Committee on Violence Against Women 1993; Australian Police Ministers' Council 1991; Australian Law Reform Commission 1986; Joint Select Committee Upon Gun Law Reform 1991; New South Wales Domestic Violence Committee 1991a,b,c; Queensland Domestic Violence Task Force 1988; Task Force on Domestic Violence (WA) 1986; Women's Policy Coordination Unit 1985; Parliament of Victoria, Social Development Committee 1988; Law Reform Commission of Victoria 1991).

The most important review had been by the National Committee on Violence (NCV), established in 1988 in the wake of two mass shootings. After hearing evidence around the country over the course of a year, the NCV made some 20 recommendations for firearms regulation (National Committee on Violence 1990). It called for national uniform gun laws and uniform guidelines for their enforcement; and for the development of a national gun control strategy aimed at (a) reducing the number of firearms in Australia and (b) preventing access to firearms by individuals who were not "fit and proper persons."

Ultimately the National Firearms Agreement contained almost all the measures recommended by the NCV and sought by the NCGC. One recommendation notably omitted from the Agreement was that handguns be required to be stored at pistol clubs.

The New Laws

The National Firearms Agreement is summarized in Table 15.1 (Australasian Police Ministers' Council 1996).

Once the National Firearms Agreement was settled, campaigners pushed for rapid implementation. As time passed and media interest waned, politicians

Table 15.1   National Firearms Agreement (1996) Australia

Ban on automatic and semi-automatic long arms—and buyback
- Ban on import, sale, resale, transfer, ownership, possession, manufacture and use

Nationwide registration of all firearms
- Integration of licensing and registration systems across the country

License applicants must prove 'genuine reason' for every firearm they wish to possess
- Personal protection is not a genuine reason; applicants for Category B, C, D and H must also prove 'genuine need'

Uniform basic licence requirements
- Age 18, prove genuine reason, be a 'fit and proper person', pass an adequate safety test, waiting period at least 28 days
- Photo licence showing the holder's address, the category of firearm, issued for a maximum of five years.
- Conditions include storage requirements, inspection by police, licence withdrawal/ seizure of guns in certain circumstances.
- Categories of licenses and firearms:
  - Category A: air rifles; rimfire rifles (excluding self-loading); single and double barrel shotguns
  - Category B: muzzle-loading firearms; single shot, double barrel and repeating centrefire rifles; break action shotgun/rifle combinations
  - Category C (prohibited except for certain occupational purposes, later expanded to include some clay target shooters): semi-automatic rimfire rifles with max 10-round magazine; semi-automatic shotguns with max 5-round magazine; pump action shotguns with max 5-round magazine.
  - Category D (prohibited except for official purposes): semi-automatic centrefire rifles; semi-automatic shotguns; pump action shotguns with a capacity over 5 rounds; semi-automatic rimfire rifles with capacity over 10 rounds.
  - Category H: all handguns, including air pistols.

Safety training as a prerequisite for licensing
- An accredited course required for first-time licence; a specialized course for persons employed in the security industry.

Grounds for licence refusal / cancellation and seizure of firearms, including:
- General reasons: not of good character, conviction for violence in past five years, contravene firearm law, unsafe storage, no longer genuine reason, not notifying change of address, licence obtained by deception, not in the public interest.
- Specific reasons: applicant/licence holder has had a restraining order or serious assault conviction in past 5 years.
- Mental or physical fitness: reliable evidence of a condition that would make the applicant unsuitable to possess a gun.

Permit to acquire
- Separate permits required for the acquisition of every firearm, with a waiting period of at least 28 days.

Table 15.1   (Continued)

Uniform standard for the security and storage of firearms
- Guns must be kept locked, ammunition stored separately; failure to store firearms safely is an offense.
- Specific storage requirements for different categories of firearms.
- Rules for safekeeping of firearms when temporarily away from the usual place of storage.

Recording of sales
- No private or backyard sales: all sales must be conducted by or through licensed firearm dealers.
- Dealers must ensure purchaser is licensed, and provide details of each purchase and sale to firearms registry.
- Ammunition sold only for those guns for which the purchaser is licensed; limits on the quantity that can be purchased.

No mail order sales
- Mail order only allowed from licensed gun dealer to licensed gun dealer.
- Advertising guns may only be conducted by or through a licensed gun dealer.
- The movement of Category C, D and H firearms must be in accordance with prescribed safety requirements.

became more susceptible to gun lobby pressure for a weak interpretation of the Agreement. However, within one year, all states and territories had amended or replaced their gun laws to comply.

The reform that received most publicity internationally was the buyback and destruction of the newly prohibited weapons. Owners had 12 months to surrender these guns for compensation, funded by a temporary increase in the national health levy. The financial carrot was backed up by a stick: after the buyback ended, possession of these weapons was a serious criminal offense. The stocks held by gun dealers were also bought back. Some 640,000 banned firearms were melted down in this 12-month program; though as discussed in the essay by Philip Alpers (in this volume), the final number of guns destroyed was considerably larger.

The legal reforms and buyback were accompanied by a large public awareness and information campaign. In addition, the computer systems of state and territory police forces were upgraded and linked together.

In 2002, following the shooting murder of two university students, the APMC made two more agreements on guns. The National Firearms Trafficking Policy Agreement strengthened border protection, regulation of gun dealers, and penalties for gun trafficking. The National Handgun Control Agreement restricted the types of handguns allowed for civilians.

Over the years, individual states and territories have amended their laws. There is no mechanism to maintain the uniform standard, and some cracks are beginning to emerge. In 2008 New South Wales made it easier for un-licensed individuals to have handguns at target clubs, with lethal conse-quences: in 2011 a patron walked out of a pistol club with one of the club's guns, and used it to shoot her father dead (*Sydney Pistol Club v Commissioner of Police, NSW Police Force* 2012). Campaigners point to tragedies like this as justifying further restrictions on handguns.

Overall, Australia's reforms have proved a resounding success. We have not had another mass shooting since 1996, and the firearms mortality rate today is 1/100,000—less than half what it was then (Australian Bureau of Statistics 2012), and one tenth the current United States rate.

This dramatic improvement in public safety has not stopped the United States gun lobby from misrepresenting the Australian experience as part of its campaign against firearm regulation. A National Rifle Association (NRA) infomercial video produced in 2000 claims crime rates have skyrocketed and Australia is overrun by criminals as a result of the reforms. The misinforma-tion was so outrageous that our Attorney General took the unusual step of writing a letter of complaint to Charlton Heston, then president of the NRA. Attorney General Daryl Williams wrote, "There are many things that Aus-tralia can learn from the United States. How to manage firearm ownership is not one of them . . . I request that you withdraw immediately the misleading information from your latest campaign" (Williams 2000).

The NRA ignored that request back in 2000, and now the video is once again in circulation on the Internet. But the reality is that firearm regulation has fulfilled its promise to make Australia safer. We hope our experience can help the United States find its own solutions.

REFERENCES

Alpers, Philip. 1995. "Firearm homicide in New Zealand: victims, perpetrators and their weapons 1992–1994." Paper presented at Public Health Association Confer-ence, Dunedin NZ, June 27–30.
Australian Bureau of Statistics. 2012. *Causes of Death, Australia, 2010,* 3303.0. Can-berra: Australian Bureau of Statistics.

Australian Law Reform Commission. 1986. *Domestic Violence*, Report No30. Canberra: Australian Government Publishing Service.

Australasian Police Ministers' Council. 1996. Resolutions from a Special Firearms Meeting. Canberra: APMC, May 10.

Australian Police Ministers' Council. 1991. "Draft Resolutions." October 23.

Bonney, Roseanne. 1989. *Homicide II*. Sydney: NSW Bureau of Crime Statistics & Research.

Dansys Consultants Inc. 1992. *Domestic Homicides Involving the Use of Firearms*. Ottawa: Department of Justice (Canada), March.

Gallagher, Patricia, Nguyen Da Huong, Marie Therese, and Bonney, Roseanne. 1994. *Trends in homicide 1968–1992*. Sydney: NSW Bureau of Crime Statistics & Research.

Harding, Richard. 1988. "Everything you need to know about gun control in Australia." Briefing paper prepared for the Australian Bankers' Association.

Howard, John. 2012. "Brothers in arms, yes, but the US needs to get rid of its guns." *The Age*, August 1. http://www.theage.com.au/opinion/politics/brothers-in-arms-yes-but-the-us-needs-to-get-rid-of-its-guns-20120731-23ct7.html#ixzz2HbNM2pA7

Joint Select Committee Upon Gun Law Reform. 1991. *Report of the Joint Select Committee Upon Gun Law Reform*. Sydney: NSW Parliament.

Law Reform Commission of Victoria. 1991. Homicide, Report No. 40. Melbourne: LRCV.

Moller, Jerry. 1994. "The spatial distribution of injury deaths in Australia: Urban, rural and remote areas." *Australian Injury Prevention Bulletin* Issue 8, December.

Mouzos, Jenny. 1999. *Firearm related Violence: The Impact of the Nationwide Agreement on Firearms*. Trends & Issues No. 116. Canberra: Australian Institute of Criminology.

National Committee on Violence Against Women. 1993. *National Strategy on Violence Against Women*. Canberra: Australian Government Publishing Service.

National Committee on Violence. 1990. *Violence—Directions for Australia*. Canberra: Australian Institute of Criminology.

Neal, David. 1992. "The murder mystery." *Modern Times*, June. Fitzroy, Victoria. Australian Modern Times.

NSW Domestic Violence Committee. 1991a. *Report of the NSW Domestic Violence Committee, NSW Domestic Violence Strategic Plan*. Sydney: Women's Coordination Unit.

NSW Domestic Violence Committee. 1991b. *Report on Submissions, Consultations and Forums, NSW Domestic Violence Strategic Plan*. Sydney: Women's Coordination Unit.

NSW Domestic Violence Committee. 1991c. "Submission to Joint Select Committee Upon Gun Law Reform." Sydney: Women's Coordination Unit.

Parliament of Victoria, Social Development Committee. 1988. *First Report Upon the Inquiry into Strategies to Deal with the Issue of Community Violence*. Melbourne: Jean Gordon Government Printer.

Queensland Domestic Violence Task Force. 1988. *Beyond These Walls, Report of the Queensland Domestic Violence Task Force*, Brisbane.

Strang, Heather. 1993. *Homicide in Australia, 1991–1992.* Canberra: Australian Institute of Criminology.

Sydney Pistol Club v Commissioner of Police, NSW Police Force. 2012. NSW Administrative Decisions Tribunal 121, 21.

Task Force on Domestic Violence (WA). 1986. *Break the Silence: Report of the Task Force on Domestic Violence to the Western Australian Government.* Perth: Western Australian Government.

Wallace, Alison. 1986. *Homicide: The Social Reality.* Sydney: NSW Bureau of Crime Statistics & Research.

Williams, Daryl. 2000. Letter to Charlton Heston, March 22.

Women's Policy Co-ordination Unit. 1985. *Criminal Assault in the Home: Social and Legal Responses to Domestic Violence.* Melbourne: Department of Premier & Cabinet (Victoria).

World Health Assembly. 1996. "WHA49.25 Prevention of violence: a public health priority." Geneva: Forty-Ninth World Health Assembly, May 20–25.

16

The Big Melt

How One Democracy Changed after Scrapping
a Third of Its Firearms

Philip Alpers

In recent years, several democracies have dramatically reduced the availability of firearms to private individuals. I emphasize the word *democracies* because, contrary to Internet chatter, the countries in which voters have supported gun amnesties and buybacks are not dictatorships. They include the United Kingdom, Brazil, Argentina, and Australia, which in recent years destroyed a third of its privately owned guns.

Many observers continue to cite the official tally of guns destroyed by smelting in the Australian National Firearms Buyback as 659,940 newly prohibited weapons (Australia 2002). Yet the actual number of private weapons destroyed is now estimated at well over one million. As outlined in the essay by Rebecca Peters (in this volume), in the late 1990s all Australian states and territories agreed to new uniform legislation, the primary declared purpose of which was to reduce the risk of mass shootings. Owner licensing was tightened to require proof of "genuine reason" to possess a gun; the sale and transfer of

Philip Alpers is an adjunct associate professor at the Sydney School of Public Health, the University of Sydney.

firearms was limited to licensed dealers; rapid-fire rifles and shotguns were banned, bought back, and destroyed; and remaining firearms were registered to uniform national standards (Australia 1996). Two nationwide, federally funded gun buybacks made the headlines, but until now the number of additional, voluntary, and unrecompensed surrenders for destruction remained unquantified.

In the seven years up to January 1988 and before the Port Arthur shootings in 1996, six gun massacres (five or more victims shot dead) had already claimed the lives of 40 Australians (Chapman, Alpers, et al. 2006). According to articles in the print media published during the twenty-four years that followed, we know that 38 state, territory, and federal firearm amnesties ran for a minimum combined total of 3,062 weeks. From the reports in which numbers were published, a total of 948,388 firearms were surrendered to police for destruction. Of these, 67,488 (7.1%) were collected before the federal long-gun buyback which followed the 1996 Port Arthur tragedy. In the 1996–97 National Firearms Buyback of rapid-fire long guns (mainly semi-automatic rifles but also self-loading and pump-action shotguns) and in the 2003 National Handgun Buyback which followed, Australians gave up for destruction 728,667 newly prohibited firearms in return for market-value compensation.

Having measured the scale of the Australian experiment with more accuracy, I have found that at least 219,721 additional firearms were surrendered for destruction—a number which until now has been untallied and largely unrecognized. Although the Australian initiative was most often described as a "buyback" in which gun owners received cash compensation, of all the weapons handed in for destruction since 1988, nearly one in four yielded no financial return to its owner (Alpers and Wilson 2013). Such was the swing in public opinion that large numbers of gun owners sent lawfully held firearms to the smelter, even when there was no obligation to do so.

This tally of just under a million weapons destroyed is conservative. In published reports of 20 gun amnesties we found no count of firearms collected and so were unable to include the numbers handed in for destruction (Alpers and Wilson 2013). In addition, many firearms seized by police and destroyed, for example by court order, are not included in amnesty totals. Two small "weapon" amnesties included non-firearms in their published totals without separation. Taking into account these uncertainties, it seems likely that Australia collected and destroyed well over a million firearms—

that is, between five and six firearms per 100 people. A commonly accepted estimate of the number of firearms in Australia at the time of the Port Arthur shootings is 3.2 million (Reuter and Mouzos 2003, 130). This suggests that post-massacre destruction efforts reduced the national stock of firearms by one-third. If we accept a frequently cited estimate of 270 million privately owned guns in the United States (Karp 2007, 47), a similar effort in that country would require the destruction of 90 million firearms.

This is not to say that such a massive reduction in the national stockpile could be effected in the United States. Because no two jurisdictions share the same problems or legislative or social settings—let alone attitudes—none can claim to have discovered the magic bullet. The Australian experience also suggests that a reduction in the availability of firearms might only be temporary, as removal of several types of newly banned firearms was followed by a surge of replacement buying.

Australia no longer has a firearm manufacturing industry. Gun dealers source their stock from overseas—mainly from the United States. In the year of the main Australian buyback, firearm imports briefly doubled as owners replaced their banned, surrendered multi-shot rifles and shotguns with new single-shot replacements. But in the two years that followed, annual gun imports crashed to just 20 percent of that 1996–97 peak. For two years the trade remained stagnant and then began to recover. By mid-2012, following a steady ten-year upward trend in gun buying, Australians had restocked the national arsenal of private guns to pre–Port Arthur levels. They did this by importing 1,055,082 firearms, an average of 43,961 each year since destruction programs began (Alpers, Wilson, and Rossetti 2013) (this total excludes 52,608 handguns imported for law enforcement and other non-civilian use). To this should be added the national stock of illicit firearms, which by definition cannot be counted. Although claims of large-scale gun smuggling to Australia are common, almost all such stories are evidence-free. But a recent study from the Australian Institute of Criminology, recounting a cross-governmental effort to trace firearms seized in crime, confirms a more influential source. Smuggled guns represent a much smaller proportion of recovered illicit firearms in this island nation than do legally imported firearms that were subsequently diverted or lost to the black market by lawful owners (Bricknell 2012, 41–43).

A range of public health benefits has been both observed and disputed. As policy changes took effect in the wake of the Port Arthur massacre, the risk of an Australian dying by gunshot fell more than 50 percent and stayed at that level (Alpers, Wilson, and Rossetti 2013a). The number of gun homicides fell from 69 in 1996 (this total excludes the 35 victims shot dead at Port Arthur) to 30 in 2012 (Alpers, Wilson, and Rossetti 2013b). In the decade before the country's change of direction, 100 people died in eleven mass shootings (Chapman, Alpers, et al. 2006). Following the 1996 announcement of legislation specifically designed to reduce gun massacres, Australia has seen no more mass shootings. Firearm-related deaths that attract smaller headlines still occur, yet the national rate of gun homicide—which before Port Arthur was already one-fifteenth the U.S. rate—has now plunged to 0.13 per 100,000, or 27 times lower than that of the United States (Alpers, Wilson, and Rossetti 2013c).

The most comprehensive impact study of the Australian interventions found that "the buyback led to a drop in the firearm suicide rates of almost 80%, with no significant effect on non-firearm death rates. The effect on firearm homicides is of similar magnitude but is less precise." Important for any discussion of causality, the authors also found that "the largest falls in firearm deaths occurred in states where more firearms were bought back." This study went on to cite survey results to suggest that Australia had nearly halved its number of gun-owning households and then estimated that, by withdrawing firearms on such a scale, this nation of nearly 23 million people had saved itself 200 deaths by gunshot and US$500 million in costs each year (Leigh and Neill 2010).

The evidence is clear that following gun law reform, Australians became many times less likely to be killed with a firearm (Alpers, Wilson, and Rossetti 2013a). That said, causality and standards of proof are as contentious in Australia as in any community polarized by the gun debate. Central to the differing interpretations is that Australia's gun death rates were already declining prior to its major public health interventions. Taking this into account, one study concluded nevertheless that "the rates per 100,000 of total firearm deaths, firearm homicides and firearm suicides all at least doubled their existing rates of decline after the revised gun laws" (Chapman, Alpers, et al. 2006).

A countervailing study interpreted essentially the same empirical findings to conclude the opposite, namely that "the gun buy-back and restrictive legislative changes had no influence on firearm homicide in Australia" (Baker and McPhedran 2007). In an article for the National Rifle Association of America, one of the coauthors of this study was quoted as saying "The findings were clear . . . the policy has made no difference. There was a trend of declining deaths which has continued" (Smith 2007). A third paper relied on different tests to find that Australia's new gun laws "did not have any large effects on reducing firearm homicide or suicide rates" (Lee and Suardi 2010). These two "little or no effect" studies and their methodology have since been heavily criticized (Neill and Leigh 2007, Hemenway 2009, 2011).

To date, one conclusion has gone uncontested. In finding "no evidence of substitution effect for suicides or homicides," the initial study of impacts showed that Australia's interventions were not followed by displacement from firearms to other methods (Chapman, Alpers, et al. 2006).

The Australian experience, catalyzed by 35 deaths in a single shooting spree, marked a national sea change in attitudes, both to firearms and to those who own them. Led by a conservative government, Australians saw that, beliefs and fears aside, death and injury by gunshot could be as amenable to public health intervention as were motor vehicle–related deaths, drunk driving, tobacco-related disease, and the spread of HIV/AIDS. The obstructions to firearm injury prevention are nothing new to public health. An industry and its self-interest groups focused on denial, the propagation of fear, and quasi-religious objections—we've seen it all before. But the future is also here to see (Mozaffarian, Hemenway, and Ludwig 2013). With gun violence, as with HIV/AIDS, waste-of-time notions such as evil, blame, and retribution can with time be sluiced away to allow long-proven public health procedures. Given the opportunity and the effort, gun injury prevention can save lives as effectively as restricting access to rocket-propelled grenades and explosives or mandating child-safe lids on bottles of poison.

ACKNOWLEDGMENTS

The author thanks Belinda Gardner and Amélie Rossetti, skilled and willing researchers at GunPolicy.org.

REFERENCES

Alpers, Philip, and Marcus Wilson. 2013. *Australian Firearm Amnesty, Buyback and Destruction Totals: Official Tallies and Media-reported Numbers, 1987–2012.* Sydney: GunPolicy.org, Sydney School of Public Health. http://www.gunpolicy.org

/documents/doc_download/5337-alpers-australian-firearm-amnesty-buyback
-and-destruction-totals.

Alpers, Philip, Marcus Wilson, and Amélie Rossetti. 2013. *Guns in Australia: Facts, Figures and Firearm Law (Imports)*. Sydney: GunPolicy.org, Sydney School of Public Health. http://www.gunpolicy.org/firearms/compareyears/10/firearm_imports_number.

Alpers, Philip, Marcus Wilson, and Amélie Rossetti. 2013a. *Guns in Australia: Facts, Figures and Firearm Law (Total Number of Gun Deaths)*. Sydney: GunPolicy.org, Sydney School of Public Health. http://www.gunpolicy.org/firearms/compareyears/10/total_number_of_gun_deaths.

Alpers, Philip, Marcus Wilson, and Amélie Rossetti. 2013b. *Guns in Australia: Facts, Figures and Firearm Law (Number of Gun Homicides)*. Sydney: GunPolicy.org, Sydney School of Public Health. http://www.gunpolicy.org/firearms/compareyears/10/number_of_gun_homicides.

Alpers, Philip, Marcus Wilson, and Amélie Rossetti. 2013c. *Guns in Australia: Facts, Figures and Firearm Law (Compare Australia: Rate of Gun Homicide)*. Sydney: Gun Policy.org, Sydney School of Public Health. http://www.gunpolicy.org/firearms/compare/10/rate_of_gun_homicide/31,66,69,87,91,128,178,192,194.

Australia. 1996. *Resolutions from a Special Firearms Meeting*. Canberra: Australian Police Ministers Council.

Australia. 2002. *The Australian Firearms Buyback: Tally for Number of Firearms Collected and Compensation Paid*. Canberra: Commonwealth Attorney-General's Department.

Baker, Jeanine, and Samara McPhedran. 2007. Gun Laws and Sudden Death: Did the Australian Firearms Legislation of 1996 Make a Difference? *British Journal of Criminology* 47:455–69.

Bricknell, Samantha. 2012. *Firearm Trafficking and Serious and Organised Crime Gangs*. Canberra: Australian Institute of Criminology Research and Public Policy Series 116.

Chapman, Simon, Philip Alpers, Kingsley Agho, and Michael Jones. 2006. Australia's 1996 Gun Law Reforms: Faster Falls in Firearm Deaths, Firearm Suicides and a Decade without Mass Shootings. *Injury Prevention* 12:365–72.

Hemenway, David. 2009. How to Find Nothing. *Journal of Public Health Policy* 30:260–68.

Hemenway, David. 2011. The Australian Gun Buyback. Boston: Harvard Injury Control Research Center *Bulletins* 4.

Karp, Aaron. 2007. Completing the Count: Civilian Firearms. In *Small Arms Survey 2007: Guns and the City*, 38–71. Cambridge: Cambridge University Press.

Lee, Wang-Sheng, and Sandy Suardi. 2010. The Australian Firearms Buyback and Its Effect on Gun Deaths. *Contemporary Economic Policy* 28:65–79.

Leigh, Andrew, and Christine Neill. 2010. Do Gun Buybacks Save Lives? Evidence from Panel Data. *American Law and Economics Review* 12(2):462–508.

Mozaffarian, Dariush, David Hemenway, and David S. Ludwig. 2013. Curbing Gun Violence: Lessons from Public Health Successes. *Journal of the American Medical Association* 1–2. Published online: Jan. 7, 2013. doi:10.1001/jama.2013.38

Neill, Christine, and Andrew Leigh. 2007. Weak Tests and Strong Conclusions: A Re-analysis of Gun Deaths and the Australian Firearms Buyback. Canberra: The

Australian National University, Centre for Economic Policy Research. *EPS Journal*, Discussion Paper 555.

Reuter, Peter, and Jenny Mouzos. 2003. Australia: A Massive Buyback of Low-risk Guns. In *Evaluating Gun Policy: Effects on Crime and Violence*, edited by Jens Ludwig and Philip J. Cook. Washington, DC: The Brookings Institution.

Smith, Blaine. 2007. Dim Bulb! *America's 1st Freedom*. Fairfax, VA: National Rifle Association of America, 8(2):34–54.

17

Brazil

Gun Control and Homicide Reduction

Antonio Rangel Bandeira

Brazil accounts for 13% of the world's firearm homicides, despite having only 2.8% of the world's population. Brazil holds the sad world record for the highest number of annual deaths by firearms in absolute numbers. Faced with such deplorable rates of death by gun violence, Brazil has started reversing this trend by implementing a series of controls on these lethal products. The results have been impressive. According to the national Ministry of Justice, Brazil has reduced deaths by firearms from 39,284 in 2003 to 34,300 in 2010—a saving of 5,000 lives.[1] This essay analyzes the steps that have been taken.

Guns in Brazil

The research organization Viva Rio found that Brazil has about 16 million guns in circulation, half of which are illegal.[2] Recent gun control reforms have made it more difficult to qualify to buy weapons. This has resulted in a dramatic

Antonio Rangel Bandeira is the Coordinator of Firearms Control Programs at Viva Rio in Rio de Janeiro.

decrease in the annual sale of guns from 155,834 in 2010 to 93,334 in 2011 and down to 12,530 as of July 2012.[3] To offset this decrease in domestic sales, the Brazilian gun industry has expanded its international exports by 370% since 2000. The country is now the fourth biggest firearm exporter, just behind the USA, Italy, and Germany, selling $314 million worth of weapons internationally in 2010.[4] In 1981, the Brazilian gun maker Taurus S.A. established a manufacturing facility in Florida. This plant and the exports from Brazil account for 20% of the pistols and revolvers sold in the North American market.[5]

Scientific Facts versus Myths

Nineteen years ago, faced with growing urban violence in Rio de Janeiro, Viva Rio sought to implement policies within the classical progressive paradigm focusing on unemployment, social inequality and illiteracy. It soon became clear that this was not enough; reducing urban violence required both gun control *and* reforms to the police force. The proliferation of weapons, which initially was viewed as a secondary cause of violence, turned out to be the key. This factor explained why personal conflicts that did not result in fatalities in other countries so often proved deadly in Rio de Janeiro. It became necessary to understand the universe of firearms.

At that time very little research had been done on gun markets, the use of guns by civilians, or their impact. Viva Rio had to create a research methodology to analyze the dynamics of arms and ammunition. (Researchers were fortunate to have as a colleague Dr. Pablo Dreyfus, an expert from Argentina, who had done field research on drug trafficking before becoming a researcher for the Small Arms Survey. He was a brilliant pioneer in this new field and his work influenced research on guns elsewhere, both in developing and developed countries. Sadly he died in the Air France crash on June 1, 2009.)

We found that guns belong to a nebulous, almost secret world. Those who profit from the production and sale of guns have no interest in sharing information with outside analysts. In Latin America gun control authorities frequently are co-opted by those who profit from the firearms trade. The arms market had never been studied in a serious manner in Latin America and usually governments did not share data with independent experts.

In 1999 a progressive city government gave us information on 250,000 weapons seized by police in Rio de Janeiro. Our analysis of this data drastically altered the public perspective about guns in Brazil. The prevailing belief was that most illegal weapons were smuggled in from abroad, but we discovered that no more than 14% were imported[6] (and we later showed that the figure was only 10% nationwide).[7] Thus the overwhelming majority of guns used in crime had been manufactured and originally sold legally in Brazil.

Furthermore, it had been assumed that most of the guns used in crime were large caliber rifles and machine guns, but we showed that 83% were actually revolvers and pistols. In other words, because of a lack of research, the police were battling the illegal arms trade based on completely erroneous information. Our analysis provided the foundation for better policies based on factual knowledge rather than myths and ideology.

New Law on Arms and Ammunition

With the data showing that illegal guns originated from the poorly controlled legal market, we began a campaign for stronger regulations. Those opposed to our efforts did not present research, only ideological arguments like those of the National Rifle Association (NRA). Despite having support from the major media organizations, we initially had no luck with members of the national Congress. The arms industry in Brazil, as in the United States, donates money to election campaigns for many politicians. We tried unsuccessfully to persuade them to reform the weak gun law which had been originally enacted under the influence of the arms industry and the former military dictatorship.

It was clear that in order to change the law we needed to gain the support of the electorate, to exert popular pressure on Congress for reform. We identified strategic allies (churches, women, social groups victimized by guns, physicians, academics and sympathetic journalists and politicians, and unions). With their support, we toured the country disseminating our research and countering myths about weapons and disarmament. As public awareness increased, hundreds of thousands of people marched in the major cities demanding tougher gun laws. When the polls showed that 81% of Brazilians favored a new gun law,[8] the climate changed in the Congress. Although the arms industry had the money, the voters were on our side. In December 2003 our bill was approved by all political parties. President Lula signed the Disarmament Statute into law as a Christmas gift to the people of Brazil.[9]

The new law is very advanced and is serving as inspiration for several other countries. The law banned the carrying of weapons by civilians, prohibited

guns above .38 caliber for civilians, raised the minimum age for gun purchases to 25 years, and added 15 requirements to the process of qualifying to
buy a gun, including evidence of psychological stability and knowledge of
gun safety. A national database was set up to monitor gun ownership, and
ammunition sold to the police and armed forces is now marked to enable
tracing. (The marking of ammunition sold to civilians is now also under discussion, with the same objective.) Once marked, cartridges left at the scene of
crimes or confrontations can be traced. This procedure was used to prove
that police officers were responsible for the 2009 killing of Patricia Acioli, a
young judge who took a stand against organized crime and corrupt police, in
Rio de Janeiro.

Myths about Firearms

The campaign for gun control drew on research to challenge widely held but
mistaken beliefs about firearms.[10] For example:

- A firearm is a good instrument for attack, but not for defense.
  The attacker uses the element of surprise and thus controls the
  circumstances of the attack.[11]
- Of the nearly 30 countries that have promoted voluntary disarmament,
  none is a dictatorship. Democracies seek to reduce the level of
  armament in their society, depending instead on good police and a
  strong rule of law to achieve public safety. Democratic regimes may
  be overthrown by military coups, but it is an illusion to imagine that
  citizens with guns can defend democracy against tanks and aircraft.
  We Latin Americans know what we're talking about, having suffered
  military coups and dictatorships.
- It is a simplistic analysis to merely consider the polarization between
  "good guys and bad guys" or "good guns and bad guns." This represents
  just a small part of the discussion of self-defense. In Brazil, as well as
  in most countries with high levels of gun homicides, interpersonal
  conflicts represent more than 80% of murders perpetrated with
  firearms. If we add together men killing women; fights between
  neighbors, in nightclubs, and in traffic jams; fired employees fighting
  against former bosses; and suicides and accidents involving children,
  these deaths represent many more casualties than those inflicted by

bandits and burglars. All reliable research demonstrates that, when there is a lack of governmental gun control, the most accurate sentiment is that "good guys kill good guys," usually with legal weapons. This situation represents a major part of the problem. Although the use of guns for self-defense sometimes results in successful self-protection, public policies cannot be established based on exceptions; they must be built on the facts of daily life.

- The old slogan says "Guns don't kill people. People kill people." In reality, "People with guns kill people."

Public Destruction of Weapons

The campaign coincided with the request by the United Nations that countries publicly destroy their surplus firearms. In July 2001, on the eve of the United Nations Conference on Small Arms, the Rio de Janeiro government, with technical support from Viva Rio and the army, carried out a public destruction of 100,000 weapons. It also highlighted the danger created by the police stockpiling huge quantities of surplus weapons that are often diverted to organized crime.

Voluntary Programs to Hand in Weapons

Another aspect of Brazil's attempt to stem gun violence has been a series of voluntary weapons buybacks. The first buyback in 2004 to 2005 saw Brazilians hand in 459,855 weapons, which were then destroyed.[12] Some of the country's largest advertising agencies worked on the campaign pro bono, and famous performers and football stars donated their services as well. Feminist and women's organizations also played an important role in changing the culture. Ad campaigns were implemented in which grandmothers, mothers, and girlfriends urged men to get rid of their guns, while pretty female soap opera stars ridiculed "insecure men who need firearms to prove their masculinity." These initiatives were especially well-received among young people. The campaign slogan was *Choose Gun Free. It Is Your Weapon or Me!* The campaign symbol was a tube of lipstick, which appeared to look like a bullet.

In addition, the 2004 to 2005 campaign featured significant involvement by community groups and the nonprofit sector (churches, NGOs, unions, etc.), which oversaw buyback locations for guns and ammunition. These sites were numerous and easily accessible, particularly for groups reluctant to trust the police. The guns were damaged with a small hammer upon receipt; a cheap and efficient way to immediately improve public safety by eliminating the risk of diversion or reuse. Citizens were paid between US$50 and US$150 for their guns, depending on the caliber. (The amounts paid were deliberately modest to reduce the likelihood that recipients would use the money to buy new guns, as happened in Australia and Haiti.) The exchanges were anonymous and amnesty was offered to owners of illegal weapons.

From 2008 to 2009, the Brazilian government launched a second campaign involving the police, but at this time without the participation of civil society. Compared with the 2004 to 2005 effort, the results were modest: only 30,721 weapons were received.[13] Then in May 2011, a month after the Realengo School shooting in Rio de Janeiro (where 12 teenagers were killed by a former student), the government announced another buyback, which continues today.

Before the 2011 launch, an international conference was convened to review the results of successful exchange programs from Angola, Argentina, Colombia, Mozambique, and Brazil. This analysis led to several improvements on our previous campaigns. Participants were paid within 24 hours, whereas previously there had been a three-month delay. And although only 18% who turn in guns do so for the money,[14] compensation was increased to between US$80 and US$225.

The new campaign's slogan is *Hand in Your Weapon. Protect Your Family*, to counter the misguided practice of arming oneself to defend family and loved ones. Activities include programs exchanging toy guns for peaceful toys. The current campaign has some shortcomings—including not compensating for ammunition (as Argentina does, with excellent results) and a continued lack of involvement by the community sector. In a period of 19 months, about 65,144 weapons were handed in.[15]

According to the Ministry of Health, the following measures have reduced firearm homicides significantly: half a million guns were removed from circulation, public carrying of firearms was outlawed, and police reform was initiated.[16] Gun deaths have dropped by more than 70% in São Paulo and by 30% in Rio de Janeiro.[17] In addition, a process of "pacification" of the largest favelas of Rio de Janeiro has taken place over the past few years, which has contributed to the decrease. (Pacification refers to the institution of community-based police forces in the favelas, which were previously dominated by the drug traffickers and by improved investments in health, education, and urban development.)

Parliamentary Oversight of Weapons and Ammunition

In 2004, a Parliamentary Commission of Inquiry (PCI) was formed to investigate Brazil's illicit arms trade. Among other things, the Commission investigated Brazil's international borders and was able to identify major smuggling points for arms and ammunition. Viva Rio supplied expert technical support and performed the field work for this endeavor.[18] The PCI also forced Brazilian gun manufacturers to identify the initial purchasers of 36,000 weapons that had been seized by the Rio de Janeiro police, which revealed that most weapons used in organized crime had been diverted from initially legal sources.[19] These included guns bought by civilians from gun shops, guns purchased by private security companies, private police and military officers guns, guns stolen from legal owners, and guns diverted from police stocks by corrupt police officers. The court system also turned out to be a significant source of diversion of guns to the criminal market, as hundreds of thousand of guns are stored in court evidence rooms. The PCI's final report has been called a pioneering document—mapping the previously unexplored world of one country's illegal arms trade.[20]

A permanent Subcommittee on Control of Arms and Munitions was established in the Parliament in 2007, created with our influence and support, to oversee the implementation of the Disarmament Statute, conduct research on weapons and ammunition, and propose new control measures. Last year the parliamentary gun lobby got control of the Subcommittee and has been trying to revoke the Disarmament Statute.

In response to the PCI's work, the International Latin American Parliamentary group, PARLATINO, asked Viva Rio and an international team of experts to draft a model law. The Model Law on Firearms, Ammunition and Related Materials was developed from this effort, to assist other countries with improved gun control measures.[21]

The Disarmament Statute mandated a referendum be held on the question of whether all sales of guns and ammunitions to civilians should be banned in Brazil. The referendum was held in October 2005, and our side lost. Although public support for strong gun control was extremely high, 64% of voters voted against the total ban. Analysts suggested several possible reasons for our defeat. Institutions receiving funds from abroad were barred from campaigning, preventing the participation of historically active groups such as most churches and nongovernmental organizations. Also relevant was the strong financial support provided by the gun lobby to the other side, as well as a slump in popularity of the Lula government, which had been accused of corruption around the time of the referendum. Even so, national support for gun control remained above 80%.

In addition to the voluntary disarmament program, the Brazilian government decided to organize an arms legalization campaign. This campaign was aimed at the large number of people who were not "criminals," but who held weapons illegally (i.e., without a license). In 2008 to 2009 the government, with support from the gun dealers, shooting clubs and pro-gun associations, secured the registration of 1,408,285 weapons[22]—a good start toward regulating 4 million illegal weapons estimated to be in the hands of non-criminals. The legalization initiative included suspending the license fee and providing an amnesty for these gun owners.

The International Agenda—and Soccer

Trafficking arms and ammunition is an international phenomenon which requires a correspondingly international approach. The agenda for international action is clear but remains largely on paper. It includes harmonizing laws within and among countries (we recommend the Model Law as a starting point). Bilateral and multilateral agreements, regionally and internationally (like the Arms Trade Treaty) are necessary for collaboration between police in different countries. An important new regional initiative is the centralization of information about arms and ammunition in the database operated by the Observatory on Citizen Security, run by the Organization of American States.[23]

In 2014 the Soccer World Cup will be in Brazil and the social theme of the tournament will be "disarmament." Soccer fans will be able to hand in guns in exchange for tickets to the matches. Whenever the Brazilians play they will display a banner supporting disarmament, as they did before their game against the United States in Washington, DC, in May 2011. We want to unite the sporting spirit of fraternity with the culture of peace and disarmament. We invite the United States to organize gun hand-in programs during the Cup, joining other nations that have already made the commitment. We do not want a violent society where people are armed, but rather a peaceful one where people are protected against guns.

NOTES

1. Brazilian Minister of Justice Declaration, Brasília, December 10, 2010.
2. Purcena and Nascimento, *Estoques*, 23.
3. Bergamo, "Venda de Armas no Brasil Despenca."
4. Guerra, "Fabricantes de Armas Triplicam Receita no Brasil em Apenas Cinco Anos."
5. Author's conversation with ATF officials, during their visit to Viva Rio's office, 2000.
6. Bandeira and Bourgeois, *Armas de Fogo*, 168–171.
7. Purcena and Nascimento, *Seguindo a Rota das Armas*, 20.
8. Instituto Sensus, June 2003, cited by Bandeira and Bourgeois, *Armas de Fogo*, 200.
9. *Estatuto do Desarmament.*
10. For more detailed analysis, see Bandeira, "Armas Pequeñas y Campañas de Desarme."
11. Cano, *Pesquisa sobre Vitimização nos Roubos.*
12. Secretaria Nacional de Segurança Pública (Brasilia: Ministry of Justice, January 2006).
13. Idem (January 2010).
14. Viva Rio's research, cited by Bandeira and Bourgeois, *Armas de Fogo*, 206.
15. Secretaria Nacional de Segurança Pública (Brasilia, Ministry of Justice, January 2013).
16. Based on Sistema Nacional de Saúde (SUS), Secretaria Nacional de Segurança Pública (Brasília: Ministry of Justice, December 2010).
17. Instituto de Segurança Pública (Rio de Janeiro, Secretaria de Segurança Pública, July 2012).
18. Dreyfus and Bandeira, *Watching the Neighborhood.*
19. Jungmann, *Comissão Parlamentar.*
20. Ibid.
21. Parliamentary Forum on Small Arms and Light Weapons and CLAVE.
22. Sistema Nacional de Armas e Munições (SINARM), Federal Police Department, cited by Purcena and Nascimento, *Estoques*, 39.
23. Bandeira, "Gun Control in Brazil," 38.

REFERENCES

Bandeira, Antonio. "Armas Pequeñas y Campañas de Desarma. Matar los Mitos y Salvar las Vidas." In *Seguridad Regional en América Latina y el Caribe*, ed. Hans Mathieu and Catalina Niño Guarnizo. Bogotá: Friedrich Ebert Stiftung, 2012.

Bandeira, Antonio. "Gun Control in Brazil and International Agenda." In *Report on Citizen Security in the Americas—2012*. Washington. DC: Secretariat for Multidimensional Security, OAS, 2012. www.alertamerica.org

Bandeira, Antonio, and Bourgeois, Josephine. *Armas de Fogo: Proteção ou Risco?* Rio de Janeiro: Viva Rio, 2005. http://www.comunidadesegura.org/files/active/0/armas%20de%20fogo%20protecao%20ou%20risco_port1.pdf

Bandeira, Antonio, and Bourgeois, Josephine. *Firearms: Protection or Risc?* Stockholm: Parliamentary Forum on Small Arms and Light Weapons, 2006. http://parliamentaryforum.org/sites/default/files/firearms%20protection%20or%20risk.pdf

Bergamo, Monica. "Venda de Armas no Brasil Despenca." *Folha de São Paulo*, August 14, 2012.

Cano, Ignácio. *Pesquisa sobre Vitimização nos Roubos*. Rio de Janeiro: ISER, 1999.

Dreyfus, Pablo, and Bandeira, Antonio. *Watching the Neighborhood: An Assessment of Small Arms and Ammunition "Grey Market Transactions" on the Borders Between Brazil and Paraguay, Bolivia, Uruguay and Argentina*. Rio de Janeiro: Viva Rio, 2006. http://www.comunidadesegura.org/files/active/0/Watching_Neighborhood_ing.pdf

Estatuto do Desarmamento, Law N. 10.826/2003. Brasília: Congresso Nacional, 2003. http://www.planalto.gov.br/ccivil_03/Leis/2003/L10.826.htm

Godnick, William, and Bustamente, Julián. *El Tráfico de Armas en América Latina y el Caribe: Mitos, Realidades y Vacios en la Agenda Internacional de Investigación*. Lima: UNLIREC, 2012.

Guerra, Natália. "Fabricantes de Armas Triplicam Receita no Brasil em Apenas Cinco Anos." *R7*, September 23, 2012.

ISER. *Referendo do Sim ao Não: Uma Experiência da Democracia Brasileira*. Rio de Janeiro: ISER, 2006. http://www.comunidadesegura.com.br/files/referendodosimaonao.pdf

Jungmann, Raul. *Comissão Parlamentar de Inquérito Sobre Organizações Criminosas do Tráfico de Armas, Sub-Relatoria de "Indústria, Comércio e C.A.C. (Colecionadores, Atiradores e Caçadores)."* Brasília: Congresso Nacional, 2006. http://www.comunidadesegura.org/files/active/0/Relatorio%20sub-relatoria%20de%20industria%20comercio%20e%20cac.pdf

Parliamentary Forum on Small Arms and Light Weapons and CLAVE (Coalición latinoamericana para la prevención de la violencia armada). *Model Law on Firearms, Ammunition and Related Materials*. Stockholm: Parliamentary Forum on Small Arms and Light Weapons, CLAVE, Swedish Fellowship of Reconciliation, and Parlatino, 2008. http://parliamentaryforum.org/sites/default/files/model_law_on_firearms_ammunition_and_related_materials_final.pdf

Purcena, Julio Cesar, and Nascimento, Marcelo. *Estoques e Distribuição de Armas de Fogo no Brasil*. Rio de Janeiro: Viva Rio, 2010. http://www.vivario.org.br/publique/media/Estoques_e_Distribuição.pdf

Purcena, Julio Cesar, and Nascimento, Marcelo. *Seguindo a Rota das Armas: Desvio, Comércio e Tráfico Ilícitos de Armamento Pequeno e Leve no Brasil*. Rio de Janeiro: Viva Rio, 2010. http://www.vivario.org.br/publique/media/Seguindo_a_Rota_das_Armas.pdf

Part V / Second Amendment

The Scope of Regulatory Authority under the Second Amendment

Lawrence E. Rosenthal and Adam Winkler

The Second Amendment to the U.S. Constitution provides: "A well regulated Militia, being necessary to the security of a free State, the right of the people to keep and bear Arms, shall not be infringed." In *District of Columbia v. Heller*,[1] the U.S. Supreme Court ruled that the District of Columbia's prohibition on handguns and requirement that long guns in the home be kept inoperable at all times violated this provision. In *McDonald v. City of Chicago*,[2] the Court subsequently held that the Second Amendment applies equally to federal and state laws burdening the right to keep and bear arms.

The "inherent right of self-defense has been central to the Second Amendment," the Court explained in *Heller,* and D.C.'s "handgun ban amounts to a prohibition on an entire class of 'arms' that is overwhelmingly chosen by American society for that lawful purpose. The prohibition extends, moreover, to the home, where the need for defense of self, family, and property is most acute." "Few laws in the history of our Nation," the Court wrote, "have

Lawrence E. Rosenthal, JD, is a professor at Chapman University School of Law in Orange, California. Adam Winkler, JD, MA, is a law professor at the University of California, Los Angeles.

come close to the severe restriction of the District of Columbia's handgun ban." Nevertheless, the Court cautioned, "[l]ike most rights, the right secured by the Second Amendment is not unlimited." Indeed, "[f]rom Blackstone through the 19th-century cases," the Court recounted, "commentators and courts routinely explained that the right was not a right to keep and carry any weapon whatsoever in any manner whatsoever and for whatever purpose." For example, "the majority of 19th-century courts to consider the question held that prohibitions on carrying concealed weapons were lawful under the Second Amendment or its state analogues." The Court added that "nothing in our opinion should be taken to cast doubt on longstanding prohibitions on the possession of firearms by felons or the mentally ill, or laws forbidding the carrying of firearms in sensitive places such as schools and government buildings, or laws imposing conditions and qualifications on the commercial sale of arms." The Court characterized such firearms regulations as "presumptively lawful," while also noting its list of presumptively permissible regulations "does not purport to be exhaustive." Accordingly, while the precise boundaries of the Second Amendment remain somewhat opaque, it is settled that many forms of gun control are consistent with the right of the people to keep and bear arms.

In this chapter, we consider the constitutionality under the Second Amendment of a number of gun control reforms that might be adopted in the wake of the tragic shooting at Sandy Hook Elementary School in Newtown, Connecticut. Discussion to date has focused on a number of potential reforms, such as universal background checks for gun purchasers, restrictions on "assault weapons," and restrictions on high-capacity ammunition magazines. While the permissibility of any reform hinges on its details, we can nevertheless begin to identify what sorts of laws are likely to be constitutional under the Second Amendment.

Since the decision in *Heller*, the lower courts have ruled on hundreds of Second Amendment challenges to a wide variety of laws. Although the overwhelming majority of these cases have upheld the challenged laws, the courts have invalidated a few held to be unusually severe burdens on the right to possess or use a firearm for self-defense. From the reasoning and language of *Heller*, *McDonald*, and the subsequent cases, we can discern an emerging jurisprudential framework for analyzing the constitutionality of gun control laws.

This emerging framework involves what the courts have called a "two-pronged approach to Second Amendment challenges."[3] The first question courts must ask is whether a challenged law burdens conduct within the scope of the Second Amendment.[4] In *Heller*, the Court defined the right to "keep" arms as the right to possess them,[5] and the right to "bear" arms as the right to "carry[ ] for a particular purpose—confrontation."[6] The Court offered no explicit definition of what amounted to an unconstitutional infringement of these rights, but treated as unconstitutional laws that effectively nullified the core interest at the heart of the Second Amendment—the right of a law-abiding citizen to have in his or her home a functional firearm suitable for personal protection. To determine whether other conduct is within the ambit of the Second Amendment, the lower courts have since *Heller* looked to the limitations recognized in *Heller* and the historical tradition of gun rights and gun regulation.

When a law burdens conduct within the scope of the Second Amendment, courts then ask a second question: does the government have adequate justification for the law? Not all regulations restricting guns burden the right to keep and bear arms, and not all regulations that do burden the right are unconstitutional.

Scope of the Second Amendment

The threshold inquiry asks whether a gun law burdens conduct within the scope of the Second Amendment. Although, as we have seen, the Second Amendment protects a right to possess and carry "Arms," *Heller* also makes clear that not every regulation is an unconstitutional infringement of the right to keep and bear arms.

There is a well-established historical tradition of gun regulation, which has been a prominent feature of the law since the birth of America. In the framing era, not only were portions of the population barred from owning guns—including law-abiding citizens unwilling to swear allegiance to the Revolution, in addition to slaves and free blacks—but the founding generation also had laws requiring the safe storage of firearms and gunpowder.[7] In the 1820s and 1830s, laws prohibiting the carrying of concealed firearms became commonplace;[8] as the Court in *Heller* recognized, a majority of nineteenth-century courts upheld these laws.

After the Civil War, the same Congress that drafted the Fourteenth Amendment, which was designed in part to make the Second Amendment applicable to state and local laws, abolished the militia in most southern states because such armed groups had proven "dangerous to the public peace and to the security of

Union citizens in those states."[9] This legislation was one of a series of gun control measures undertaken at the time in an effort to suppress violence in the then-turbulent South. In the early twentieth century, Congress in the National Firearms Act of 1934 severely restricted access to machine guns and sawed-off shotguns.[10] Meanwhile, many states passed laws restricting the public possession of firearms, imposed waiting periods on the purchase of certain firearms, and barred violent felons from possessing guns.[11] Thus, the right to keep and bear arms has been understood to permit lawmakers considerable leeway to regulate.

It seems equally clear that in determining the scope of the Second Amendment right, lawmakers are not restricted to enacting only the regulations in place when the Second Amendment was adopted. For example, the laws characterized as presumptively valid in *Heller*—bans on possession by felons and the mentally ill, restrictions on guns in sensitive places like schools and government buildings, and commercial sale qualifications—did not exist at the time of ratification.[12] Instead, the history of innovation in firearms regulation since the framing has led courts to conclude that legislatures are not limited to framing-era regulations.[13] One approach to assessing the permissibility of regulation is to inquire whether the challenged law comports with historical traditions broadly defined. For example, the ban on possession by felons and the mentally ill reflects a longstanding tradition of restricting access to firearms by people deemed dangerous to public safety. So, too, do laws barring possession of firearms by people convicted of domestic violence misdemeanors or subject to a domestic violence restraining order, which have been consistently upheld even though no such restrictions existed at the framing.[14]

Nothing in the text of the Second Amendment suggests that the government's power to regulate guns is limited to those regulations common in the framing era or even of long standing. As we have seen, its preamble contemplates a "well regulated Militia," which *Heller* explained meant not a formal military organization but rather "the body of all citizens capable of military service, who would be expected to bring the sorts of lawful weapons that they possessed at home to militia duty." The Court wrote that the Second Amendment's preamble is properly consulted to clarify the meaning of the Second Amendment, adding that "well regulated" meant "the imposition of proper training and discipline." The Second Amendment therefore contemplates a body of citizens that is subject to whatever regulations are warranted to impose proper discipline on those qualified to keep and bear arms. Accordingly, the Second Amendment's preamble offers textual support for a variety of limitations on the ability of individuals to possess or carry firearms that are justified in terms of contemporary exigencies.[15]

If, after examining the history and tradition of gun regulation, a court determines a challenged law burdens only conduct outside of the protection of the Second Amendment, the inquiry is over and the law upheld. Only if a challenger can show that the law does create such a burden will the courts proceed to the next step: scrutiny of the law's burdens and justifications.

Judicial Scrutiny of Burdens and Justification

The second step of the emerging Second Amendment jurisprudence asks whether a challenged regulation can be sufficiently justified in light of the burden it imposes on the interests protected by the Second Amendment.

In *Heller*, the Court declined to decide what types of justification are required to sustain a challenged regulation on access to or use of firearms. Nonetheless, it did hold that rational basis review, the weakest and most deferential level of judicial scrutiny, was inappropriate, as was the "freestanding 'interest-balancing' approach" proposed in Justice Stephen Breyer's dissent.[16] The Court's rejection of Justice Breyer's approach, however, does not mean that no standard of review is ever appropriate in Second Amendment cases. The Court explicitly distinguished Justice Breyer's unique formulation from "the traditionally expressed levels (strict scrutiny, intermediate scrutiny, rational basis)."[17]

The most rigorous form of judicial scrutiny is strict scrutiny, which requires that a challenged law be "justified by a compelling government interest" and "narrowly drawn to serve that interest."[18] Because of the requirement of narrow tailoring, strict scrutiny forbids regulations that are overinclusive—covering more conduct than necessary—or underinclusive—covering less.[19] The vast majority of courts to consider strict scrutiny have rejected it as inconsistent with the language and reasoning of *Heller*.[20] After all, *Heller* characterizes a wide variety of prophylactic regulations as presumptively lawful, which is contrary to strict scrutiny's traditional presumption of unconstitutionality. Moreover, the Second Amendment's text explicitly contemplates regulation. At the same time, *Heller* also explains that the most severe burdens on the core right of armed self-defense on the part of law-abiding persons are invalid on their face. Second Amendment jurisprudence must accommodate both points.

The prevailing view in the lower courts is that a form of intermediate scrutiny, inquiring whether a challenged law is substantially related to an important governmental objective, is appropriate for laws that impose something less than the most serious burdens on the core right of armed self-defense recognized in *Heller*.[21] Other courts have taken something of a "sliding scale" approach, concluding that laws imposing more onerous burdens on the right to keep or bear firearms should be subject to concomitantly more demanding scrutiny.[22]

These two approaches are united by consideration of the aggregate burden imposed by a challenged regulation rather than its impact on a particular individual. Laws prohibiting convicted felons from possessing firearms, for example, impose an absolute burden for the affected individuals on their right to keep and bear arms. Yet, they were treated as presumptively valid in *Heller*, and such laws have been consistently sustained, even when they also reach other categories of high-risk individuals such as convicted domestic violence misdemeanants or those subject to a domestic violence order of protection.[23] Similarly, a statute prohibiting individuals from carrying handguns in public unless they could demonstrate a special need entitling them to a carry permit was sustained, even though it imposed an absolute prohibition on those unable to qualify for the permit.[24]

Most gun control laws to date have satisfied the requirement that they be substantially related to the government's objective of enhancing public safety.[25] As the Supreme Court explained in the context of the First Amendment, where this same test often applies, "substantial deference to the predictive judgments" of the legislature is warranted.[26] Yet courts do not require lawmakers to have overwhelming proof before they act; reliable studies may not always be available, especially for innovative reforms. Courts ordinarily look to the legislative record and available empirical data to assess whether there is sufficient reason to credit the legislature's judgment.[27]

In the wake of the Newtown shooting, a number of different types of gun control laws have been proposed to reduce the likelihood of mass shootings and gun crime more generally. In this section, we consider the constitutionality of some particular reforms: universal background checks for gun purchases and regulation of trafficking and restrictions on "assault weapons" and high-capacity magazines. In our assessment, most of the types of reforms being considered are capable of surviving judicial review under the prevailing standards.

Universal Background Checks and Regulation of Dealers

Under current federal law, background checks are only required on people who seek to purchase a firearm from a federally licensed gun dealer. Yet, because people without a federal license are permitted to sell firearms, a significant percentage of gun transfers occur with no background check. A law designed to close this loophole, and to ensure that firearms are transferred only by licensed dealers who can perform background checks and are subject to regulatory oversight, would almost certainly be constitutional. The Supreme Court has already made clear that prohibiting felons and the mentally ill from possessing arms is not an infringement of the right to keep and bear arms. Background checks are preventative measures designed for a compelling governmental interest: to ensure that people prohibited from possessing firearms cannot lawfully purchase them. Universal background checks and comprehensive regulation of firearms sales substantially further this governmental interest. Moreover, given the instantaneous verification offered by the federal National Instant Criminal Background Check System, or NICS, a background check imposes only a minor, incidental burden on lawful gun purchasers. This is no more of a burden than we impose on numerous other fundamental rights including the right to vote, which allows states to require preregistration, and the right to marry, which allows states to require a marriage license. Using the moment of sale to confirm the eligibility of a person to possess firearms is also appropriate given the Supreme Court's approval of "laws imposing conditions and qualifications on the commercial sale of arms."

"Assault Weapons"

One measure Congress may consider is the reenactment of the federal ban on the sale of "assault weapons." Although this terminology has been controversial, for purposes of this essay we'll accept the definition included in the 1994 assault weapons law, which applied generally to semi-automatic firearms with a detachable ammunition magazine and military-style features, like a bayonet fitting or a pistol grip.[28]

A restriction on the sale or possession of assault weapons would likely be constitutional because such firearms may not be "Arms" under the meaning of the Second Amendment. In *Heller*, the Court held that the Second Amendment preserves access to firearms that are "in common use" and are not "dangerous or unusual." The "Arms" protected include "weapons that were not specifically designed for military use and were not employed in a military capacity," including those arms "typically possessed by law-abiding citizens for lawful purposes" such as "self-defense within the home." This construction is consistent with historic traditions, in which "dangerous and unusual weapons" have long been subject to heavy restriction. Handguns, by contrast, were held to be constitutionally protected because they are "the most popular weapon chosen by Americans for self-defense in the home."

Arguably, assault weapons do not meet *Heller*'s definition of a protected arm. While such firearms may be commonplace, they are primarily used for recreational purposes, not self-defense. Because of their size, they can be difficult to maneuver in a tight space, and they propel bullets with such force as to travel easily through residential walls, endangering family members or neighbors. Of course, one can use an assault weapon, like any firearm, for self-defense. Yet more is required under the Second Amendment. Just as "dangerous and unusual weapons" like machine guns, which can also be used for self-defense, can be restricted consistent with the Second Amendment, so can assault weapons.

Heller's language may be read to compel an alternate conclusion. On one reading, *Heller* protects any arm that is typically used for any "lawful purpose," even if that purpose isn't personal protection. While assault weapons are not primarily used for self-defense in the home, they may be typically used for other lawful purposes, like recreational shooting and hunting. Yet, there are reasons to believe this reading is too broad; machine guns, too, can be used for lawful purposes, like recreational shooting.

Another potential constitutional difficulty with an assault weapons ban is that it may not meet the requirements of means–ends scrutiny. The 1994 law was easily evaded by manufacturers who simply eliminated the distinguishing military-style features, like bayonet fittings and pistol grips, and sold what were essentially the same guns. These legal firearms may have been just as dangerous as the prohibited assault weapons, with the same lethality and firepower. Unless lawmakers can show that military-style features like bayonet fittings and pistol grips make a weapon unusually dangerous, and a sufficiently comprehensive law is enacted that limits the possibility of evasion, it will be difficult to prove that the government's interest in public safety is substantially furthered when effectively similar guns remain legal.

Even so, the emerging jurisprudential framework provides reason to believe an assault-weapon ban could be sustained. In light of the availability of many other firearms, including handguns, characterized by *Heller* as the "quintessential self-defense weapon," it may be that a prohibition on assault-type weapons places a sufficiently modest burden on the right of armed self-defense that it would require only modest justification. Indeed, the U.S. Court of Appeals for the District of Columbia Circuit recently held that a ban on assault rifles was constitutional. In that case, the court ruled that, while assault rifles may be "in common use," a prohibition on such firearms "does not effectively disarm individuals or substantially affect their ability to defend themselves." Furthermore, the court wrote, "the evidence demonstrates a ban on assault weapons is likely to promote the Government's interest in crime control in the densely populated urban area that is the District of Columbia."[29]

High-Capacity Ammunition Magazines

An analysis similar to that for assault weapons applies to high-capacity ammunition magazines. The District of Columbia Circuit that upheld the ban on assault weapons also upheld D.C.'s prohibition on magazines that carry more than ten rounds of ammunition. Although the court said that high-capacity magazines may be in common use, a prohibition on such magazines does not significantly burden self-defense. In fact, the court held that high-capacity magazines may be unusually dangerous when used in self-defense because so many rounds can be fired unnecessarily.[30] As with a prohibition on assault weapons, the burden imposed on the core right of armed self-defense by this type of restriction is modest.

Moreover, restricting ammunition magazines substantially furthers the government's important interest in public safety. Mass shooters and criminals prefer high-capacity magazines in order to maximize the threat they pose without having to reload. While people with malicious intent can carry multiple magazines and reload their weapons, magazine size restrictions can force them to take the two or three seconds pause necessary to reload. Even this short pause, the D.C. Circuit held, can be a "critical benefit to law enforcement," affording officers, potential victims, or bystanders the opportunity to intercede. Requiring mass shooters to pause even an instant can be the difference between life and death for intended victims; indeed, bystanders stopped the man who shot Rep. Gabrielle Giffords when he was forced to reload his weapon. Thus, a restriction on high-capacity magazines may substantially serve the government's interest in public safety without significantly burdening the ability of law-abiding individuals to defend themselves.

The Second Amendment leaves Congress and the state and local governments significant regulatory power, at least when they do not compromise the core right recognized in *Heller* and regulate with substantial justification. Indeed, in conducting this inquiry, there is a strong case to be made for judicial modesty. As one federal appellate tribunal put it: "This is serious business. We do not wish to be even minutely responsible for some unspeakably tragic act of mayhem because in the peace of our judicial chambers we miscalculated as to Second Amendment rights."[31]

NOTES

1. 554 U.S. 570 (2008).

2. 130 S. Ct. 3020 (2010).

3. United States v. Greeno, 679 F.3d 510, 518 (6th Cir. 2012) (quoting United States v. Marzzarella, 614 F.3d 85, 89 (3d Cir. 2010)).

4. *See, e.g.*, Nat'l Rifle Ass'n of Am., Inc. v. BATFE, 700 F.3d 185, 194 (5th Cir. 2012); GeorgiaCarry.Org, Inc. v. Georgia, 687 F.3d 1244, 1260 n.34 (11th Cir. 2012); Greeno, 679 F.3d at 518; Heller v. District of Columbia, 670 F.3d 1244, 1252 (D.C. Cir. 2011); Ezell v. City of Chicago, 651 F.3d 684, 701–04 (7th Cir. 2011); United States v. Chester, 628 F.3d 673, 680 (4th Cir. 2010); United States v. Reese, 627 F.3d 792, 800–01 (10th Cir. 2010); United States v. Marzzarella, 634 F.3d 85, 89 (3d Cir. 2010); People v. Alvarado, 964 N.E.2d 532, 547 (Ill. App. Ct. 2011); Pohlabel v. State, 268 P.3d 1264, 1266–67 (Nev. 2012); Johnston v. State, 2012 WL 6595935 * 6 (N.C. App. Ct. Dec. 18, 2012).

5. 554 U.S. at 582.

6. *Id.* at 584.

7. *See, e.g.*, Adam Winkler, Gunfight: The Battle over the Right to Bear Arms in America 115–17 (2011); Saul Cornell & Nathan DeDino, *A Well-Regulated Right: The Early American Origins of Gun Control*, 73 FORDHAM L. REV. 487, 506–08, 510–12 (2005).

8. *See, e.g.*, Saul Cornell, A Well-Regulated Militia: The Founding Fathers and the Origins of Gun Control in America 138–44 (2006); Clayton E. Cramer, Concealed Weapon Laws of the Early Republic: Dueling, Southern Violence, and Moral Reform 2–3, 139–41 (1999); WINKLER, *supra* note 7, at 166–69.

9. Cong. Globe, 39th Cong., 1st Sess. 1849 (1866) (Sen. Lane). *Accord id.* at 1848–49 (Sen. Wilson). *See* Carole Emberton, *The Limits of Incorporation: Violence, Gun Rights, and Gun Regulation in the Reconstruction South*, 17 Stan. L. & Pol'y Rev. 615, 621–23 (2006).

10. *See* Pub.L. 474, 48 Stat. 1236 (1934).

11. *See* Winkler, *supra* note 7, at 209–12; C. Kevin Marshall, *Why Can't Martha Stewart Have a Gun?*, 32 Harv. J.L. & Pub. Pol'y 695, 698–728 (2009).

12. *See, e.g.*, Carlton F.W. Larson, *Four Exceptions in Search of a Theory:* District of Columbia v. Heller *and Judicial Ipse Dixit*, 60 Hastings L.J. 1371, 1373–79 (2009); Nelson Lund, *The Second Amendment,* Heller, *and Originalist Jurisprudence*, 56 UCLA L. Rev. 1343, 1356–62 (2009); Marshall, *supra* note 11 at 698–728.

13. *See, e.g.*, Nat'l Rifle Ass'n, Inc. v. BATFE, 700 F.3d 185, 196–97 (5th Cir. 2012); United States v. Skoien, 614 F.3d 638, 641 (7th Cir. 2010) (en banc).

14. *See, e.g.*, United States v. Chapman, 666 F.3d 220, 227–31 (4th Cir. 2012); United States v. Staten, 666 F.3d 154, 160–67 (4th Cir. 2012); United States v. Booker, 644 F.3d 12, 25 (1st Cir. 2011) (same); United States v. Reese, 627 F.3d 792, 800–04 (10th Cir. 2010); *Skoien*, 614 F.3d at 641–42.

15. On the role of the preamble in determining permissive gun regulation, *see* Lawrence Rosenthal, *Second Amendment Plumbing after* Heller: *Of Standards of Scrutiny, Incorporation, Well-Regulated Militias, and Criminal Street Gangs*, 41 Urb. Law. 1, 80–81 (2009).

16. *See id.* at 629 n.27, 634–35.

17. *Id.* at 634.

18. Brown v. Entertainment Merchants Association, 131 S. Ct. 2729, 2738 (2011).

19. *See, e.g., id.* at 2738–42; Church of the Lukumi Babalu Aye, Inc. v. City of Hialeah, 508 U.S. 520, 546 (1993); Arkansas Writers' Project, Inc, v. Ragland, 481 U.S. 221, 231–32 (1987); First Nat'l Bank of Boston v Bellotti, 435 U.S. 765, 786, 792–94 (1978).

20. *See, e.g.*, Heller v. District of Columbia, 670 F.3d 1244, 1252, 1256–57 (D.C. Cir. 2011).

21. *See, e.g.*, Schrader v. Holder, 2013 WL 135246 * 8–10 (D.C. Cir. Jan. 11, 2013) (upholding prohibition on possession of firearms by individuals convicted of misdemeanors punishable by more than two years' imprisonment); *Heller*, 670 F.3d at 1260–64 (upholding ordinance prohibiting possession of semi-automatic rifles and large-capacity magazines); United States v. Staten, 666 F.3d 154, 160–67 (4th Cir. 2012) (upholding statute prohibiting possession of firearms by individuals convicted of misdemeanor domestic violence), United States v. Booker, 644 F.3d 12, 25 (1st Cir. 2011) (same); United States v. Reese, 627 F.3d 792, 800–04 (10th Cir. 2010) (upholding statute prohibiting possession of firearms by individuals under a domestic violence order of protection); United States v. Skoien, 614 F.3d 638, 641–42 (7th Cir. 2010) (en banc) (upholding statute prohibiting possession of firearms by individuals convicted of misdemeanor domestic violence); United States v. Marzzarella, 614 F.3d 85, 95–99 (3d Cir. 2010) (upholding statute prohibiting possession of firearms with obliterated serial number).

22. *See, e.g.*, Moore v. Madigan, 2012 WL 6156062 * 6–7 (7th Cir. Dec. 11, 2012) (invalidating a statute prohibiting carrying readily operable firearms in public); Kachalsky v. County of Westchester, 701 F.3d 81, 93–97 (2d Cir. 2012) (upholding statute prohibiting

carrying firearms absent a permit issued on a showing of special need); Nat'l Rifle Ass'n, Inc. v. BATFE, 700 F.3d 185, 195–98 (5th Cir. 2012) (upholding statute prohibiting the sale of handguns to persons under age 21); United States v. DeCastro, 682 F.3d 160, 166–68 (2d Cir. 2011) (upholding statute prohibiting purchasing firearms in another state and transporting them to state of residence); Ezell v. City of Chicago, 651 F.3d 684, 707–09 (7th Cir. 2011) (granting preliminary injunction against ordinance prohibiting firing ranges within city).

23. *See, e.g.*, United States v. Chapman, 666 F.3d 220, 227–31 (4th Cir. 2012); United States v. Staten, 666 F.3d 154, 160–67 (4th Cir. 2012); United States v. Booker, 644 F.3d 12, 25 (1st Cir. 2011) (same); United States v. Reese, 627 F.3d 792, 800–04 (10th Cir. 2010); United States v. Skoien, 614 F.3d 638, 641–42 (7th Cir. 2010) (en banc).

24. *See* Kachalsky v. County of Westchester, 701 F.3d 81, 99–101 (2d Cir. 2012).

25. For a representative sample, see cases cited *supra* at notes 21–22.

26. Turner Broad. Sys., Inc. v. FCC, 520 U.S. 180, 195 (1997).

27. *See, e.g.*, *Kachalsky*, 701 F.3d at 97–99.

28. *See* 18 U.S.C. § 921(a)(30)(B) (1994), *repealed by* Pub. L. No. 103-322, tit. XI, § 11015(2), 108 Stat. 2000 (1994).

29. Heller v. District of Columbia, 670 F.3d 1244, 1262–63 (D.C. Cir. 2011).

30. *Id.* at 1263–64.

31. United States v. Masciandaro, 638 F.3d 458, 475 (4th Cir. 2011).

Part VI / Public Opinion on Gun Policy

Public Opinion on Proposals to Strengthen U.S. Gun Laws

Findings from a 2013 Survey

Emma E. McGinty, Daniel W. Webster, Jon S. Vernick, and Colleen L. Barry

In the aftermath of the tragedy at Sandy Hook Elementary School in New town, Connecticut, policy proposals to reduce gun violence are being actively considered and debated at the national, state, and local levels. Within weeks of the mass shooting in Newtown, public opinion data emerged indicating some shift in views among Americans toward greater support for strengthening gun laws. For example, a Gallup survey conducted December 19 through December 22, 2012, found that 58% of Americans supported stricter gun laws, compared with only 43% in support of stricter gun laws in an October 2011 poll.[1]

By and large, these opinion data focused on general attitudes about gun policy rather than public support for specific policy proposals to reduce gun

Emma E. McGinty, MS, is a research assistant and fourth-year PhD candidate in Health Policy and Management at the Johns Hopkins Bloomberg School of Public Health. Daniel W. Webster, ScD, MPH, is a professor in the Department of Health Policy and Management at the Johns Hopkins Bloomberg School of Public Health. Jon S. Vernick, JD, MPH, is an associate professor and associate chair in the Department of Health Policy and Management at the Johns Hopkins Bloomberg School of Public Health. Colleen L. Barry, PhD, MPP, is an associate professor and associate chair for Research and Practice in the Department of Health Policy and Management at the Johns Hopkins Bloomberg School of Public Health.

violence. For example, a national survey conducted December 17 through December 19, 2012, by the Pew Center for the People and the Press examined trends in public views about whether it was more important to control gun ownership or to protect gun rights, but examined public support for only four specific policies: bans of handguns, semi-automatic guns, high-capacity ammunition magazines, and exploding bullets, respectively.[2] The December 19–22, 2012, Gallup survey assessed support for four policies: requiring background checks at gun shows and banning handguns, semi-automatic guns, and high-capacity ammunition magazines.[3] Another survey by YouGov conducted December 21 and 22, 2012, examined public attitudes about the National Rifle Association (NRA) but did not examine specific gun policies beyond support for armed guards in schools.[4]

Following the Sandy Hook shooting, experts are recommending and policymakers are considering a much wider range of gun policy options than those assessed in recent public opinion polls. In addition, most recent polls did not examine how public opinion varied by gun ownership or by political party affiliation, and none oversampled gun owners to obtain more precise estimates of policy attitudes among this group. Prior evidence has shown that attitudes about gun policies vary significantly by gun ownership and by partisanship.[5,6]

It has been nearly 15 years since research studies have examined attitudes among the American public about a broad set of public policies aimed at curbing gun violence.[7,8,9] Given the fast-moving pace of deliberations over gun policy, it is critical to understand how the American public views specific proposals to strengthen gun laws and how policy support varies across important subgroups. To fill these gaps, we fielded the Johns Hopkins National Survey of Public Opinion on Gun Proposals in 2013 from January 2 to 14, 2013. This survey examined support for 33 different policies to reduce gun violence in America. These measures were chosen in conjunction with the policy options analyzed by gun violence experts at the 2013 Johns Hopkins Summit on Reducing Gun Violence in America and reported on in this volume.

Data and Methods

We used the survey research firm GfK Knowledge Networks (GfK KN) to conduct this study. GfK KN has recruited a probability-based online panel of 50,000 adult members older than 18, including persons living in cell phone only households, using equal probability sampling with a sample frame of residential addresses covering 97% of U.S. households. The survey was pilot-tested between December 28 and 31, 2012. In order to avoid priming, the specific nature of the survey was not described to respondents. They were asked to answer "some questions about public affairs," and there was no mention of the Sandy Hook school shooting. Policy item order was randomized. The survey completion rate was 69%.[10] To compare rates stratified by gun ownership, we oversampled gun owners and non-gun owners living in households with guns. We tested differences in proportions by group using the Pearson's chi square test. To make estimates representative of the U.S. population, all analyses used survey weights adjusting the sample for known selection deviations and survey nonresponse. This study was approved as exempt by the Johns Hopkins School of Public Health Institutional Review Board (#4850).

Results

Consistent with recent data reported elsewhere,[11,3] we found that 33% of Americans reported having guns in their home or garage. Twenty-two percent of Americans identified the guns as personally belonging to them (referred to henceforth as gun owners), and 11% identified as non-gun owners living in a household with a gun. Among gun owners, 71% reported owning a handgun, 62% owned a shotgun, and 61% owned a rifle. The remaining 67% of Americans identified as non-gun owners living in non-gun households (referred to henceforth as non-gun owners).

Table 19.1 indicates that a majority of Americans supported banning the sale of military-style semi-automatic assault weapons, banning large-capacity ammunition magazines, and a range of measures to strengthen background checks and improve oversight of gun dealers. In the case of assault weapon and ammunition policies, public views differed substantially by gun ownership. Although 69% of the public overall supported banning assault weapon sales, a much higher proportion of non-gun owners (77%) and non-gun owners living in households with guns (68%) than gun-owners (46%) or self-reported NRA members (15%) supported this policy. Sixty-eight percent of the general public supported banning the sale of large-capacity ammunition magazines that allow some guns to shoot more than 10 bullets before reloading, and this policy was supported by most non-gun owners (76%), most non-gun owners living in households with guns (69%), a near majority of gun-owners

Table 19.1 Percentage of people who favor gun policies, overall and by gun ownership

Item	Overall (N = 2,703)	Non-gun owners[a] (n = 913)	Non-gun owner, gun in household (n = 843)	Gun owners (n = 947)	NRA members (n = 169)
Assault weapon and ammunition policies					
Banning the sale of military-style, semi-automatic assault weapons that are capable of shooting more than 10 rounds of ammunition without reloading?	69.0	77.4	67.7**	45.7***	14.9***
Banning the sale of large-capacity ammunition clips or magazines that allow some guns to shoot more than 10 bullets before reloading?	68.4	75.5	69.2*	47.8***	19.2***
Banning the sale of large-capacity ammunition clips or magazines that allow some guns to shoot more than 20 bullets before reloading?	68.8	75.6	69.9	49.4***	19.9***
Banning the possession of military-style, semi-automatic assault weapons that are capable of shooting more than 10 rounds of ammunition without reloading if the government is required to pay gun owners the fair market value of their weapons?	56.0	63.3	52.6**	36.9***	17.0***
Banning the possession of large-capacity ammunition clips or magazines that allow some guns to shoot more than 10 bullets before reloading if the government is required to pay gun owners the fair market value of their ammunition clips?	55.0	61.9	51.6**	37.0***	22.9***

Prohibited person policies

Prohibiting a person convicted of two or more crimes involving alcohol or drugs within a three-year period from having a gun for 10 years?	74.8	76.1	74.8	70.5*	64.2
Prohibiting a person convicted of violating a domestic violence restraining order from having a gun for 10 years?	80.8	82.9	79.1	75.6**	61.5**
Prohibiting a person convicted of a serious crime as a juvenile from having a gun for 10 years?	83.1	84.4	81.3	80.0	70.0
Prohibiting a person under the age of 21 from having a handgun?	69.5	76.4	63.6***	52.3***	42.3***
Prohibiting a person on the terror watch list from having a gun?	86.0	87.5	85.6	82.2*	75.5
Prohibiting people who have been convicted of each of these crimes from having a gun for 10 years:					
Public display of a gun in a threatening manner excluding self-defense	71.1	69.8	78.7**	71.3	58.5
Domestic violence	73.7	72.4	80.4**	73.7	61.4
Assault and battery that does not result in serious injury or involve a lethal weapon	53.0	54.6	53.4	48.5*	33.1
Drunk and disorderly conduct	37.5	39.7	36.6	32.1*	29.1*
Carrying a concealed gun without a permit	57.8	60.3	61.3	49.0***	43.3**
Indecent exposure	25.9	28.1	23.7	21.2*	27.1*
Background check policies					
Requiring a background check system for all gun sales to make sure a purchaser is not legally prohibited from having a gun?	88.8	89.9	91.5	84.3**	73.7*

(Continued)

Table 19.1 (Continued)

Item	Overall (N = 2,703)	Non-gun owners[a] (n = 913)	Non-gun owner, gun in household (n = 843)	Gun owners (n = 947)	NRA members (n = 169)
Increasing federal funding to states to improve reporting of people prohibited by law from having a gun to the background check system?	66.4	67.8	65.5	63.4	60.9
Allowing law enforcement up to five business days, if needed, to complete a background check for gun buyers?[b]	76.3	79.8	79.2	67.0***	47.1***
Policies affecting gun dealers					
Allowing the U.S. Bureau of Alcohol, Tobacco, Firearms and Explosives to temporarily take away a gun dealer's license if an audit reveals record-keeping violations and the dealer cannot account for 20 or more of the guns?	84.6	86.4	84.1	78.9**	64.0**
Allowing cities to sue licensed gun dealers when there is strong evidence that the gun dealer's careless sales practices allowed many criminals to obtain guns?	73.2	77.0	72.2	62.9***	43.5***
Allowing the information about which gun dealers sell the most guns used in crimes to be available to the police and the public so that those gun dealers can be prioritized for greater oversight?	68.8	74.1	64.3**	56.5***	41.2***
Requiring a mandatory minimum sentence of two years in prison for a person convicted of knowingly selling a gun to someone who cannot legally have one?	76.0	77.7	76.3	70.7**	69.8**

Other gun policies					
Requiring a person to obtain a license from a local law enforcement agency before buying a gun to verify their identity and ensure that they are not legally prohibited from having a gun?	77.3	83.5	76.4**	59.4***	37.6***
Providing government funding for research to develop and test "smart guns" designed to fire only when held by the owner of the gun or other authorized user?	44.2	47.4	43.4	35.3***	23.0***
Requiring by law that people lock up the guns in their home when not in use to prevent handling by children or teenagers without adult supervision?	67.2	75.3	62.6***	44.4***	32.2***

Note: We asked respondents whether they favored or opposed each policy using a 5-point Likert scale (strongly favor, somewhat favor, neither favor nor oppose, somewhat oppose, strongly oppose). We coded strongly favor and somewhat favor responses as being in support of a given policy.

$*p < .05$, $**p < .01$, $***p < .001$

[a]Responses among non-gun owners with a gun in their household, gun owners, and NRA members were compared with responses among non-gun owners (no gun in household) using chi-square tests.

[b]Question informed respondents that under current federal law, most background checks for gun buyers are completed in just a few minutes. But if law enforcement needs additional time to determine if a gun buyer is not legally allowed to have a gun, they may only take up to a maximum of three business days to complete the check.

(48%), but by few NRA members (19%). Support levels did not differ meaningfully for a policy banning the sale of large-capacity ammunition magazines that allow some guns to shoot more than 20 bullets. As expected, support was lower for policies banning the possession (as opposed to the sale) of assault weapons and large-capacity ammunition magazines even if the government was required to pay gun owners their fair market value.

For many policies, differences in policy support between gun and non-gun owners were smaller in magnitude than might have been expected. Majorities of gun owners supported all policies bolstering background checks and strengthening oversight of gun dealers and almost all policies prohibiting gun ownership by certain types of persons deemed to be dangerous. A majority of NRA members supported many of these categories of policies, as well. For example, 84% of gun owners and 74% of NRA members supported requiring a background check system for all gun sales; 71% of gun owners and 64% of NRA members supported prohibiting a person convicted of two or more crimes involving alcohol or drugs from having a gun for 10 years; and 71% of gun owners and 70% of NRA members supported requiring a mandatory minimum sentence of two years in prison for a person convicted of selling a gun to someone who cannot legally have a gun. These measures were supported by large majorities of non-gun owners, as well.

We found larger differences in support between non-gun owners and gun owners for policies prohibiting handguns for those under age 21 (76% versus 52%) and requiring gun owners to lock guns when not in use to prevent handling by children or teens without adult supervision (75% versus 44%). Support for government funding to develop and test smart guns designed to fire only when held by the owner or authorized user also differed between non-gun owners and gun owners (47% versus 35%). Support among non-gun owners and gun owners was similar on those policies attracting overall low levels of support, such as prohibiting individuals with misdemeanor convictions for drunk and disorderly conduct (40% versus 32%) or indecent exposure (28% versus 21%) from having guns.

For many policies, the views of non-gun owners living in households with guns were aligned more closely with other non-gun owners than they were with gun owners. For instance, 76% of non-gun owners living in households with guns supported requiring a person to obtain a license from a local law enforcement agency before buying a gun (versus 84% of other non-gun owners and 59% of gun owners). Seventy-nine percent of non-gun owners living in households with guns supported allowing law enforcement up to five business days to complete a background check for gun buyers (versus 80% of other non-gun owners and 67% of gun owners).

As Table 19.2 indicates, policies specifically targeting gun access by persons with mental illness received widespread public support. Most of these policies were supported by a large majority of non-gun owners and gun owners. Eighty-five percent of the general public supported requiring states to report to the background check system individuals who are prohibited from having guns due to either involuntary commitment or having been declared mentally incompetent by a court. While these mental health–related prohibitions have been in place since before the implementation of the background check system in 1998, many states do not report mental health records due to concerns about confidentiality and lack of data systems to track mental health records at the state level.[12] Seventy-five percent of the public supported requiring health care providers to report people who threaten to harm themselves or others to the background check system for a period of six months, and 79% supported requiring the military to report persons rejected from service for mental health or substance abuse reasons to the background check system to prevent them from having a gun. Public support was lower for a policy allowing police officers to search for and remove guns without a warrant from persons they believe to be dangerous due to mental illness or a tendency toward violence (53%), and only 32% of the public supported restoring the right to have a gun to people with mental illness who are determined no longer to be dangerous.

In addition to supporting policies to limit gun access among persons with mental illness, the majority of the public supported increasing government spending on mental health screening and treatment as a strategy to reduce gun violence (60%). However, far fewer supported increasing government spending on drug and alcohol abuse screening and treatment as a violence reduction strategy (44%).

Table 19.3 indicates that, in most cases, Republicans were less likely than Independents and Democrats to support gun violence prevention policies. However, support for most policies prohibiting certain persons from having guns, bolstering background checks, and strengthening oversight of gun dealers was high regardless of political party identification. For example, 77% of Republicans, 79% of Independents, and 85% of Democrats supported prohibiting a person convicted of violating a domestic violence restraining order

Table 19.2 Percentage who favor gun policies affecting persons with mental illness, overall and by gun ownership

Item	Overall ($N = 2,703$)	Non-gun owners[a] ($n = 913$)	Non-gun owner, gun in household ($n = 843$)	Gun owners ($n = 947$)	NRA members ($n = 169$)
Background check policies					
Requiring states to report a person to the background check system who is prohibited from buying a gun due either to involuntary commitment to a hospital for psychiatric treatment or to being declared mentally incompetent by a court of law?	85.4	85.3	86.5	85.6	80.7
Requiring health care providers to report people who threaten to harm themselves or others to the background check system to prevent them from having a gun for six months?	74.5	75.4	76.1	72.0	66.0
Requiring the military to report a person who has been rejected from service due to mental illness or drug or alcohol abuse to the background check system to prevent them from having a gun?	78.9	79.6	79.7	76.2	67.5

Other gun policies

Allowing police officers to search for and remove guns from a person, without a warrant, if they believe the person is dangerous due to a mental illness, emotional instability, or a tendency to be violent?	52.5	55.3	53.4	43.6***	31.1**
Allowing people who have lost the right to have a gun due to mental illness to have that right restored if they are determined not to be dangerous?	31.6	31.6	28.9	34.0	41.6

Government spending

Increasing government spending on mental health screening and treatment as a strategy to reduce gun violence?	60.4	61.8	60.6	55.1*	57.2
Increasing government spending on drug and alcohol abuse screening and treatment as a strategy to reduce gun violence?	43.5	46.6	44.2	35.0***	36.6***

Note: We asked respondents whether they favored or opposed each policy using a 5-point Likert scale (strongly favor, somewhat favor, neither favor nor oppose, somewhat oppose, strongly oppose). We coded strongly favor and somewhat favor responses as being in support of a given policy.

$*p < .05, **p < .01, ***p < .001$

[a]Responses among non-gun owners with a gun in their household, gun owners, and NRA members were compared with responses among non-gun owners (no gun in household) using chi-square tests.

Table 19.3 Percentage who favor gun policies by political party affiliation

Item	Democrats[a] (n = 788)	Independents (n = 1,121)	Republicans (n = 794)
Assault weapon and ammunition policies			
Banning the sale of military-style, semi-automatic assault weapons that are capable of shooting more than 10 rounds of ammunition without reloading?	86.6	63.9***	51.6***
Banning the sale of large-capacity ammunition clips or magazines that allow some guns to shoot more than 10 bullets before reloading?	83.2	65.6***	51.0***
Banning the sale of large-capacity ammunition clips or magazines that allow some guns to shoot more than 20 bullets before reloading?	82.8	66.7***	51.9***
Banning the possession of military-style, semi-automatic assault weapons that are capable of shooting more than 10 rounds of ammunition without reloading if the government is required to pay gun owners the fair market value of their weapons?	72.1	51.3***	40.2***
Banning the possession of large capacity ammunition clips or magazines that allow some guns to shoot more than 10 bullets before reloading if the government is required to pay gun owners the fair market value of their ammunition clips?	68.6	52.4***	38.9***
Prohibited person policies			
Prohibiting a person convicted of two or more crimes involving alcohol or drugs within a three-year period from having a gun for 10 years?	79.4	72.2*	75.2*
Prohibiting a person convicted of violating a domestic violence restraining order from having a gun for 10 years?	85.1	79.2*	77.3*
Prohibiting a person convicted of a serious crime as a juvenile from having a gun for 10 years?	88.5	79.2**	82.0*
Prohibiting a person under the age of 21 from having a handgun?	83.6	66.1***	54.5***
Prohibiting a person on the terror watch list from having a gun?	88.3	84.0	86.3

Prohibiting people who have been convicted of each of these crimes from having a gun for 10 years:			
Public display of a gun in a threatening manner excluding self-defense	70.7	71.1	71.7
Domestic violence	76.1	73.5	70.2
Assault and battery that does not result in serious injury or involve a lethal weapon	58.2	50.4*	49.9*
Drunk and disorderly conduct	42.3	33.7*	37.4
Carrying a concealed gun without a permit	64.2	56.8*	50.0***
Indecent exposure	28.4	24.7	24.4
Background check policies			
Requiring a background check system for all gun sales to make sure a purchaser is not legally prohibited from having a gun?	92.1	87.5	86.3*
Increasing federal funding to states to improve reporting of people prohibited by law from having a gun to the background check system?	76.2	64.0***	56.1***
Allowing law enforcement up to five business days, if needed, to complete a background check for gun buyers?[b]	87.3	70.8***	71.1***
Policies affecting gun dealers			
Allowing the U.S. Bureau of Alcohol, Tobacco, Firearms and Explosives to temporarily take away a gun dealer's license if an audit reveals record-keeping violations and the dealer cannot account for 20 or more of the guns?	88.5	83.3	80.9*
Allowing cities to sue licensed gun dealers when there is strong evidence that the gun dealer's careless sales practices allowed criminals to obtain guns?	82.2	69.5***	66.5***
Allowing the information about which gun dealers sell the most guns used in crimes to be available to the police and the public so that those gun dealers can be prioritized for greater oversight?	79.5	65.3***	58.8***
Requiring a mandatory minimum sentence of two years in prison for a person convicted of knowingly selling a gun to someone who cannot legally have a gun?	81.1	73.4*	73.0*

(Continued)

Table 19.3 (Continued)

Item	Democrats[a] (n=788)	Independents (n=1,121)	Republicans (n=794)
Other gun policies			
Requiring people to obtain a license from a local law enforcement agency before buying a gun to verify their identity and ensure that they are not legally prohibited from having a gun?	87.8	73.5***	68.7***
Providing government funding for research to develop and test "smart guns" designed to fire only when held by the owner of the gun or other authorized user?	51.4	43.8*	34.1***
Requiring by law that people lock up the guns in their home when not in use to prevent handling by children or teenagers without adult supervision?	80.8	65.3***	49.5***

Note: We asked respondents whether they favored or opposed each policy using a 5-point Likert scale (strongly favor, somewhat favor, neither favor nor oppose, somewhat oppose, strongly oppose). We coded strongly favor and somewhat favor responses as being in support of a given policy. $N=2,703$.

$*p<.05$, $**p<.01$, $***p<.001$

[a] Responses among Independents and Republicans were compared with responses among Democrats using chi-square tests.

[b] Question informed respondents that under current federal law, most background checks for gun buyers are completed in just a few minutes. But if law enforcement needs additional time to determine if a gun buyer is not legally allowed to have a gun, they may only take up to a maximum of three business days to complete the check.

from having a gun for two years. Similarly, 82% of Republicans, 79% of Independents, and 89% of Democrats supported prohibiting a person convicted of a serious crime as a juvenile from having a gun for 10 years. A large majority of Republicans (86%) also supported universal background checks for gun sales (versus 88% among Independents and 92% among Democrats) and requiring a mandatory minimum sentence of two years in prison for a person convicted of making an illegal gun sale (73% among Republicans, 73% among Independents, and 81% among Democrats). A wider gradient of support across party affiliation was evident for assault weapon and ammunition policies. Fifty-two percent of Republicans supported banning the sale of assault weapons, compared with 64% of Independents and 87% of Democrats. A similar gradient of support was observed for banning the sale of large-capacity magazines capable of holding 10 or more ammunition rounds (51% among Republicans, 66% among Independents, and 83% among Democrats).

As Table 19.4 indicates, we did not find large differences by political party affiliation in support for policies aimed at restricting access to guns by persons with mental illness. Like Democrats and Independents, Republicans were supportive of bolstering background check policies and resistant to allowing people who had lost their right to have a gun due to mental illness to have that right restored if they were determined not to be dangerous. Republicans and Independents were significantly less willing than Democrats to allow police officers to search for and remove a gun from a person, without a warrant, if they believed the person was dangerous due to mental illness, emotional instability, or a tendency to be violent. A wider gradient of support by party affiliation was also evident for increasing government spending on mental health treatment and on drug and alcohol abuse treatment as a strategy to reduce gun violence. We found that 50% of Republicans, 57% of Independents, and 71% of Democrats were in support of increased spending on mental health screening and treatment as a strategy for reducing gun violence. In contrast, 33% of Republicans, 41% of Independents, and 53% of Democrats supported increased spending on substance abuse treatment to reduce to gun violence.

Discussion

Findings from this national survey indicate high support—including among gun owners, in most cases—for a range of policies aimed at reducing gun

Table 19.4   Percentage who favor gun policies affecting persons with mental illness, by political party affiliation

Item	Democrats[a] (n = 788)	Independents (n = 1,121)	Republicans (n = 794)
Background check policies			
Requiring states to report a person to the background check system who is prohibited from buying a gun due either to involuntary commitment to a hospital for psychiatric treatment or to being declared mentally incompetent by a court of law?	87.1	84.5	84.5
Requiring health care providers to report people who threaten to harm themselves or others to the background check system to prevent them from having a gun for six months?	80.0	71.3**	72.1*
Requiring the military to report a person who has been rejected from service due to mental illness or drug or alcohol abuse to the background check system to prevent them from having a gun?	84.7	74.9**	77.5*
Other gun policies			
Allowing police officers to search for and remove guns from a person, without a warrant, if they believe the person is dangerous due to a mental illness, emotional instability, or a tendency to be violent?	60.7	47.9***	48.5**
Allowing people who have lost the right to have a gun due to mental illness to have that right restored if they are determined not to be dangerous?	31.1	30.7	33.8
Government spending			
Increasing government spending on mental health screening and treatment as a strategy to reduce gun violence?	71.1	57.2**	50.0***
Increasing government spending on drug and alcohol abuse screening and treatment as a strategy to reduce gun violence?	53.4	41.1**	32.7***

Note: We asked respondents whether they favored or opposed each policy using a 5-point Likert scale (strongly favor, somewhat favor, neither favor nor oppose, somewhat oppose, strongly oppose). We coded strongly favor and somewhat favor responses as being in support of a given policy.

$*p < .05, **p < .01, ***p < .001$

[a]Responses among Independents and Republicans were compared with responses among Democrats using chi-square tests.

violence. All but 5 of the 33 gun policies assessed were supported by a majority of the American public. The most feasible policies from a political perspective include 19 with support by majorities of the public regardless of gun ownership or political party identification. These policies would require a universal background check system and strengthen how the system operates, help curtail dangerous sales practices by gun dealers, require firearm licensing by law enforcement, and restrict gun access to certain groups that are not currently prohibited under federal law from possessing firearms, including individuals with a range of serious criminal convictions and on the terror watch list. Other policies supported by a majority of Americans and across all partisan affiliations, including bans on the sale of assault weapons and large-capacity magazines, had support among a majority or close to a majority of gun owners but few NRA member gun owners. These findings suggest that policymakers have a large range of options for curbing gun violence to choose from that are supported by the majority of the American public.

Among the most popular policies were those affecting access to guns by persons with mental illness. The majority of Americans also supported increasing government spending on mental health treatment as a strategy to reduce gun violence. Given substantial rates of undertreatment of mental health problems in the United States,[13] it is worth considering whether gun policies targeting persons with mental illness might negatively affect treatment-seeking behavior. This may be of particular concern if there are efforts to broaden how mental illness is defined for the purpose of screening potentially dangerous individuals from having guns.

As with all research studies, our study findings should be assessed within the context of our methodological approach. While web-based panels provide an attractive alternative to the increasing challenges of national telephone surveys, methodological issues related to their use should be considered with some care. GfK KN uses probability-based recruitment consistent with established standards.[14] We assessed these data by comparing detailed respondent socio-demographic characteristics (both weighted and unweighted) with national rates to confirm their representativeness of the U.S. population (available upon request from authors). In addition, as with all public opinion survey research, differences in question wording can lead to differences in respondent ratings about the same policy across survey instruments; therefore, it is critical to interpret all public opinion studies with a careful eye to the language used to describe policy items.

Conclusion

The tragic mass shooting at Sandy Hook Elementary School appears to have shifted the policy debate about gun violence in America. These 2013 national public opinion data collected three weeks after the Sandy Hook massacre suggest that the American public is supportive of a range of policy options for reducing gun violence. Time will tell how public sentiments about proposals to strengthen U.S. gun laws translate into policy action in Washington, D.C., and in state capitals around the country.

ACKNOWLEDGMENTS

The authors gratefully acknowledge funding to conduct this study from an anonymous donor to the Johns Hopkins Center for Gun Policy and Research.

NOTES

1. Gun Control Support Soars in New Polls. http://www.huffingtonpost.com/2012/12/27/gun-control-support-poll_n_2370265.html

2. After Newtown Modest Change in Opinion about Gun Control. http://www.people-press.org/2012/12/20/after-newtown-modest-change-in-opinion-about-gun-control/

3. Americans Want Stricter Gun Laws, Still Oppose Bans. http://www.gallup.com/poll/159569/americans-stricter-gun-laws-oppose-bans.aspx

4. Sides J. Gun Owners vs. the NRA: What the Polling Shows. Washington Post, December 23, 2012. http://www.washingtonpost.com/blogs/wonkblog/wp/2012/12/23/gun-owners-vs-the-nra-what-the-polling-shows/

5. New Poll of NRA Members by Frank Luntz Shows Strong Support for Common-Sense Gun Laws, Exposing Significant Divide between Rank-and-File Members and NRA Leadership. http://www.mayorsagainstillegalguns.org/html/media-center/pr006-12.shtml

6. Stricter Gun Control. http://today.yougov.com/news/2011/01/20/stricter-gun-control/

7. Vernick JS, Teret SP, Howard KA, Teret M, and Wintemute GJ, "Public Opinion Polling on Gun Policy," *Health Affairs* 12, no.4 (1993): 198–208.

8. Blendon RJ, Young JT, and Hemenway D, "The American Public and the Gun Control Debate," *Journal of the American Medical Association* 275, no. 22 (1996): 1719–1722.

9. Teret SP, Webster DW, Vernick JS, et al., "Support for New Policies to Regulate Firearms," *New England Journal of Medicine* 339, no.12 (1998): 813–818.

10. We report a sample completion rate rather than a sample response rate as is standard for online survey research panels. Given that we used an online panel based on probability sampling at the first stage of recruitment, it is important to note the GfK KN panel recruitment response rate of 16.6%.

11. Davis JA and Smith TW, General Social Surveys, 2010. Principal Investigator, James A. Davis; Director and Co-Principal Investigator, Tom W. Smith; Co-Principal Investigator, Peter V. Marsden, NORC ed. Chicago: National Opinion Research Center.

12. Schmidt MS, Gaps in FBI Data Undercut Background Checks for Guns. New York Times, December 20, 2012. http://www.nytimes.com/2012/12/21/us/gaps-in-fbi -data-undercut-background-checks-for-guns.html?pagewanted=all&_r=0

13. Frank RG and Glied, SA, *Better but not well: Mental health policy in the United States.* Baltimore: Johns Hopkins University Press, 2006

14. American Association for Public Opinion Research (AAPOR) Standards Committee. AAPOR Report on Online Panels. March 2010. http://www.aapor.org/AM /Template.cfm?Section=AAPOR_Committee_and_Task_Force_Reports&Template= /CM/ContentDisplay.cfm&ContentID=2223+

Consensus Recommendations for Reforms to Federal Gun Policies

On January 14 and 15, 2013, the Johns Hopkins University brought together more than 20 global leaders in gun policy and violence—representing the fields of law, medicine, public health, advocacy and public safety—for the Summit on Reducing Gun Violence in America.

The purpose was to distill the best research, analysis, and experience from these experts into a set of clear and comprehensive policy recommendations to prevent gun violence. By summarizing both new and prior research relevant to a number of policies, and issuing policy recommendations, the outcomes of the Summit can contribute to the prevention of gun violence through more informed legislative and regulatory proposals.

The researchers identified the policy recommendations described below as the most likely to reduce gun violence in the United States.*

---

* These recommendations represent the consensus of the experts presenting at the Johns Hopkins Summit on Reducing Gun Violence in America. However, it may not be the case that every expert endorsed every specific recommendation.

Background Checks

Fix the background check system by doing the following:

- Establish a universal background check system, which would require a background check for all persons purchasing a firearm (with an exception for inheritance transfers).
- Facilitate all sales through a federally licensed gun dealer. This would have the effect of mandating the same record keeping for all firearm transfers.
- Increase the maximum amount of time for the FBI to complete a background check from 3 to 10 business days.
- Require all firearm owners to report the theft or loss of their firearm within 72 hours of becoming aware of its loss.
- Subject even those persons who have a license to carry a firearm, permit to purchase, or other firearm permit to a background check when purchasing a firearm.

Prohibiting High-Risk Individuals from Purchasing Guns

Expand the conditions for firearm purchase:

- Persons convicted of a violent misdemeanor would be prohibited from firearm purchase for a period of 15 years.
- Persons who committed a violent crime as a juvenile would be prohibited from firearm purchase until 30 years of age.
- Persons convicted of two or more crimes involving drugs or alcohol within a three-year period would be prohibited from firearm purchase for a period of 10 years.
- Persons convicted of a single drug-trafficking offense would be prohibited from gun purchase.
- Persons determined by a judge to be a gang member would be prohibited from gun purchase.
- Establish a minimum of 21 years of age for handgun purchase or possession.
- Persons who have violated a restraining order issued due to the threat of violence (including permanent, temporary and emergency) would be prohibited from purchasing firearms.

- Persons with temporary restraining orders filed against them for violence or threats of violence would be prohibited from purchasing firearms.
- Persons who have been convicted of misdemeanor stalking would be prohibited from purchasing firearms.

Mental Health

- Focus federal restrictions on gun purchases by persons with serious mental illness on the dangerousness of the individual.
- Fully fund federal incentives for states to provide information about disqualifying mental health conditions to the National Instant Criminal Background Check System for gun buyers.

Trafficking and Dealer Licensing

- A permanent director for ATF should be appointed and confirmed.
- ATF should be required to provide adequate resources to inspect and otherwise engage in oversight of federally licensed gun dealers.
- Restrictions imposed under the Firearm Owners' Protection Act limiting ATF to one routine inspection of gun dealers per year should be repealed.
- The provisions of the Firearm Owners' Protection Act which raise the evidentiary standard for prosecuting dealers who make unlawful sales should be repealed.
- ATF should be granted authority to develop a range of sanctions for gun dealers who violate gun sales or other laws.
- The Protection of Lawful Commerce in Arms Act, providing gun dealers and manufacturers protection from tort liability, should be repealed.
- Federal restrictions on access to firearms trace data, other than those associated with ongoing criminal investigations, should be repealed.
- Federal law mandating reporting of multiple sales of handguns should be expanded to include long guns.
- Adequate penalties are needed for violations of the above provisions.

Personalized Guns

- Congress should provide financial incentives to states to mandate childproof or personalized guns.
- The Federal Consumer Product Safety Commission should be granted authority to regulate the safety of firearms and ammunition as consumer products.

Assault Weapons

- Ban the future sale of assault weapons, incorporating a more carefully crafted definition to reduce the risk—compared with the 1994 ban—that the law would be easily evaded.

High-Capacity Magazines

- Ban the future sale and possession of large-capacity (greater than 10 rounds) ammunition magazines.

Research Funding

- The federal government should provide funds to the Centers for Disease Control and Prevention, the National Institutes of Health, and the National Institute of Justice adequate to understand the causes and solutions of gun violence, commensurate with its impact on the public's health and safety.
- The Surgeon General of the United States should produce a regular report on the state of the problem of gun violence in America and progress toward solutions.

Biographies of Contributors

Ted Alcorn, MA, MHS, is a senior policy analyst in the Office of the Mayor of New York City. He contributes frequent public health reporting to *The Lancet* and has also published work in the *International Herald Tribune, The Financial Times, Guernica,* and the *American Journal of Tropical Medicine and Hygiene.* He earned an MHS from the Johns Hopkins Bloomberg School of Public Health and MA from the Johns Hopkins School for Advanced International Studies (SAIS), and then lived in Beijing, China, as a Henry Luce Scholar.

Philip Alpers is an adjunct associate professor at the Sydney School of Public Health, The University of Sydney. Alpers analyzes the public health effects of armed violence, firearm injury prevention, and small arms proliferation. His website GunPolicy.org compares armed violence and gun laws across more than 200 jurisdictions. Accredited to the United Nations small arms Programme of Action since 2001, Alpers participates in the United Nations process as a member of the Australian government delegation. Relevant work includes a 20-nation regional study (*Small Arms in the Pacific*), field work with users and traffickers (*Gunrunning in Papua New Guinea: From Arrows to Assault Weapons in the Southern Highlands*), a 10-year impact analysis of the world's largest firearm buyback (*Australia's 1996 Gun Law Reforms: Faster Falls in Firearm Deaths, Firearm Suicides, and a Decade without Mass Shootings*) and the disposal of military small arms (Papua New Guinea: small numbers, big fuss, real results).

Deborah Azrael, PhD, has been a member of the firearms research group at the Harvard School of Public Health for more than 20 years, working collaboratively with her colleagues David Hemenway, Matthew Miller, and Cathy Barber throughout that time. Dr. Azrael's academic training is in statistics and evaluative sciences. Much of her work over the past decades has been in designing and building injury surveillance systems, including the pilot for the National Violent Death Reporting System (of which she was co-director, with Cathy Barber), and the Boston Data System, a surveillance system designed to track youth violence at the neighborhood level in Boston (which she continues to direct). Her academic work has focused, often in collaboration with David Hemenway and Matt Miller, on the relationship between firearm availability and injury-related mortality. She has also worked extensively on studies that have used ecologic- and individual-level data to understand risk of suicide across and within populations, e.g., suicide in the Veterans Administration, suicide among young African American men, and the effects of psychotropic medications on suicide risk.

Antonio Rangel Bandeira is coordinator for Firearms Control, Viva Rio, Brazil. Mr. Bandeira has served as an advisor for the Parliamentary Front for Disarmament for the new firearms control law, the Disarmament Statute (2003). He also serves as the civil society coordinator for the National Buy-Back Small Arms and Light Weapons (SALW) Campaign and has been a member of the Brazilian government delegation for the UN Conference on Illicit Traffic of SALW. In addition, he has advised the governments of Mozambique, Bolivia, Angola, El Salvador, Venezuela, and the province of Buenos Aires, Argentina, on SALW public policy and ammunition control and buy-back disarmament campaigns. Mr. Bandeira is a former vice-minister of Welfare in the Brazilian government and advisor to the president of Brazil. He is a founding member of the International Network on Small Arms. He earned an MA in Political Science from York University.

Colleen L. Barry, PhD, MPP, is an associate professor and associate chair for Research and Practice in the Department of Health Policy and Management at the Johns Hopkins Bloomberg School of Public Health. Dr. Barry's research focuses on policy and regulation affecting often-stigmatized health conditions with a focus on mental illness, substance use disorders, and obesity. She teaches courses in health policy and politics and public opinion research. She is principal investigator of an NIMH R01 to understand the effects of implementation of the recent federal mental health and addiction parity law, and is principal investigator on a NIDA R01 to evaluate the effects of regulations aimed at increasing rates of use of new treatments for substance use disorders. Dr. Barry has been involved with a number of projects examining the implications of various aspects of the Affordable Care Act (ACA) on mental illness and addiction treatment. She is also principal investigator on two Robert Wood Johnson Foundation Healthy Eating Research grants, studying how news media messages used to frame the issue of childhood obesity affect public attitudes about food-marketing regulation, and testing how media messages affect public opinion about sugar-sweetened beverage taxes. She received a PhD in Health Policy from Harvard University and a master's degree in public policy from the John F. Kennedy School of Government at Harvard.

Michael R. Bloomberg is the 108th Mayor of the City of New York. He began his career in 1966 at Salomon Brothers, and after being let go in 1981, he began Bloomberg LP, a global media company that today has over 310,000 subscribers to its financial news and information service. As his company grew, Michael Bloomberg started directing more of his attention to philanthropy. He has sat on the boards of numerous charitable institutions, including Johns Hopkins University, where he helped build the Bloomberg School of Public Health into one of the world's leading institutions of public health research and training. In 2001 he ran for mayor of the City of New York and, in a major upset, won the election. In office, Mayor Bloomberg has cut crime more than 35 percent and created jobs by attracting new investment and supporting small business growth. He has implemented ambitious public health strategies, including the ban on smoking in restaurants and bars, and expanded support for arts and cultural organizations. His education reforms have driven graduation rates up 40 percent since 2005. The City has weathered the national recession much better than most other places. Since October 2009, the nation has gained back only one out of every four jobs that were lost in the recession. Meanwhile, New York City has gained back nearly all of its lost jobs. Michael Bloomberg attended Johns Hopkins University and received an MBA from Harvard Business School. He is the father of two daughters, Emma and Georgina.

Anthony A. Braga, PhD, is the Don M. Gottfredson Professor of Evidence-Based Criminology in the School of Criminal Justice at Rutgers University and a senior research fellow in the Program in Criminal Justice Policy and Management at Harvard University. He is also a member of the University of Chicago Crime Lab and a Senior Fellow in the Chief Justice Earl Warren Institute on Law and Social Policy at the University of California, Berkeley. He is currently the President and an elected Fellow of the Academy of Experimental Criminology. Dr. Braga's research involves collaborating with criminal justice, social service, and community-based organizations to address illegal access to firearms, reduce gang and group-involved violence, and control crime hot spots. Since 1995, Braga has worked closely with criminal justice practitioners in Boston to reduce youth gun violence. He was a member of the Boston Gun Project that implemented the Operation Ceasefire gang violence reduction strategy that was associated with a 63% reduction in youth homicides in Boston. Dr. Braga's research has been published in top criminal justice, medical, and public health journals. He received his MPA from Harvard University and his PhD in Criminal Justice from Rutgers University.

Philip J. Cook, PhD, is ITT/Sanford Professor of Public Policy and Professor of Economics and Sociology at Duke University. He has conducted research on crime and criminal justice throughout his career, with a sustained focus on gun violence and gun policy. He serves as co-organizer of the NBER Workshop on the Economics of Crime. He has served as consultant to the U.S. Department of Justice (Criminal Division) and to the U.S. Department of Treasury (Enforcement Division). His service with the National Academy of Science includes membership on expert panels dealing with alcohol-abuse prevention, injury control, violence, school rampage shootings, underage drinking, and the deterrent effect of the death penalty. Dr. Cook is a member of the Institute of Medicine of the National Academy of Sciences and an honorary Fellow in both the American Society of Criminology and of the Academy of Experimental Criminology. Dr. Cook completed his PhD in economics at the University of California, Berkeley, in 1973.

Ronald J. Daniels, JD, LLM, is 14th president of The Johns Hopkins University. Previously, he was provost and professor of law at the University of Pennsylvania and dean and James M. Tory Professor of Law at the University of Toronto. Since arriving at Johns Hopkins, Daniels has focused his leadership on three overarching themes: enhanced interdisciplinary collaboration, individual excellence, and community engagement. Under his leadership, a number of cross-school collaborations have emerged, including efforts related to individual health and the science of learning; significant investments have been made in undergraduate and graduate education and financial aid; and the university has strategically deepened its commitment to Baltimore, as evidenced by the new Elmer A. Henderson School in East Baltimore and the $10 million Homewood Community Partners Initiative. Daniels's research focuses on the intersections of law, economics, development, and public policy, and he has also has engaged on a range of policy issues from corporate governance and anti-terrorism legislation in Canada, to risk and disaster policy in the United States. Daniels received an LLM from Yale University and a BA and JD from the University of Toronto.

Shannon Frattaroli, PhD, MPH, is an associate professor at the Johns Hopkins Bloomberg School of Public Health where she is affiliated with the Center for Gun Policy and Research. Dr. Frattaroli's research in the area of gun violence prevention focuses on understanding and improving how policies are implemented and enforced, with particular attention to those that aim to limit batterers' access to guns. The role of policy makers, law enforcement, the courts, and advocates in assuring that laws designed to prevent gun violence are realized through implementation and enforcement strategies is a common theme in her work. Dr. Frattaroli is currently serving as a member of the Maryland Task Force to Study Access of Mentally Ill Individuals to Regulated Firearms.

Linda K. Frisman, PhD, is a research professor at the University of Connecticut School of Social Work and a senior research scientist with the Connecticut Department of Mental Health and Addiction Services. Dr. Frisman holds a PhD in Social Policy from the Heller School of Brandeis University and was a postdoctoral fellow in mental health services research at Yale University. She has been the principal investigator of several federally funded studies testing interventions that address homelessness, co-occurring mental health and substance use disorders, and criminal justice populations with behavioral health disorders. Currently she is the principal investigator of the Connecticut Criminal Justice Drug Abuse Treatment Studies Center funded by NIDA and co-principal investigator of an NIMH study regarding the impact of connection to entitlements by prisoners with mental illness who are being released.

Peter L. Gagliardi is senior vice president for Forensic Technology Inc. He has more than 40 years of experience extracting useful investigative information from crime guns and related evidence in both the public and private sectors. He spent 30 of those years in law enforcement, most of which were focused on the investigation of firearms and explosives-related crimes with ATF. In 1999, Mr. Gagliardi retired from ATF as the Special Agent in Charge of the New York Field Division. During his tenure in New York, he was responsible for managing all of ATF's law enforcement and regulatory operations within the New York/New Jersey metropolitan area. While assigned to ATF headquarters in Washington, DC, he served as the agency's principal liaison to Congress, the deputy assistant director of Science and Technology, the deputy assistant director of Law Enforcement Programs, and the chief of Strategic Planning. In 2010, he authored the book, *The 13 Critical Tasks: An Inside-Out Approach to Solving More Gun Crime,* which Forensic Technology makes available at no cost to criminal justice agencies and educators. He currently serves on the Firearms Committee of the International Association of Chiefs of Police (IACP).

David Hemenway, PhD, is an economist and professor at Harvard School of Public Health (HSPH) and a former James Marsh Visiting Professor at Large at the University of Vermont. He is director of the Harvard Injury Control Research Center. He received the Excellence in Science award from the Injury and Violence Section of the American Public Health Association and fellowships from the Pew, Soros, and Robert Wood Johnson foundations. Dr. Hemenway was recognized in 2012 by the Centers for Disease Control and Prevention as one of the 20 "most influential injury and violence professionals over the past 20 years." He has written more than 165 journal articles and is sole author of five books. Recent books include *Private Guns Public Health* (2006; University of Michigan Press) and *While We Were Sleeping: Success Stories in Injury and Violence Prevention* (2009; University of California Press). Dr. Hemenway has received 10 HSPH teaching awards.

Michael J. Klag, MD, MPH, is dean of the Johns Hopkins Bloomberg School of Public Health. Dr. Klag is an internist and kidney disease epidemiologist whose scientific contributions have been in the prevention and epidemiology of kidney disease, hypertension, and cardiovascular disease. He was one of the earliest investigators to apply epidemiologic methods to the study of kidney disease. For eight years, he was Director of the Division of General Internal Medicine and was the first Vice Dean for Clinical Investigation at the Johns Hopkins School of Medicine, where he instituted new policies and procedures for oversight of human subject research. He was the Editor-in-Chief of the *Johns Hopkins Family Health Book*, and from 1988 to 2011 he directed one of the longest running longitudinal studies in existence, the Precursors Study, which began in 1946. Dr. Klag received his medical degree from the University of Pennsylvania and his MPH degree from the Bloomberg School.

Christopher S. Koper, PhD, is an associate professor in the Department of Criminology, Law and Society at George Mason University and a senior fellow and co-director of the evidence-based policing research program in George Mason's Center for Evidence-Based Crime Policy. Dr. Koper has more than 20 years of experience conducting criminological research at the Police Executive Research Forum, the University of Pennsylvania, the Urban Institute, the RAND Corporation, the Police Foundation, and other organizations, where he has written and published extensively on issues related to firearms, policing, federal crime prevention efforts, and other topics. His research on firearms, much of which he has conducted for the U.S. Department of Justice, has included studies of illegal gun markets, law enforcement strategies to reduce gun crime, trends in criminal weaponry, the 1994 federal assault weapons ban, and other federal and state policies to reduce firearms violence. He holds a PhD in criminology and criminal justice from the University of Maryland.

Hsiu-Ju Lin, PhD, is an associate research professor in the School of Social Work at the University of Connecticut and the principal data analyst for the Research Division at the Connecticut Department of Mental Health and Addiction Services. Dr. Lin plans and oversees data analyses of all the Division's quantitative work, including several federally funded studies. Her areas of specialization include longitudinal data analysis, multilevel modeling, structural equation modeling, and health behavior studies. She holds a doctorate in social/personality psychology from the University of Albany, State University of New York.

Jens Ludwig, PhD, MA, is the McCormick Foundation Professor of Social Service Administration, Law, and Public Policy at the University of Chicago, director of the University of Chicago Crime Lab, and co-director of the University of Chicago Urban Education Lab. He is also a non-resident senior fellow at the Brookings Institution, research associate of the National Bureau of Economic Research (NBER), co-director of the NBER's Working Group on the Economics of Crime, and member of the MacArthur Foundation's research network on housing and families. His research has been published in leading scientific journals across a range of disciplines, including *Science, New England Journal of Medicine, Journal of the American Medical Association, American Economic Review,* and *American Journal of Sociology.* He is co-author with Philip J. Cook of *Gun Violence: The Real Costs* (2000; Oxford University Press), co-editor with Cook of *Evaluating Gun Policy* (2003; Brookings Institution Press), and co-editor with Cook and Justin McCrary of *Controlling Crime: Strategies and Tradeoffs* (2011; University of Chicago Press). In 2012, he was elected to the National Academy of Science's Institute of Medicine. Ludwig received his BA in economics from Rutgers College and his MA and PhD in economics from Duke University.

Emma E. McGinty, MS, is a research assistant and fourth-year PhD candidate in Health Policy and Management at the Johns Hopkins Bloomberg School of Public Health. Her research interests include mental illness, gun violence, and the role of the news media in public policy. Her dissertation research examines the effects of news media coverage of gun violence by persons with serious mental illness, the public's support for gun control policies, and stigma toward persons with serious mental illnesses, such as schizophrenia and bipolar disorder. At the Center for Gun Policy and Research, she is collaborating on studies on the effects of minimum legal age restrictions for firearm purchasers and possessors on gun violence and the effects of state gun sales policies on interstate trafficking of guns. She also serves as a resource on mental illness and gun violence. Prior to coming to the Bloomberg School as a Sommer Scholar in 2009, she worked for the Centers for Disease Control and Prevention. She received an MS in Health and Behavior Science from Columbia University in 2006.

Adam D. Mernit, an undergraduate senior Public Health Studies major at Johns Hopkins University, is applying to the Master of Science in Public Health (MSPH) program at the Bloomberg School of Public Health. A native of Huntington, New York, he recently began working with Stephen Teret in the field of gun policy. He plans to continue along the path of gun policy research and study the impact of health research on legislative action.

Matthew Miller, MD, ScD, MPH, is deputy director of the Harvard Injury Control Research Center and associate professor of Injury Prevention and Health Policy at the Harvard School of Public Health. Dr. Miller, a physician with training in internal medicine, medical oncology, medical ethics, health policy and management, epidemiology, and pharmacoepidemiology, has authored more than 100 journal articles and op-ed articles on suicide, interpersonal violence, and unintentional injuries, many of which focus on the relationship between firearms and lethal violence. He has been recognized as an outstanding teacher at Harvard's School of Public Health and at Harvard College, most recently in 2011 when he received both the Burke Award from the Harvard Initiative for Global Health for teaching injury and violence prevention to undergraduates and the Harvard School of Public Health's annual Teaching Award for his graduate school course on suicide prevention. He is also the recipient of the 2011 Excellence in Science Award, an honor bestowed annually by the Injury Control and Emergency Health Services Section of the American Public Health Association.

Michael A. Norko, MD, MAR, is a forensic psychiatrist and serves as director of Forensic Services for the Connecticut Department of Mental Health and Addiction Services (DMHAS), where he oversees all public sector forensic services. He manages DMHAS reporting to the FBI of persons ineligible for gun purchase due to mental health adjudications. Dr. Norko is also an associate professor of psychiatry, Law & Psychiatry Division at Yale University School of Medicine. He served on the APA Task Force on the Assessment of Violence Risk. Dr. Norko collaborated in writing legislative proposals for the "Relief from Disabilities" provision required by the NICS Improvement Amendments Act.

Michael J. North, PhD, was a faculty member in Biochemistry at the University of Stirling in Scotland when, in March of 1996, his only daughter was killed in a mass shooting at Dunblane Primary School. Following that event, he became a tireless advocate for gun control. He participated in the Snowdrop Campaign for a handgun ban and helped to launch the Gun Control Network (GCN) to campaign for tighter gun legislation in the UK. He remains involved with the GCN and recently served on a panel advising the Scottish government on airgun legislation. He has participated in a number of international meetings relating to gun violence and public safety and has spoken about gun control in the UK to audiences in Europe, North America, and Australia. Until recently, he was on the board of the International Action Network on Small Arms.

Rebecca Peters is a violence prevention specialist who has worked for more than 20 years on arms control, women's rights, public health, and human security. A lawyer and a journalist, she was the first director of the International Action Network on Small Arms (IANSA), the global movement against gun violence. She previously worked for the Open Society Institute and was a Soros Senior Justice Fellow at the Johns Hopkins School of Hygiene and Public Health. In the 1990s, she led the grassroots campaign in Australia that secured the overhaul of all state and territory gun laws. (Gun death rates in Australia have subsequently dropped by 50%.) For this work, she received the Australian Human Rights Medal, her country's highest human rights award. She is currently working for Surviving Gun Violence, a project aiming to increase assistance to survivors. A member of the IANSA Board and the Fundacio per la Pau's International Council, she is also a consultant to the University of Sydney and the Centre for Humanitarian Dialogue.

Allison Gilbert Robertson, PhD, MPH, is assistant professor in the Department of Psychiatry and Behavioral Sciences at Duke University School of Medicine. Dr. Robertson's interests span several areas of mental health law, policy, and services research, in particular the problems of co-occurring substance abuse and the intersection between these disorders and criminal justice involvement. She is currently an investigator on several projects including the multisite study on gun control laws, mental illness, and prevention of violence led by Dr. Jeffrey Swanson. She is principal investigator on a study funded by the Robert Wood Johnson Foundation Program on Public Health Law Research examining the effects of legal practices used in jail diversion programs for persons with serious mental illness that aim to improve participants' access to treatment and reduce recidivism. She received a PhD in Health Policy and Management from the University of North Carolina at Chapel Hill and an MPH in Health Management and Policy from the University of Michigan at Ann Arbor.

Lawrence E. Rosenthal, JD, is a professor at Chapman University School of Law in Orange, California. Previously, he was deputy corporation counsel for Counseling, Appeals and Legal Policy with the City of Chicago's Department of Law. In this capacity, he argued three cases before the U.S. Supreme Court and supervised a large volume of complex litigation, as well as legislative and policy matters. He entered the practice of law as an assistant U.S. attorney for the Northern District of Illinois, specializing in organized crime and public corruption prosecutions. He brought the first racketeering case involving insider trading, and secured the longest sentence–200 years–in the history of the District in an organized crime case. He clerked for Judge Prentice Marshall of the U.S. District Court for the Northern District of Illinois and for Justice John Paul Stevens of the U.S. Supreme Court. He graduated from Harvard Law School, where he won the Fay Diploma and was an editor of the Harvard Law Review. He continues to engage in litigation before the Supreme Court and other appellate courts, usually on a pro bono basis.

Jeffrey W. Swanson, PhD, is a professor in Psychiatry and Behavioral Sciences at Duke University School of Medicine. He is a medical sociologist with expertise in psychiatric epidemiology, mental health services research, and mental health law and policy studies. Dr. Swanson is principal investigator of a multisite study on gun control laws, mental illness and prevention of violence, cosponsored by the National Science Foundation and the Robert Wood Johnson Foundation's Program on Public Health Law Research (PHLR).

He received the 2011 Carl Taube Award from the American Public Health Association for outstanding career contributions to mental health research.

Marvin S. Swartz, MD, is professor and head of the Division of Social and Community Psychiatry and director of Behavioral Health for the Duke University Health System. Dr. Swartz's major research and clinical interests are in improving the care of mentally ill individuals. He has been extensively involved in policy issues related to the organization and care of mentally ill individuals at the state and national level. He was a Network Member in the MacArthur Foundation Research Network on mandated community treatment examining use of legal tools to promote adherence to mental health treatment, and led the Duke team studying the use of assisted outpatient treatment in New York. He co-led a North Carolina study examining the effectiveness of psychiatric advance directives and co-led the Duke team investigating the role of antipsychotics in treatment outcomes in schizophrenia as part of the landmark NIMH-funded Clinical Antipsychotics Trials of Intervention Effectiveness study. He is a co-investigator of a study of the cost of criminal justice involvement of mentally ill individuals and the effectiveness of gun laws in reducing gun-related deaths. Dr. Swartz is also director of the National Resource Center on Psychiatric Advance Directives and recipient of the 2011 American Public Health Association's Carl Taube Award and American Psychiatric Association's Senior Scholar, Health Services Research Award for career contributions to mental health services research.

Stephen P. Teret, JD, MPH, is a professor of Health Policy and director of the Johns Hopkins Center for Law and the Public's Health. Professor Teret holds joint faculty appointments in Pediatrics and in Emergency Medicine at the Johns Hopkins School of Medicine. He began his career working as a poverty lawyer and a trial lawyer in New York. Since 1979, he has been a full-time faculty member at the Johns Hopkins Bloomberg School of Public Health. His work includes research, teaching, and public service in the areas of injury prevention, vaccine policy, tobacco policy, food policy, preparedness, and, generally, public health law. Professor Teret's work has also focused on the understanding and prevention of violence, with an emphasis on gun policy. Teret is recognized as one of the first persons to write about and advocate for the use of litigation as a tool for protecting the public's health. Professor Teret is a frequent lecturer at major universities and has served as a consultant to the President, the Attorney General, the U.S. Congress, federal agencies, state legislatures, and health departments. Professor Teret is the recipient of distinguished career awards from the American Public Health Association, and the Association of Trial Lawyers of America.

Jon S. Vernick, JD, MPH, is an associate professor and associate chair in Health Policy and Management at the Johns Hopkins Bloomberg School of Public Health. He is co-director of the Johns Hopkins Center for Gun Policy and Research. In addition, Vernick is co-director of the Johns Hopkins Center for Law and the Public's Health and deputy director of the Center for Injury Research and Policy. His work has concentrated on ways in which the law and legal interventions can improve the public's health. He is particularly interested in epidemiology, policy, and legal and ethical issues associated with firearm and motor vehicle injuries. He has also examined aspects of numerous other public health issues including tobacco control, preparedness and health advocacy. Vernick is also committed to graduate education, serving as an associate chair of the Johns Hopkins MPH Program. He received a BA from Johns Hopkins University, a law degree cum laude from George Washington University, and an MPH from the Johns Hopkins School of Hygiene and Public Health.

Katherine A. Vittes, PhD, MPH, is a research associate at the Johns Hopkins Center for Gun Policy and Research. Her research focuses on evaluating policies designed to prevent gun violence. She has published numerous articles on adolescent gun violence and gun use in intimate partner violence. In addition to having presented at more than a dozen professional conferences, Vittes has been called upon to testify in front of the Maryland legislature. Prior to joining the Bloomberg School faculty in 2008, Dr. Vittes earned her MPH and PhD at the UCLA School of Public Health and completed a post-doc at the University of Pennsylvania.

Daniel W. Webster, ScD, MPH, is a professor in Health Policy and Management at the Johns Hopkins Bloomberg School of Public Health. He serves as director of the Johns Hopkins Center for Gun Policy and Research, as well as deputy director of research for the Center for the Prevention of Youth Violence. He is also affiliated with the Johns Hopkins Center for Injury Research and Policy. Webster is the author of numerous articles on the prevention of gun violence and firearm policy. His current research interests include evaluating the effects of various efforts to reduce violence, including state gun and alcohol policies, policing strategies focused on deterring gun violence, a community gun violence prevention initiative (Safe Streets) and Maryland's Lethality Assessment Program for reducing the recurrence of intimate partner violence.

Adam Winkler, JD, MA, is a law professor at the University of California, Los Angeles. He is a specialist in American constitutional law, known primarily for his research on the right to bear arms and on corporate political speech. His work has been cited by the U.S. Supreme Court and numerous federal and state courts. His recent book, *Gunfight: The Battle Over the Right to Bear Arms,* was called "provocative" and "illuminating" by *The New York Times;* "a fascinating survey of the misunderstood history of guns and gun control in America" by *The Wall Street Journal;* and "an antidote to so much in the gun debate that is one-sided and dishonest" by the *Los Angeles Times.* A contributor to *The Daily Beast* and *The Huffington Post,* his commentary has been featured on NBC Nightly News, CNN, *The New York Times, The Wall Street Journal, Newsweek, The Atlantic, The New Republic,* and SCOTUSblog. He edited, along with Pulitzer Prize–winning historian Leonard Levy, the *Encyclopedia of the American Constitution.* He is a graduate of the Georgetown University School of Foreign Service and New York University School of Law. He also holds a master's degree in political science from UCLA.

Garen J. Wintemute, MD, MPH, is the inaugural Susan P. Baker-Stephen P. Teret Chair in Violence Prevention and director of the Violence Prevention Research Program at the University of California, Davis. He practices and teaches emergency medicine at UC Davis Medical Center, Sacramento (a level I regional trauma center), and is professor of emergency medicine at the UC Davis School of Medicine. Dr. Wintemute's research focuses on the nature and prevention of violence and on the development of effective violence prevention measures and policies. Selected studies include assessments of risk for criminal activity and violent death among legal purchasers of handguns, evaluations of the effectiveness of denying handgun purchase to felons and violent misdemeanants, in-depth studies of gun dealers who are disproportionate sources of crime guns, and the first empirical study of gun shows. He is the author of two books: Ring of Fire (1994), a study of the handgun makers of Southern California, and Inside Gun Shows: What Goes on When Everybody Thinks Nobody's Watching (2009). He has testified before committees of Congress and state and local legislatures as an expert on firearm violence and its prevention. In 1997 he was named a Hero of Medicine by Time magazine.

April M. Zeoli, PhD, MPH, is an assistant professor in the School of Criminal Justice at Michigan State University. In her research, she uses public health methods and models to increase the understanding of violence and homicide. Her main field of investigation is the prevention of intimate partner violence and homicide through public health policy.

Index

"Access Denied" (Mayors Against Illegal Guns), xiv
access to guns, restrictions on, 144
accidental deaths, related to guns, 174–75
Acioli, Patricia, 216
alcohol, consumption of, laws relating to, 70
alcohol abuse: federal denial criteria and, 68–69, 72, 78, 88; gun purchase and possession and, 79; personal gun ownership and, 82–83; as risk factor for gun-related violence, 82, 83. *See also* drunk driving
ammunition, marking of, 216
amnesty programs, 205
Argentina, supporting gun amnesties and buybacks, 205
Armatix GmbH, 177–78
Arms Trade Treaty, 220
assault weapons, 143; associated with drug trafficking and organized crime, 161; ban on, Americans' support of, 241–44; as crime guns, 162–64; JHU Summit recommendations on, 262; mass shootings and, 161; as percentage of guns recovered by police, 164; prices for, 162–63; prohibitions on, constitutionality of, 230–33; restrictions on, public support for, 168
assault weapons ban, federal, xii–xiii, 157; effects of, 162–65; exemptions in, 158, 160; features test provision of, 159, 160; impact on gun violence, 165–66; LCMs and, 159–60; lessons and implications from, 168–69; mixed effects of, 158; passage of, 161; provisions of, 159–61
ATF. *See* U.S. Bureau of Alcohol, Tobacco, Firearms and Explosives
Aurora (CO), mass shootings at, 158

Australasian Police Ministers' Council (APMC), 195, 201–2
Australia: battle in, over gun regulation, 196–98; effects in, of gun policy changes, 207–9; gun manufacturing industry gone from, 207; guns in, 196; lunatic fringe in, 198; Port Arthur, mass shooting at, 195; restocking, following gun legislation, 207; supporting gun amnesties and buybacks, 205, 206–7; weapons destroyed in, 205–7
Australian Institute of Criminology, 207
AWs. *See* assault weapons
Azrael, Deborah, 6

background checks, xii, xiii, 22, 27, 35; avoiding, 104; comprehensive requirements for, potential effects of, 103–5; constitutionality of, 230–31; costs of, 90; criminal records accessible for, 28–29; effectiveness of, 45, 57, 102–3; extending, to misdemeanor convictions and alcohol-related offenses, 89; improvements in, 60; JHU Summit recommendations on, 260; mentally ill people and, 36; nondomestic violence convictions and, 56–57; results of, 78, 79; speed of, 96; state regulation of, 97; strengthening, Americans' support of, 241, 246–47; universal system for, 29; usefulness of, dependent on related databases, 90; waiving, 97. *See also* Brady Act, the
Badger Guns and Ammo, 137, 138, 147
BATF. *See* U.S. Bureau of Alcohol, Tobacco, Firearms and Explosives (ATF)
batterers: convicted, prohibited from buying or possessing guns, 55, 56; prohibiting gun access for, 68; using weapons to threaten, 54.

batterers (*continued*)
  See also domestic violence; domestic violence
    restraining orders; intimate partner
    homicides
Behavioral Risk Factor Surveillance System
  (BRFSS), 6, 9, 82
Biden, Joseph, xi, xiii
Bird, Derrick, 192
Bloomberg, Michael R., 126
Blose, J., 78
Boston, gun market disruption strategy in,
  146–47
Brady, James, 23
Brady, Sarah, 23
Brady Act, the (Brady Handgun Violence
  Prevention Act), 23, 25, 110; background
  check requirement of, 28; gun running and,
  25; homicide rates and, 22–23, 26–27, 78, 88;
  linked with decrease in crime gun imports,
  147; not applicable to secondary-market
  transactions, 148; private-sale loophole in, 28
  (*see also* private-sales loophole); risk of violent
  crime and, 44–45; suicide rates and, 22–23,
  26; waiting periods and, 23, 26
Braga, Anthony A., 28, 146
Brazil: arms industry in, 214, 215; arms
  legalization campaign in, 220; buyback
  programs in, 217–18; destroying weapons in,
  217, 218; dispelling myths in, about guns,
  216–17; gun control reforms in, 213–15; as gun
  exporter, 214; gun homicides in, 213; gun
  regulation in, 219–20; illegal gun trade in,
  219; pacification efforts in, 218–19; public
  opinion in, on gun control, 205, 219–20
Breyer, Stephen, Justice, 229
British Medical Association, 189
Bureau of Alcohol, Tobacco and Firearms. *See*
  U.S. Bureau of Alcohol, Tobacco, Firearms
  and Explosives (ATF)
Bush, George W., 179
Bush (George W.) administration, 152
buyback programs, 201, 205, 208, 217–18

California: allowing seizure of guns from the
  dangerous mentally ill, 48–49; background
  checks and recordkeeping policies in, 98–99;

denying gun purchases for violent misdemeanor convictions, 79–81; gun market in,
  90, 99; gun shows in, 102; juvenile offenders
  in, gun possession and, 71
California Armed and Prohibited Persons
  System, 61
CAP laws. *See* child access prevention (CAP)
  laws
Centers for Disease Control and Prevention
  (CDC), xiv, 152, 262
Chicago, 146; action in, against gun dealers,
  124–25, 136; crime guns in, 25
child access prevention (CAP) laws, 70
childproof guns. *See* personalized guns; youth
children. *See* youth
Clinton, Bill, 22, 177
Clinton administration, 152
college students, gun ownership among, 69
Colt's, 177
concealed weapon permits, 90
Connecticut, NICS reporting in, 37–38,
  40–44, 45
Conservative Party (UK), 186–87, 190–91
consignment sales, 99
Consumer Product Safety Commission, 180, 262
Cook, Philip J., 8, 28, 78, 95, 146, 175
countermarketing, 130
crime guns, 143; ATF definition of, 115; assault
  weapons as, 162–64; in Brazil, 215; exporting
  of, to other states, 114–17; illegally diverted
  from legal commerce, 144; purchase of, 28;
  regional processing protocols for, 150;
  sources of, 100, 114–15, 118, 119, 124, 133–34;
  trace data on, unavailable from ATF, 129,
  130; tracing of, national report on, 151–52
crime rates, drop in (U.S., 1990s), 24
criminals: demand of, for guns, xiii, 28, 39–40,
  143; guns diverted to, 112–18; guns of, sources
  for, 110–11, 123, 145–46; with mental illness,
  preventing gun violence among, 49; selling
  guns to, 99–101, 105
Cullen, Lord W. Douglas, 187
Cullen Report, 188, 190–91

dealers, licensed, 101–2, 105, 110–11; constitutionality of regulating, 231; effect of, on the

illicit market, 124; increasing oversight of, Americans' support of, 241; inspections of, 134–35, 138; interventions on, 134; JHU Summit recommendations on, 261; lawsuits against, 136; licensing of, 134; regulation and oversight of, 112, 124, 133–34; revocation of license for, 135; role of, in gun trafficking, 123; stings against, 136; supplying crime guns, 133–34. *See also* private-party sellers

deaths: firearms-related, in the U.S., xv, 3–5; unintentional, firearms-related, 5, 13; violent, linked with gun prevalence, 13. *See also homicide, mortality, and suicide entries*

Democrats, supporting gun violence prevention policies, 247–54

denial criteria: based on prior felony conviction, effectiveness of, 85–87; federal, for gun purchase and possession, 77–78; including violent misdemeanors, 78–79, 88; support for expanding, 89–90

denials, delayed, 89, 104

depression: evidence-based treatment for, 50; suicide and, 49

Detroit, actions against gun dealers in, 124–25, 136, 146

disarmament, as social theme for 2014 World Cup, 220–21

Disarmament Statute (Brazil), 215, 219

disqualified individuals, removing guns from, 58, 59

District of Columbia, handgun ban in, 225–26

District of Columbia v. Heller, 225–30, 232–34

diversion of guns: to criminals, 111–13, 117–19, 125, 129–30, 134; to the illegal market, 123, 124

document falsification violations, gun sales and, 149

domestic violence, 79, 198; alcohol and, 68; gun prohibitions and, implementing and enforcing, 61; guns and, 54; increased risk of IPH and, 66; state-level gun legislation and, 55–56

domestic violence restraining orders (DVROs), 54–56; associated with lower IPH rates, 68; gun laws and, 57–61; improving public safety through, 59–60; laws relating to, and

reducing IPH risk, 57–58; permanent, 55; service of, 59; state-level gun prohibitions and, 87–88; temporary, 55–56, 60–61; violation of, 61

Dreyfus, Pablo, 214

drug abuse: associated with violent and criminal behavior, 66, 72; suicide and, 66

drunk drivers, 69

Dunblane Primary School (Scotland), shootings at, 185, 187–91, 192

Dunblane Snowdrop Petition, 189

DVROs. *See* domestic violence restraining orders

Eddie Eagle GunSafe Program, 174

federal firearms license (FFL), 22. *See also* dealers, licensed; sellers

felons, committing subsequent violent crimes, 66

FFL. *See* federal firearms license

Firearm Owners' Protection Act (FOPA), 97, 135, 138, 148–49, 261

firearms. *See assault weapons and guns entries*

Firearms Act (UK), 186

firearms convictions, data regarding, usefulness of, 38

firearms disabilities program, federal, relief from, 71–72

Firearms Transaction Record, 96

Fix Gun Checks Act, 104–5

FN Manufacturing, 177

FOPA. *See* Firearm Owners' Protection Act

Forsyth, Michael, 187

Fox, Gerald, 176

Fox Carbine, 176

Gallup, 239, 240

Gary (IN), stings of gun dealers in, 136

GCA. *See* Gun Control Act of 1968

GCN. *See* Gun Control Network

General Social Survey (GSS), 5–6, 89

Giffords, Gabrielle, 158

Great Britain: gun control movement in, 192; gun legislation in, 186; gun ownership in, 188; handgun ban in, 185, 187–92. *See also* United Kingdom

grip recognition, 179
grip safety, 176
GSS. *See* General Social Survey
Gun Control Act of 1968 (GCA), 22, 35,
    71–72; amendments to, 55, 72; applicability
    of, 97
Gun Control Network (GCN), 189, 192
gun shows, 96, 98, 99, 100, 101–3, 112; gun show
    loophole, 104; oversight of, 29

Hamilton, Thomas, 185, 186, 188, 189
Handgun Control, Inc., 23
Hemenway, D., 8
high-capacity magazines. *See* large-capacity
    magazines
high-risk individuals, gun purchases by, JHU
    Summit recommendations on, 260–61
highway fatalities, reduction in, 173–74
History of Smith & Wesson (Jinks), 175
homicide rates: Brady Act and, 22–23, 26–27,
    78, 88; dropping, 24; pre-*Brady* trends in,
    25; women's, 8, 10–11; young people
    and, 70
homicides, 3–4; ages of victims, 24; alcohol
    and, 68; cyclical rates of, 4; demographics of,
    4; gun ownership and, 6–10; guns and, 174,
    192, 198, 208–9, 213; increased risk of, among
    violent intimates, 54; perpetrators of, and
    prior felony convictions, 28. *See also* intimate
    partner homicides (IPHs)
Howard, John, 197, 198
Hungerford (Berkshire, UK), mass shooting at,
    186, 187, 188, 189

iColt, 177
Independents, supporting gun violence
    prevention policies, 247–54
Indiana, dangerous persons law in, 48–49
integrity tests, of private-party sellers, 101
International Crime Survey, 8
intimate partner homicides (IPHs), 53; declines
    in, for women, 87–88; effects on, of limiting
    gun access, 57; guns and, 54; and laws
    prohibiting purchase or possession, 57,
    58; risk of, reducing, 57–58; risk factors for,
    54, 56

intimate partners, defining, 55, 56, 61
IPHs. *See* intimate partner homicides

Jersey City (NJ), handgun attacks in, 167
Jinks, Roy G., 175
Johns Hopkins Bloomberg School of Public
    Health, xv, 176
Johns Hopkins Center for Gun Policy and
    Research, xix, 179
Johns Hopkins National Survey of Public
    Opinion on Gun Proposals, 240–53
Johns Hopkins University Summit on
    Reducing Gun Violence in America,
    recommendations of, 259–62
judicial scrutiny, of Second Amendment
    cases, 229–30
junk guns, 111, 118–19, 137
juveniles. *See* youth

Kellermann, A. L., 9, 10
Killias, M., 8
Knight, Brian G., 114

Labour Party (UK), 187, 191
large-capacity magazines (LCMs): Americans'
    support of ban on, 241; ban on, 158–60;
    constitutionality of bans on, 230–31, 233–34;
    JHU Summit recommendations on, 262;
    limiting availability of, xii; mass shootings
    and, 161; ownership of, 161; restrictions on,
    168; used in gun crimes, 162, 164–65
life, value of, 29
litigation: against gun makers and sellers, 125;
    deterring certain gun sales practices, 124;
    diminished effectiveness of, 136; of NYC gun
    dealers' activities, 125–30
Ludwig, Jens, 28, 146
Lula (Luiz Inácio Lula da Silva), 215
Lula government, 220

magazine capacity, restricting, 168. *See also*
    large-capacity magazines
MAIG. *See* Mayors Against Illegal Guns
Maryland, banning junk guns, 118–19
Massachusetts, juvenile offenders in, gun
    possession and, 71

mass shootings, xxv, 157–58, 161, 185, 186, 192, 195, 206, 218; as catalyst for assault weapons debates, 166; effect on, of the federal assault weapons ban, 166; rarity of, by disturbed persons, 34

Mayors Against Illegal Guns, xi–xii, xiv, 114, 135

McChrystal, Stanley, xii

McClure-Volkmer Act. *See* Firearm Owners' Protection Act (FOPA)

McDonald v. City of Chicago, 225, 226

means–ends scrutiny, 232–33

mental health: JHU Summit recommendations on, 261; rates of adjudication, 45–48; revising federal criteria for prohibitions on guns and, 48

mental illness: assumptions about, 36; and disqualification from buying guns, 39–40, 44; firearms prevalence and, 12; gun policy and, 34, 35–36; violence and, 34, 36; violent crime and, 38–44, 48

Mercy, J. A., 57

military, U.S., suicides in, xv

military-style weapons, limiting availability of, xii

militias, 227–29

Miller, Matthew, 6, 8, 9

Ministry of Health (Brazil), 218

Ministry of Justice (Brazil), 213

misdemeanors: convictions for, and future arrest rates, 81–82; nonviolent, and new offenses, 81. *See also* violent misdemeanors

Missouri, PTP licensing in, repeal of, 112–14, 117

"Model Handgun Safety Standard Act," 179

Model Law on Firearms, Ammunition and Related Materials (Latin America), 219, 220

mortality rate, gun-related, Australia vs. U.S., 196, 202, 208

National Academies' Committee to Improve Research Information and Data on Firearms, 145

National Ballistics Intelligence Service (Nabis), 192

National Coalition for Gun Control (NCGC; Australia), 196–99

National Committee on Violence (NCV; Australia), 199

National Crime Victimization Survey (NCVS), 175

National Criminal History Improvement Program (NCHIP), 28–29

National Firearms Act of 1934, 228

National Firearms Agreement (Australia), 195–96, 199–201

National Firearms Buyback (Australia), 205–6

National Firearms Survey, 96, 101–2

National Firearms Trafficking Policy Agreement (Australia), 201–2

National Handgun Buyback (Australia), 206

National Handgun Control Agreement (Australia), 202

National Instant Criminal Background Check System (NICS), 23, 29, 35, 96, 231, 261; comprehensive state reporting to, of mental health records, 45; Connecticut's reporting to, 37–38, 40–44, 45; reach of reporting, extending, 36–37; reporting effect of, 40–44, 45

National Institute of Justice (NIJ), 152, 158, 177, 262

National Institutes of Health (NIH), xiv, 152, 262

National Integrated Ballistics Information Network (NIBIN), 150, 151

National Rifle Association (NRA), 151, 174; members of, responding to gun proposals, 90, 246; misrepresenting the Australian experience, 202

National Survey of Private Ownership of Firearms, 96, 101

NCGC. *See* National Coalition for Gun Control

NCHIP. *See* National Criminal History Improvement Program

NCV. *See* National Committee on Violence

NCVS. *See* National Crime Victimization Survey

Nevada, gun shows in, 102

New Jersey: personalized gun law in, 179–80; possession laws in, 67

New Jersey Institute of Technology, 179

Newtown (CT). *See* Sandy Hook Elementary School, shooting at
New York, state of, enacting penalties for illegal handgun possession, xvi
New York City: litigating gun dealers' activities, 125–30; murders in, dropping numbers of, xvi; stings and lawsuits in, against gun dealers, 136–37
NIBIN. *See* National Integrated Ballistics Information Network
NICS. *See* National Instant Criminal Background Check System
NIH. *See* National Institutes of Health
NIJ. *See* National Institute of Justice
North, Mick, 186
North Carolina, DVRO gun law in, 58
Northern Ireland, gun legislation in, 186

Obama, Barack, xi
Observatory on Citizen Security, 220
Office of Legislative Research (CT), 38
one-gun-per-month limits, 115, 119
Organization of American States, 220
out-of-state residents, sales to, 100
ownership of guns: and increased risk for alcohol abuse, 69; minimum federal standards for, 67; state laws relating to, differences in, 67

pacification, 218–19
PARLATINO, 219
Parliamentary Commission of Inquiry (PCI; Brazil), 219
Pennsylvania: juvenile offenders in, gun possession and, 71; prohibiting gun purchase by repeat DUI offenders, 69
permit holders, exempting, from background checks, 104–5
permit-to-purchase (PTP) licensing, 112–18
personalized guns, 174, 246; achieving, 179–80; history of, 175–77; JHU Summit recommendations on, 262; need for, 174–75; presently available, 177–79; technology for, 176–79
Pew Center for the People and the Press, 240
Philip, J. C., 6

PLCAA. *See* Protection of Lawful Commerce in Arms Act
Port Arthur (Australia), mass shooting at, 195
possession of guns, federal prohibitory criteria for, 65–66
Powell, Colin, xii
private-party sales, xii, 36, 102, 144, 147–48
private-party sellers, 96–97, 99–101, 103–5, 110
private-sales loophole, 28–29, 60, 149, 231
product liability litigation, gun makers immune from, 179
products, countermarketing of, 130
Protection of Lawful Commerce in Arms Act (PLCAA), 125, 136, 139, 179, 180, 261
psychiatric illness. *See* mental illness
psychological testing, for handgun ownership, 189
PTP. *See* permit-to-purchase licensing
public health issues, 173–74: death-by-gunshot, 209; gun ownership as, 228
public safety, gun control laws related to, 230
purchases of guns, multiple, extending mandatory reporting for, 148

Realengo School (Rio de Janeiro), mass shooting at, 218
recidivism, criminal, 71, 88
record-of-sale databases, 59–60
registries: for gun ownership, 60; for handguns, 29
regulation of guns, linked with firearm prevalence, 7
Republicans, supporting gun violence prevention policies, 247–54
research funding, JHU Summit recommendations on, 262
retail outlets, supplying criminals with guns, 146
retailers, licensed. *See* dealers, licensed
Richmond (VA), LCM use in, 165
rights: balancing, with safety, 48; of law-abiding citizens, 65
Rio de Janeiro, violence in, 214, 218
robbery, gun availability and, 8–9
robbery–murder, gun availability and, 8–9
Rossi, Peter H., 146

safety of guns, U.S. Consumer Product Safety
Commission prohibited from addressing, 179
sales of guns: consignments, 99; to criminals,
99–101; differing laws among states, 111–12,
118; federal double standard for, 96–97;
primary market for, 95; private, regulation
of, 112; process for, 96; secondary market for,
95–96; special reports of, 96; state regulation
of, 97–99. *See also* dealers; private-party sellers
sale-to-crime intervals, 113–14
Sandy Hook Elementary School (Newtown,
CT): mass shooting at, xi, 158; policy
response to shooting at, 33–34; U.S. public
opinion after, on gun policy, 239, 256
Saturday Night Specials. *See* junk guns
Second Amendment, 225–26; "arms" in,
meaning of, 232; challenges of, 226–27; core
interest of, 227; gun lobby's concern over,
xiii; limits on, constitutionality of, 226; lower
courts' rulings on, 226; preamble of, 228–29;
scope of, 227–29; "well-regulated militia" in,
228–29
secondary-market transactions, 147
selective prohibition, as approach to gun
ownership, 21–22. *See also* Brady Act, the
sellers. *See* dealers, licensed; private-party sellers
semi-automatic weapons: attacks with, effects
of, 166–67; legal, under assault weapons ban,
159; rifles, 143
Sheley, Joseph, 146
shooting organizations (UK), 187, 189–90, 191
Shooting Sports Retailer, 103
SISCF. *See* Survey of Inmates in State
Correctional Facilities
smart guns. *See* personalized guns
Smith & Wesson, 175–76, 177
Squires, Peter, 186
stalking, 54, 61
state-level gun dealer's licenses, 138
state regulation, 97–99, 102
states: assault weapons bans in, 161; gun dealer
licensing requirements in, 134; gun export
rates among, 116–17, 135; gun sales laws in,
111–12, 118
sting operations, against gun sellers, 112, 124,
126, 136

straw purchases, xvi, 103, 112, 117, 124, 125, 127,
134, 148
Subcommittee on Control of Arms and
Munitions (Brazil), 219
substitution effect, 209
suicide rates, 49; Brady Act and, 22–23, 26, 29;
CAP laws and, 70
suicides, xv, 3, 4–5; alcohol and, 68; demographics of, 5; depression and, 49; drug abuse
and, 66; and guns obtained from FFLs,
30–31n6; gun ownership and, 6–7, 11–13; guns
and, 174, 198, 208–9; mental illness and, 49
Sunday Mail (Scotland), 189
supply-side approach to violence, support for, 152
supply-side interventions, 144, 147
Survey of Inmates in State Correctional
Facilities (SISCF), 110

Taurus S.A., 214
theft of guns, 175
Tiahrt, Todd, xiv, 137
Tiahrt Amendment, xiv, 137–38, 139, 152
trace data, 144–45; limiting the release of,
137–38; utility of, 137
traces: for assault weapons, 163; difficult
procedure for, 148
traffickers, charged with other crimes, 150
trafficking of guns, xii, 96, 97; Brady Act and,
25; indicia of, 137; international, 220;
interstate, 135; intrastate, 124, 135, JHU
Summit recommendations on, 261; licensed
dealers and, 102, 111; no federal laws regarding, 148; private-party sales and, 100;
reduced by enhanced dealer oversight, 135;
revisiting sentencing guidelines for, 149–50;
routes for, 145–46
transfer agents, 98, 102
TriggerSmart, 178–79
Truscott, Carl, 151

underground markets for guns, frictions in, 146
United Kingdom: criminal recidivism in, 89;
gun legislation in, 186–87; Public Inquiries
in, following disasters, 187; supporting gun
amnesties and buybacks, 205. *See also* Great
Britain

United States: female homicide victims in, 8, 10–11; gun homicides in, compared with other nations, xvii; gun laws in, dividing the population, 21; gun deaths in, 3–5, 15; gun ownership in, 5–7, 241; gun proposals in, responses from gun owners and non-gun owners, 246–48; gun regulation in, historical tradition of, 227–28; murders in, with guns, xi–xii; policy change in, driven by public sentiment, xx; premature mortality in, xxv, 3, 4; public opinion in, 239–40; regulation of gun sales in, 119; suicide rates in, compared with other nations, 4–5; violence in, compared with other nations, 3–4; violent deaths in, linked to gun prevalence, 13–15

U.S. Bureau of Alcohol, Tobacco, Firearms and Explosives (ATF), xiv, 72, 96, 97, 100, 110, 111, 113, 115, 124, 134, 135, 159; approach of, to gun trafficking crimes, 148; granting permission for sale of personalized handguns, 178; JHU Summit recommendations on, 261; responsibility of, 147; sanctioning authority for, 138; strengthening, 150–51; tactics of, questioned, 151; trace data and, 136, 137, 144–45

U.S. Congress, and gun lobby, xiv, xv

U.S. Constitution, Second Amendment. *See* Second Amendment

U.S. Consumer Product Safety Commission, 179, 180

U.S. Court of Appeals (D.C. Circuit), and assault rifle ban, 233–34

U.S. Department of Justice, xiii, 147, 177

U.S. Supreme Court, Second Amendment rulings of, xiii, 78, 225–34

U.S. Surgeon General, JHU Summit recommendations for, 262

Vigdor, E. R., 57

violence: alcohol and, 68; drug abuse and, 66; as public health problem, 198; rates of, in developed nations, 8

violence with guns: societal costs of, 167; trends in, after expiration of the federal assault weapons ban, 165–66

violent crime: Brady Act prohibitions and, 44–45; correlated with illegal gun usage, 38;

effects on, of background checks, 45; factors associated with, 44; increasing in adolescence and early adulthood, 67; mental illness and, 38–44, 48; risks of committing, 44–45

Violent Crime Control and Law Enforcement Act of 1994, 159, 161

violent misdemeanors: federal denial criteria and, 77, 78, 85, 88; and new offenses, 79–80; state treatment of, and gun purchase and possession, 79

Virginia Tech, mass shootings at, 158

Viva Rio, 213, 214, 217, 219

waiting periods, 23, 26; and dealers, licensed, 99; ending, before completion of background checks, 89; extending, in individual cases, 89; lifting, 104

Walmart, gun sales practices of, 130

weapon accessories, ban on, 159

weapons, threatening with, associated with increased homicide risk, 54

Webster, Daniel, xv–xvi, 135

Wesson, D. B., 175

Wesson, Joe, 175

Wiebe, D. J., 10

Williams, Daryl, 202

Wintemute, Garen J., 68, 174

women: domestic violence against, 54; homicide rates of, 8, 10–11; killed by intimate partners, 53; seeking justice system assistance for domestic violence, 54–55

World Cup (soccer), in Brazil, 220–21

World Health Assembly, 198

Wright, James D., 146

YouGov, 240

youth: broadening gun prohibitions for, 70, 72; committing suicide with guns, 175; deaths of, related to firearms, 13; juvenile offenders, expanding gun prohibitions for, 71, 72; purchases by, 100; restricting gun access for, 67; training, in gun safety, 174. *See also* juvenile offenders

Youth Crime Gun Interdiction Initiative, 151